Comprehensive Virology 11

Comprehensive Virology

Edited by Heinz Fraenkel-Conrat
University of California at Berkeley

and Robert R. Wagner
University of Virginia

Comprehensive

Edited by

Heinz Fraenkel-Conrat

Department of Molecular Biology and Virus Laboratory
University of California, Berkeley, California

and

Robert R. Wagner

Department of Microbiology
University of Virginia, Charlottesville, Virginia

Virology

11

Regulation and Genetics
Plant Viruses

PLENUM PRESS • NEW YORK AND LONDON

Library of Congress Cataloging in Publication Data

Fraenkel-Conrat, Heinz, 1910-
  Regulation and genetics, plant viruses.

  (Their Comprehensive virology; v. 11)
  Includes bibliographies and index.
  1. Plant viruses. 2. Viral genetics. 3. Genetic regulation. I. Wagner, Robert R.,
1923-   joint author. II. Title. III. Title: Plant viruses. IV. Series: Fraenkel-
Conrat, Heinz, 1910-   Comprehensive virology; v. 11.
QR357.F72 vol. 11 [QR351]   576'.64'08s   77-7908
                                                   [576'.6483]

ISBN-13: 978-1-4684-2723-3   e-ISBN-13: 978-1-4684-2721-9
DOI: 10.1007/978-1-4684-2721-9

© 1977 Plenum Press, New York
A Division of Plenum Publishing Corporation
227 West 17th Street, New York, N.Y. 10011

Foreword

The time seems ripe for a critical compendium of that segment of the biological universe we call viruses. Virology, as a science, having passed only recently through its descriptive phase of naming and numbering, has probably reached that stage at which relatively few new— truly new—viruses will be discovered. Triggered by the intellectual probes and techniques of molecular biology, genetics, biochemical cytology, and high resolution microscopy and spectroscopy, the field has experienced a genuine information explosion.

Few serious attempts have been made to chronicle these events. This comprehensive series, which will comprise some 6000 pages in a total of about 22 volumes, represents a commitment by a large group of active investigators to analyze, digest, and expostulate on the great mass of data relating to viruses, much of which is now amorphous and disjointed, and scattered throughout a wide literature. In this way, we hope to place the entire field in perspective, and to develop an invaluable reference and sourcebook for researchers and students at all levels.

This series is designed as a continuum that can be entered anywhere, but which also provides a logical progression of developing facts and integrated concepts.

Volume 1 contains an alphabetical catalogue of almost all viruses of vertebrates, insects, plants, and protists, describing them in general terms. Volumes 2–4 deal primarily, but not exclusively, with the processes of infection and reproduction of the major groups of viruses in their hosts. Volume 2 deals with the simple RNA viruses of bacteria, plants, and animals; the togaviruses (formerly called arboviruses), which share with these only the feature that the virion's RNA is able to act as messenger RNA in the host cell; and the reoviruses of animals and plants, which all share several structurally singular features, the most important being the double-strandedness of their multiple RNA molecules.

Volume 3 addresses itself to the reproduction of all DNA-containing viruses of vertebrates, encompassing the smallest and the largest viruses known. The reproduction of the larger and more complex RNA viruses is the subject matter of Volume 4. These viruses share the property of being enclosed in lipoportein membranes, as do the togaviruses included in Volume 2. They share as a group, along with the reoviruses, the presence of polymerase enzymes in their virions to satisfy the need for their RNA to become transcribed before it can serve messenger functions.

Volumes 5 and 6 represent the first in a series that focuses primarily on the structure and assembly of virus particles. Volume 5 is devoted to general structural principles involving the relationship and specificity of interaction of viral capsid proteins and their nucleic acids, or host nucleic acids. It deals primarily with helical and the simpler isometric viruses, as well as with the relationship of nucleic acid to protein shell in the T-even phages. Volume 6 is concerned with the structure of the picornaviruses, and with the reconstitution of plant and bacterial RNA viruses.

Volumes 7 and 8 deal with the DNA bacteriophages. Volume 7 concludes the series of volumes on the reproduction of viruses (Volumes 2–4 and Volume 7) and deals particularly with the single- and double-stranded virulent bacteriophages.

Volume 8, the first of the series on regulation and genetics of viruses, covers the biological properties of the lysogenic and defective phages, the phage-satellite system P 2–P 4, and in-depth discussion of the regulatory principles governing the development of selected lytic phages.

Volume 9 provides a truly comprehensive analysis of the genetics of all animal viruses that have been studied to date. These chapters cover the principles and methodology of mutant selection, complementation analysis, gene mapping with restriction endonucleases, etc. Volume 10 also deals with animal cells, covering transcriptional and translational regulation of viral gene expression, defective virions, and integration of tumor virus genomes into host chromosomes.

The present volume deals with the considerable advances in methodology and understanding that have greatly broadened the general interest of molecular biologists in plant viruses in recent years. This volume represents the only one of the Comprehensive Virology series to deal exclusively with plant viruses, although their replication and assembly are covered in Volumes 2 and 5. The first two chapters focus on the nature of multicomponent viruses or coviruses that carry a subdivided genome distributed over separate virus particles. The third chapter concerns itself with the classical and simplest case of satellitism in viruses (a parasite of a parasite) and with other cases of defective viruses that are not completely functional. The fourth chapter deals with the mode and regulation of the first event after RNA virus infection, the translation strategy of multigenic viral RNAs. The fifth chapter describes the advantages and uses of mesophyll protoplasts in the study of plant virus replication and its regulation. Finally there is an authoritative chapter on the remarkable nature of viroids, disease causing self-replicating RNA molecules which are too small to code for proteins and may act by causing the activation of pathogenic genes carried within the host's genome.

Volume 12 will cover the general properties of special virus groups of invertebrates, algae, fungi, and bacteria. Volume 13 will be the last of the series on structure and assembly, dealing with general principles of virion structure, phage assembly, and the complete structural analyses of small RNA and DNA phage nucleic acids and proteins. Volume 14 will deal with the general properties of newly characterized groups of vertebrate viruses, such as, for example, arena-, corona-, and bunyaviruses.

Contents

Chapter 2

Plant Covirus Systems: Two-Component Systems

George Bruening

Chapter 5

Protoplasts in the Study of Plant Virus Replication

Itaru Takebe

Chapter 6

Viroids

T. O. Diener and A. Hadidi

CHAPTER 1

Plant Covirus Systems: Three-Component Systems

Lous Van Vloten-Doting and E. M. J. Jaspars

Department of Biochemistry
State University
Leiden, The Netherlands

1. INTRODUCTION

Recent developments have brought together viruses which were not previously supposed to bear any relationship except that they were simple RNA-containing plant viruses. These viruses are the spherical bromoviruses, once thought to have a very small genome (Bockstahler and Kaesberg, 1961); the small spherical cucumber mosaic virus and its relatives, which, in contrast to bromoviruses, are transmitted by aphids; the aphid-transmitted alfalfa mosaic virus, which is one of the very few small viruses with bacilliform particles; and a number of structurally not very well studied viruses among which are tobacco streak virus and citrus leaf rugose virus, which seem to have in common the possession of spherical virions of different size.

The reason for handling these viruses in one chapter is the nature of their genome. Electrophoresis in polyacrylamide gel has shown that their virions contain three RNA species with molecular weights not far from 10^6 (Fig. 1). These RNA species are in separate capsids. Infectivity studies with separated RNA species or with nucleoprotein species containing these RNAs have indicated that all three RNAs are needed for infection. With some of these viruses, these indications are much stronger than with others.

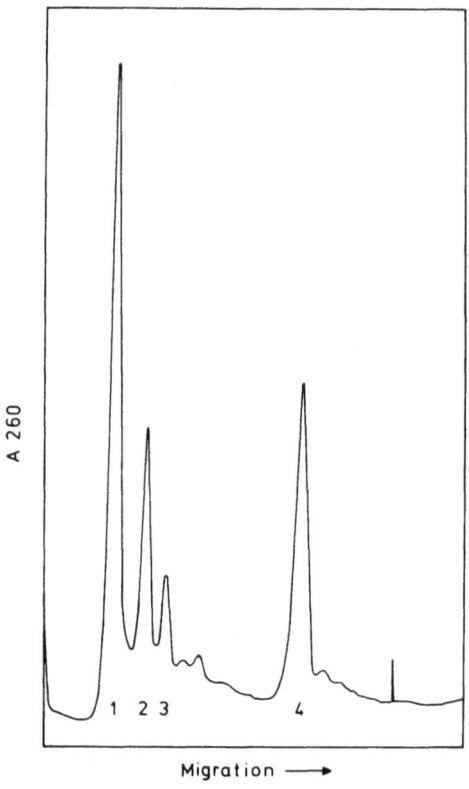

Fig. 1. Characteristic pattern of the RNAs of a plant virus with a tripartite genome (AMV) as revealed by electrophoresis in 3% polyacrylamide gel. The three peaks at the left represent the three parts of the genome. They are designated as RNAs 1, 2, and 3. Their molecular weights are not far from 10^6. RNA 4 at the right has a molecular weight of about 0.3×10^6 and comprises a cistron for the coat protein. With heterocapsidic viruses, this RNA or its translation product is needed to start an infection. Minor RNAs migrating between RNAs 3 and 4 or faster than RNA 4 are often found. With AMV they are called X- and Z-RNAs, respectively.

A further step in the argumentation in favor of a tripartite genome of these viruses was that genetic markers could be exchanged by exchanging RNA or nucleoprotein species in the test tube.

Finally, it could be demonstrated with alfalfa mosaic and brome mosaic viruses that the three RNAs have at least partly unique base sequences and that three species of double-stranded RNA occur in infected cells.

The preparations of plant viruses with tripartite genomes often contain more than three RNA species. One of these, a small RNA with a molecular weight of about 0.3×10^6, occurs very reproducibly and sometimes in appreciable amounts (Fig. 1). It is encapsidated either separately or together with the smallest genome part. With bromoviruses, cucumber mosaic virus, and alfalfa mosaic virus, it has been shown that this RNA directs in an efficient way the synthesis of viral coat protein in *in vitro* translation systems. When unfractionated RNA preparations are carefully freed from this RNA, no change in infectivity occurs in the case of bromo- and cucumoviruses, but in the case of the other viruses mentioned above infectivity is completely lost.

With the latter viruses, infectivity can be restored by adding the small RNA or by adding a small amount of its translation product, the coat protein. Apparently, with these viruses, the coat protein is necessary to start an infection. It has to be assumed that the gene for the coat protein in the genome is not available for translation, as it is in the monocistronic messenger RNA.

On the basis of the above, we can divide the tripartite genomes into protein-independent and protein-dependent genomes. Viruses of the former group have their genome parts in identical capsids and will be called here "isocapsidic viruses." Viruses of the latter group will be called "heterocapsidic viruses" since they have bacilliform or spherical capsids of different size. Apparently, the capsids are fitted to the size of the genome parts. It seems as if the coat protein is adapted to a biological function rather than to a very stringent role in particle structure. At this moment it cannot be stated with certainty whether capsid heterogeneity is always correlated with protein dependency, but for reasons of convenience we will maintain the division between isocapsidic and heterocapsidic viruses throughout this chapter.

Thus the grouping of the viruses we will handle is as shown in Table 1.

Jones and Mayo (1975) showed that BRLV is serologically related to TSV. That CLRV and the related CVV are heterocapsidic is inferred from an electron micrograph given by Garnsey (1975). Lister and Saksena (1976) have measured different particle size classes with preparations of NRSV. These authors point out that several other

TABLE 1
Grouping of Viruses with Tripartite Genomes

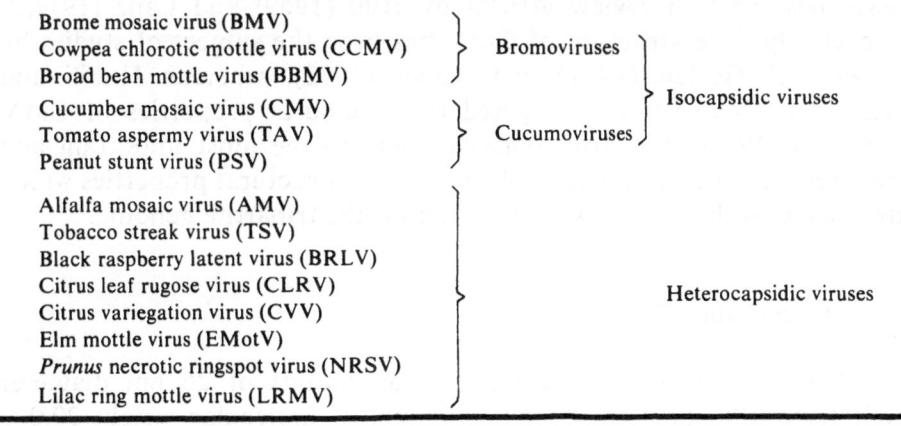

Brome mosaic virus (BMV)		
Cowpea chlorotic mottle virus (CCMV)	Bromoviruses	
Broad bean mottle virus (BBMV)		Isocapsidic viruses
Cucumber mosaic virus (CMV)		
Tomato aspermy virus (TAV)	Cucumoviruses	
Peanut stunt virus (PSV)		
Alfalfa mosaic virus (AMV)		
Tobacco streak virus (TSV)		
Black raspberry latent virus (BRLV)		
Citrus leaf rugose virus (CLRV)		Heterocapsidic viruses
Citrus variegation virus (CVV)		
Elm mottle virus (EMotV)		
Prunus necrotic ringspot virus (NRSV)		
Lilac ring mottle virus (LRMV)		

viruses may be grouped with TSV; thus Tulare apple mosaic virus (TAMV) has been shown by them to have similar particle classes and RNA species. Infectivity is greatly enhanced when particle classes are combined. Furthermore, TAMV is serologically related to CLRV (Lister, Gonsalves, and Garnsey, unpublished). Preparations of EMotV contain quasispherical particles which sediment in a sucrose density gradient in three bands. Infectivity is mainly associated with the fastest-sedimenting component, but addition of the slower-sedimenting components enhanced the infectivity about threefold (Jones and Mayo, 1973). NRSV is classified by Fulton (1968) with apple mosaic virus and rose mosaic virus in a group called ILAR viruses (isometric, labile, ringspot). Four centrifugal components comparable with those of NRSV and TAMV were detected by Lister and Saksena (1976) in preparations of apple mosaic virus. Preparations of lilac ring mottle virus (LRMV) consist of two centrifugal components. The two components have the same buoyant density but can be separated by polyacrylamide gel electrophoresis suggesting difference in particle size (Huttinga and Mosch, 1976). In the electron microscope, rather irregularly shaped isometric particles are seen (Van der Meer *et al.*, 1976).

There are indications that the genome of barley stripe mosaic virus is also tripartite (Lane, 1974*b*). However, the molecular weights of the three RNAs from this rod-shaped virus are around 1.25×10^6, and there is apparently no RNA of molecular weight 0.3×10^6.

2.   STRUCTURE AND COMPOSITION

The properties of AMV and of the bromoviruses have been extensively described in review articles by Hull (1969) and Lane (1974*a*), respectively. The structure of CMV has been the subject of studies by Kaper and Geelen (1971) and Kaper (1972), whereas Habili and Francki (1974*a,b*) have compared the structural properties of CMV and TAV. We will restrict ourselves here to the most important and most recent data. Emphasis will be on those structural properties which are related to the leitmotiv of this chapter, the tripartite genome.

2.1.   Isocapsidic Viruses

The bromoviruses have icosahedral capsids of 26 nm diameter built from 180 identical protein subunits of molecular weight 20,000

(Lane, 1974a). CMV has the same structure (Finch *et al.*, 1967), but the diameter of the particles is somewhat larger and the subunit molecular weight is close to 25,000 (Hill and Shepherd, 1972; Van Regenmortel *et al.*, 1972; Habili and Francki, 1974a). Bromovirus particles undergo swelling at pH values above 6.0 and become sensitive to ribonuclease and proteolytic enzymes in the swollen state (Lane, 1974a; Pfeiffer and Hirth, 1975). Cucumoviruses do not show such a swelling phenomenon but are nevertheless sensitive to ribonuclease (Francki, 1968; Habili and Francki, 1974b; Mink, 1975). At alkaline pH, CMV undergoes drastic structural changes (Kaper and Geelen, 1971).

All isocapsidic viruses are dissociated into protein and RNA by sodium dodecylsulfate (SDS) and high salt concentrations, which led Kaper (1972, 1973) to postulate that the structure of these viruses is mainly stabilized by protein–RNA interactions rather than by protein–protein interactions. Under proper conditions, the viruses can be reassembled from salt-prepared protein and RNA (Bancroft, 1970; Kaper and Geelen, 1971; Lane, 1974a) (see also chapter by P. P. Hung in Vol. 6 of this series).

The four main RNA species of bromo- and cucumoviruses have molecular weights of about 1.1, 1.0, 0.8, and 0.3×10^6. Somewhat higher and lower values have also been reported for the three large RNAs (Lane, 1974a; Kaper and Waterworth, 1973; Peden and Symons, 1973; Habili and Francki, 1974a; Kaper and Re, 1974). Since RNAs 3 and 4 are encapsidated together, there are only three types of virions. These three types of virions have nearly identical particle weights and sediment as single species with s values of about 86 S and 99 S in the case of bromo- and cucumoviruses, respectively (Lane, 1974a; Van Regenmortel, 1967; Mink *et al.*, 1969; Stace-Smith and Tremaine, 1973). The virion types can be partly resolved by equilibrium density gradient centrifugation. Density differences are more pronounced in bromoviruses than in cucumoviruses (Lane, 1974a; Lot and Kaper, 1973). This is probably due to the fact that in several strains of CMV an additional small RNA (RNA 5, of molecular weight 0.11×10^6, Kaper and West, 1972) is present. All nucleoprotein fractions from an RbCl density gradient contained about the same amount of RNA 5. Apparently this RNA is encapsidated with a variety of other RNAs (Lot and Kaper, 1976a,b).

Nucleotide sequence information is available only for the RNAs of BMV. From analysis of octa- and nonanucleotides of complete pancreatic ribonuclease digests of the separated RNAs, it follows that RNAs 1, 2, and 3 have at least partly unique nucleotide sequences. RNA 4 yielded two octanucleotides and three nonanucleotides, which were also present in the digest of RNA 3. RNAs 1 and 2 lacked at least some of the oligonucleotides of RNA 4, so that RNA 3 must contain the information of the subgenomic RNA 4 (Shih *et al.*, 1972).

The 3′ ends of all BMV RNAs are -GpCpCpCpA$_{OH}$ (Glitz and Eichler, 1971), which fits in well with their amino acid acceptor function (Section 5.3). Upon limited digestion by ribonuclease T_1, all RNAs yield a 160-nucleotide fragment which contains the 3′ end of the molecules (Bastin *et al.*, 1976). This fragment may well comprise a common recognition site for the replicase.

The 5′ ends of the BMV RNAs appeared to be heterogeneous in earlier studies of Fraenkel-Conrat and Fowlks (1972), but recent work (Dasgupta *et al.*, 1975, 1976) shows that they are actually all blocked by a 7-methylguanosine residue linked by 5′-p-p-p-5′ bonds to the adjacent nucleotide, as has been found in other eukaryotic messengers (Furuichi *et al.*, 1975; Adams and Cory, 1975; Keith and Fraenkel-Conrat, 1975). A sequence of 53 nucleotides at the 5′ end of RNA 4 has been determined. It appeared that the initiating AUG codon is only ten nucleotides from the 5′ end (Dasgupta *et al.*, 1975). This is the only ribosomal binding site on a eukaryotic messenger RNA that has been sequenced thus far.

The 3′ end of the CMV RNAs consists of either C or A, while the 5′ terminus is capped by $m^7G^{5'}ppp^{5'}Gp$ (Symons, 1975, 1976).

2.2. Heterocapsidic Viruses

AMV has bacilliform capsids of equal width (about 18 nm) but of different lengths (about 30–60 nm) (Hull, 1969), built from a single species of coat protein of molecular weight 24,300 (Kruseman *et al.*, 1971; Kraal *et al.*, 1972; Van Beynum *et al.*, 1975, 1977; Kraal *et al.*, 1976; Collot *et al.*, 1976).

Hull (1969) has proposed a model series for the structure of the AMV capsids. The series would start from a 60-subunit icosahedron cut across its threefold axis. In between, a tubular part, increasing in length with steps of 18 subunits arranged in a hexagonal lattice, would be interposed. Strong evidence for such a tubular structure in which the protein subunits are placed at the dyad positions of the lattice has been obtained (Heijtink, 1974; Mellema and Van den Berg, 1974; Mellema, 1975). The four major RNA species of the virus are called B-, M-, Tb-, and Ta-RNA and have molecular weights of 1.1, 0.8, 0.7, and 0.3 × 10^6, respectively. To facilitate comparison with the RNAs of the other viruses, we will designate them henceforth RNAs 1–4, respectively. The four RNAs fit capsids of 240, 186, 150, and 132 subunits, resulting in nucleoprotein components with s values of 94, 82, 73, and 66 S, respectively (Heijtink, 1974; Bol and Lak-Kaashoek, 1974). The Ta nucleoprotein contains two molecules of RNA 4 (Hull, 1969; Heijtink, 1974). Differences in buoyant density of the components in CsCl or in Cs_2SO_4 are small (Heijtink, 1974; Hull, 1976).

Electrophoresis in polyacrylamide gels reveals the presence of at least 13 minor nucleoprotein species in AMV preparations in addition to the four major species. Their RNA contents are heterogeneous: besides major RNAs, minor RNA species intermediate in molecular weight between RNAs 3 and 4 (X-RNAs) or of a molecular weight smaller than that of RNA 4 (Z-RNAs) are found. Probably these minor nucleoproteins represent other steps of the structural series (Bol and Lak-Kaashoek, 1974). Bacilliform particles longer than component B have been found in some strains of AMV, but these do not contain RNA species longer than B-RNA (Hull, 1969, 1970a; Heijtink and Jaspars, 1974).

AMV particles are sensitive to ribonuclease (Bol and Veldstra, 1969) and trypsin (Bol et al., 1974). Ribonuclease removes nucleotide material from the particles. At first, the particles remain intact, but have a lower electrophoretic mobility. Later, they degrade to smaller structures. This indicates that the RNA contributes to the surface charge of the particles and is an important factor in their structural integrity.

At slightly alkaline pH values, the sedimentation coefficients of the AMV nucleoproteins are strongly reduced, and well-defined bacilliform structures are not observed by electron microscopy. The unfolding does not necessarily lead to RNA degradation and is largely reversible (Verhagen and Bol, 1972; Verhagen, 1973; Verhagen et al., 1976).

The AMV RNAs are able to withdraw protein subunits from intact AMV particles (Van Vloten-Doting and Jaspars, 1972). TSV RNAs do the same (Van Vloten-Doting, 1975). The RNAs of the isocapsidic viruses are much less active in this respect, while the RNA from TMV or Escherichia coli ribosomal RNA is inactive (Van Boxsel, 1976). The uncoating is thought to be related to the coat protein dependency of the genomes of the heterocapsidic viruses (Section 3.4). There could be high-affinity sites on the RNAs, where the coat protein exercises its regulatory function. By titration with coat protein, the maximum number of high-affinity sites on the AMV RNAs has been estimated to be between four and eight for both RNA 1 and RNA 4 (Verhagen et al., 1976; Van Boxsel, 1976). It is uncertain whether these sites are clustered or scattered along the RNA chains. Experiments with fragments obtained from RNA 4 indicate that the protein binding region is located near the 3′ end (Houwing and Jaspars, to be published).

AMV nucleoproteins dissociate easily into protein and RNA at high salt concentrations (Hull, 1969) and in the presence of SDS (Bol *et al.*, 1971; Boatman and Kaper, 1976). Reassociation of salt-prepared protein and phenol-extracted RNA takes place under proper conditions, but bacilliform particles are scarcely found (Lebeurier *et al.*, 1969*b*; Hull, 1970*b*). However, they are formed when the particles are first dissociated by high salt and the salt is subsequently dialyzed out (Bol and Kruseman, 1969; Lebeurier *et al.*, 1969*a*).

The above observations point to a virus that is stabilized by RNA–protein rather than by protein–protein interactions.

Competitive hybridization experiments (Bol *et al.*, 1975) and sequence determination of oligonucleotide fragments in pancreatic ribonuclease digests (Pinck and Fauquet, 1975) have shown that the large AMV RNAs contain unique nucleotide sequences. Reannealing of double-stranded RNA was performed in the presence of an unfractionated ³H-labeled preparation of AMV RNAs and increasing amounts of one unlabeled purified RNA species or of mixtures of two or three unlabeled purified RNAs. It was found that RNAs 1 and 2 had at most a sequence of 180 nucleotides in common. Oligonucleotide analysis showed that the RNAs had two nona-, nine octa-, and five heptanucleotides in common out of totals of 17, 31, and 31, respectively. Both observations taken together would imply that the common sequences of 180 nucleotides are very poor in pyrimidines. The hybridization experiments demonstrated further that RNA 3 had unique nucleotide sequences since a mixture of RNAs 1 and 2 could not displace all radioactive label, whereas a mixture of the three large RNAs could. The percentage of homology between RNA 3 and the two larger RNAs could not be determined because of a contamination of the RNA 3 preparation with X-RNAs. X-RNAs were shown to contain all sequences of the AMV genome. However, oligonucleotide analysis revealed that the two nona-, six octa-, and twelve heptanucleotides of RNA 3 were not present in the digest of RNAs 1 and 2. Thus RNA 3 probably has a low degree of sequence homology, if any, with the larger RNAs.

Competitive hybridization experiments were also performed with ³H-labeled RNA 4 and increasing amounts of all four major RNAs, which were unlabeled. Some sequence homology (240 nucleotides) was detected between RNA 4 on the one hand and RNAs 1 and 2 on the other hand. The degree to which this homology actually represents RNA 4 sequences is uncertain, since the labeled RNA 4 preparation was slightly contaminated with X-RNAs. RNAs 4 and 3 were equally efficient in displacing the radioactive label. This must have been due to contamination with minor RNAs, since oligonucleotide analysis, which is less sensitive to small amounts of contamination, shows that the RNAs have only one nona-, two octa-, and four heptanucleotides in common. RNA 4 yields no unique oligonucleotides, and none of its obligonucleotides was found in the digests of RNAs 1 and 2. Thus it is clear that the information of the subgenomic RNA 4 is present in RNA 3.

The 5′ end of all four AMV RNAs was found to be capped by $m^7G^{5'}ppp^{5'}Gp$ (Pinck, 1975). From the fact that AMV RNA does not bind to an oligo (dT)-cellulose column, it follows that it does not contain an appreciable poly(A)tract (Bol *et al.*, 1976*b*).

Much less is known about the structure of spherical heterocapsidic viruses and their RNAs. Several of these viruses are only beginning to leave the realm of phytopathology. It would not be surprising if all these viruses were to apparently fit the following general outline: virions stabilized mainly by RNA–protein interactions; sensitive to high salt, SDS, ribonuclease, and trypsin; built from a single coat protein species; separable into four size classes by means of velocity centrifugation or sieve gel electrophoresis, but not by equilibrium centrifugation, the three fastest-sedimenting classes containing each a different RNA species with a molecular weight not far from 10^6 and the slowest-sedimenting class consisting of particles with two identical RNA molecules of molecular weight 0.3×10^6.

Let us now look into what is known. Particles of TSV (Van Vloten-Doting, 1975), CLRV, and CVV (Gonsalves and Garnsey, 1975*a,b*) can be dissociated at high salt concentrations. TSV is dissociated by SDS (Van Vloten-Doting, 1975; Lister and Saksena, 1976) and is sensitive to plant nucleases (Clark and Lister, 1971) and to trypsin (Van Vloten-Doting, 1975). TAMV is also sensitive to SDS. A single coat protein (with a molecular weight of about 29,000) has been found in TSV (Ghabrial and Lister, 1974), CLRV, CVV (Gonsalves and Garnsey, 1975*b*), and TAMV (Lister and Saksena, 1976). The protein of TSV has the same electrophoretic mobility in SDS gels as that of AMV (Van Vloten-Doting, 1975). The molecular weights of proteins of CLRV and CVV were estimated to be 26,000 (Gonsalves and Garnsey, 1975*b*), and that of LRMV 27,500 (Huttinga and Mosch,

1976). Four centrifugal components have been observed in preparations of TSV (113, 96, 84, and 78 S) (Lister *et al.*, 1972; Van Vloten-Doting, 1975), CLRV (106, 98, 89, and 79 S) (Garnsey, 1975), CVV (110, 93, 83, and 79 S) (Corbett and Grant, 1967; Gonsalves and Garnsey, 1975b), NRSV (Lister and Saksena, 1976), and apple mosaic virus (Lister and Saksena, 1976). However, the lightest component is often not apparent in TSV (Fulton, 1972; Lister *et al.*, 1972) and in CVV preparations (Corbett and Grant, 1967; Garnsey, 1975). NRSV preparations were found by Loesch and Fulton (1975) to consist of only three components (95, 90, and 72 S). Electrophoresis in polyacrylamide gel was performed only with TSV particles. Three components were resolved (Lister *et al.*, 1972). The three heaviest components of TSV were correlated with particles of 35, 30, and 27 nm, respectively (Lister *et al.*, 1972). The lightest TSV component has particles of 25 nm (Lister and Saksena, 1976). Mean diameters of 31, 30, and 28 nm were found for the three heaviest components of TAMV, and of 32, 30, and 27 nm for those of NRSV (Lister and Saksena, 1976). Particles in unfractionated preparations of CLRV were rather variable in size. Their mean diameter was 28 nm (Garnsey, 1975). De Sequeira (1967) found two size classes (26 and 29 nm) in preparations of apple mosaic virus. Lister *et al.* (1972) and Ghabrial and Lister (1974) have discussed the possibility of whether the different capsids of TSV could represent an icosahedral series with increasing T number. Density homogeneity has been demonstrated for the particles of TSV (Lister *et al.*, 1972), NRSV, TAMV, apple mosaic virus (Lister and Saksena, 1976), and LRMV (Huttinga and Mosch, 1976). From UV absorbance spectra it is evident that the components of CLRV do not vary much in RNA content (Garnsey, 1975).

A set of four RNA species with molecular weights close to those found with isocapsidic viruses and AMV was detected with TSV (Clark and Lister, 1971), CLRV (Gonsalves and Garnsey, 1974), CVV (Gonsalves and Garnsey, 1975b), NRSV (Loesch and Fulton, 1975), and LRMV (Huttinga and Mosch, 1976). TAMV seems to lack the smallest RNA species (Lister and Saksena, 1976). The correlation with particle classes has been demonstrated with TSV (Clark and Lister, 1971; Van Vloten-Doting, 1975) and CLRV (Gonsalves and Garnsey, 1974), although at least with TSV the correlation is apparently less stringent than with AMV (Fulton, 1970, 1972; Clark and Lister, 1971) (see Sections 4.1.2 and 4.2).

It will be evident from the above that the spherical heterocapsidic viruses have many structural properties in common with AMV. However, the shape of the particles is a very conspicuous difference. In this respect, it is of interest that component Ta and smaller nucleoproteins of AMV have spherical counterparts occurring in large amounts in the same preparations (Heijtink, 1974; Heijtink and Jaspars, 1976) and that bacilliform particles have been observed in preparations of TAMV (Fulton, 1967), rose mosaic virus (Basit and Francki, 1970), and NRSV (Lister and Saksena, 1976).

2.3. Separation Methods

The demonstration that multipartite genomes exist was dependent on separation techniques. Therefore, separation methods deserve a few remarks here. The degree of purity of a nucleoprotein or RNA species sufficient for chemical investigations may be insufficient for biological assay. The last few percent of a contamination may considerably suppress the biological effect of a combination experiment, as can be seen from infectivity experiments with preparations of varying component composition (Bruening and Agrawal, 1967; Van Vloten-Doting *et al.*, 1970). Infectivity experiments with BMV RNAs separated by velocity gradient centrifugation were first performed in 1965 by Bockstahler and Kaesberg, but the effect of combination did not surpass the effect obtained by adding, for example, ribosomal RNA and so escaped attention. That three RNAs were needed for infectivity was not detected until 1971, when gel electrophoretic separation came into use (Lane and Kaesberg, 1971).

With heterocapsidic viruses, the parts of the genome can be separated by separating the corresponding nucleoprotein species in velocity gradients. This procedure has been performed with AMV (Van Vloten-Doting *et al.*, 1970) and TSV (Fulton, 1970; Van Vloten-Doting, 1975). It is very laborious, since several cycles of centrifugation are required to obtain an adequate degree of purity of the components. The use of zonal rotors is recommended. During the purification the RNAs may degrade *in situ*. However, with AMV (Bol *et al.*, 1971) and TSV (Fulton, 1972) inactivation has been prevented by handling the components in buffers containing EDTA. EDTA was not effective with NRSV (Loesch and Fulton, 1975). With AMV, a much easier method to prepare purified nucleoproteins for biological experiments is electrophoretic separation in polyacrylamide gels (Bol and Lak-Kaashoek, 1974). When 3% gels were run for 2 days, components B, M, and Tb could sometimes be used after one cycle of purification, starting with crude preparations (J. F. Bol, personal communication).

In separating nucleoproteins, one takes the risk of contamination with particles having aberrant RNA contents. With AMV, it is very difficult to get rid of minor nucleoproteins (Bol *et al.*, 1971) which have been shown to contain RNA species different from those present in the adjacent major nucleoprotein species (Bol and Lak-Kaashoek, 1974; Heijtink and Jaspars, 1974). A certain heterogeneity with regard to RNA contents occurs with TSV nucleoproteins (Fulton, 1970, 1972; Clark and Lister, 1971) and with LRMV nucleoproteins (Huttinga and Mosch, 1976).

In general, a separation of the genome parts at the RNA level is preferable. With isocapsidic viruses, this is the only feasible method. Zones may be cut from polyacrylamide gels in which the RNA mixture has been electrophoresed (Lane and Kaesberg, 1971; Bancroft and Flack, 1972; Hull, 1972; Peden and Symons, 1973; Gonsalves and Garnsey, 1974; Mohier and Hirth, 1972), or continuous electrophoresis may be applied (Lot *et al.*, 1974). When working with RNAs, the danger of aggregation and conformational variation must not be neglected (Lane, 1974*a*). Greatly improved separations have been obtained when RNA preparations were heated before electrophoresis (Van Vloten-Doting and Jaspars, 1967; Bancroft, 1971; Harrison *et al.*, 1972).

3. INFECTIVITY

3.1. Dose–Infectivity Curves

A number of mathematical models for infectivity–dilution curves have been proposed (Kado, 1972). Most of these are rather complicated and rely on a number of assumptions.

When we simply divide the number of particles inoculated by the number of local lesions found, we would have to conclude that at least 10^4–10^6 particles are required for one infection. However, from the fact that mutants can easily be selected from a virus preparation treated with a mutagenic agent (Price, 1964), it follows that, at least with some viruses, only one particle is sufficient for an infection.

When the infectivity–dilution curves of a number of viruses are compared, a great variation in the steepness of the curves is found. Thus, when the dilution curves of AMV and TNV were compared on the same host (Van Vloten-Doting *et al.*, 1968), the curve for AMV was much steeper than that for TNV. The steepness of these curves seems to reflect the number of particles required for one infection: one for TNV and three for AMV.

However, conclusions about the constitution of the viral genome cannot be drawn from the dilution curve alone, since in some cases the slope of the dilution curve is influenced by the local lesion host (Fulton, 1967). For the bromo- and cucumoviruses, which all have a multipartite genome (Section 3.3), the infectivity–dilution curve did not deviate from the so-called one-hit curve [Fulton, 1962; Peden and Symons, 1973 (CMV); Lane, 1974a (bromoviruses)]. According to Lane and Kaesberg (1971) and Peden and Symons (1973), this could be due to the presence of dimers. An alternative explanation suggested by Peden and Symons (1973) is that one of the three essential RNA species is limiting in its contribution to infectivity relative to the other two.

In conclusion, we can say that a steep dilution curve points to a multipartite nature of a virus genome, whereas the finding of a so-called one-hit curve does not exclude this possibility.

3.2. Infectivity of Nucleoprotein Components

3.2.1. Isocapsidic Viruses

Since the nucleoprotein components of isocapsidic viruses can only partially be separated (see Section 2.3), we do not know whether they possess intrinsic infectivity. Lane and Kaesberg (1971) found that mixtures of heavy and light virions of BMV (containing RNA 1 and 2, respectively) had invariably higher specific infectivities than the isolated fractions.

3.2.2. Heterocapsidic Viruses

The nucleoprotein components of heterocapsidic viruses can be separated by sucrose density gradient centrifugation (see Section 2.3). By measuring the infectivity of each of the components alone and of all possible combinations of components, it is possible to determine the combination of components which contains the genetic information required for infectivity.

3.2.2a. AMV

Van Vloten-Doting et al. (1970) purified the four components of alfalfa mosaic virus by repeated centrifugation in a zonal rotor. None of the resulting preparations was infectious at concentrations of a few micrograms per millimeter. The twofold combinations had very low infectivities, whereas the infectivity of the combination of the three largest nucleoprotein components was comparable to that of a freshly isolated preparation. Addition of Ta to this combination did not increase the infectivity, nor could Ta replace any of the three larger components. Addition of very high concentrations of Ta to a mixture of B, M, and Tb reduces the infectivity considerably (Moed, 1966).

No indications were found in these experiments that any of the AMV components had intrinsic infectivity. However, both Desjardins and Steere (1969) and Majorana and Paul (1969) found that preparations of B which had been purified by successive cycles of centrifugation, and apparently contained less than 2–5% of M and Tb, showed considerable infectivity. This could indicate that B really possesses intrinsic infectivity. However, it must be realized that the presence of small amounts of M and Tb can have a rather large effect on the infectivity (Van Vloten-Doting *et al.*, 1970). Furthermore, B preparations may be contaminated with minor nucleoproteins which may have aberrant RNA contents (Section 2.3).

3.2.2b. TSV

For tobacco streak virus, three or four nucleoprotein components have been described. Fulton (1970) showed that the highest specific infectivity was associated with the combination of the three fastest sedimenting components. However, the two fastest sedimenting components both showed a low but significant infectivity and at least for B it was shown that this infectivity was not due to the presence of contaminating smaller components.

Van Vloten-Doting (1975) found that during purification of the nucleoprotein components the infectivity of the isolated components decreased drastically, while the combination of NP1, NP2, and NP3 (most likely corresponding to the B, M, and T of Fulton) remained infectious. From this, she concluded that probably all three components were required for infectivity. Also in this case it was found that addition of NP4 (not described by Fulton) did not further enhance the infectivity, nor could this component be substituted for any of the three larger ones.

The existence of particles with aberrant RNA contents could easily reconcile the findings of Fulton and Van Vloten-Doting. Although Van Vloten-Doting found that each component contains mainly one specific RNA species, this does not exclude the possibility that a small fraction of the components contains the "wrong" RNA together with a small piece of RNA to add up to the adequate RNA weight. Clark and Lister (1971) and Loesch and Fulton (to be published) found that at least M and T did have an RNA species in common.

3.2.2c. CLRV

Gonsalves and Garnsey (1974) found that preparations of citrus leaf rugose virus consisted of four closely sedimenting nucleoprotein components. After two cycles of sucrose density gradient centrifugation, only the fastest-sedimenting zone, comprising two components, was infectious at a concentration of a few micrograms per millimeter. Upon mixing of the different nucleoprotein preparations, the infectivity increased 2–7 times. Since the nucleoproteins sedimented rather closely, the authors thought that a better separation was not feasible and all further investigations were performed with RNA (see Section 3.3).

3.2.2d. TAMV

The components from Tulare apple mosaic virus, which is serologically related to CLRV, were separated by successive cycles of rate zonal density gradient centrifugation (Lister and Saksena, 1976). The purified components were not or were only slightly infectious, while mixtures of two components were moderately infectious and the mixtures of all three components were highly so.

3.2.2e. NRSV

Prunus necrotic ringspot virus requires cooperation of two of its three particle types to initiate infection. Top particles, although they contain nucleic acid, apparently do not function as carriers of genetic information. Addition of top particles to a mixture of the two fastest-sedimenting particles resulted in a decrease of infectivity (Loesch and Fulton, 1975).

3.2.2f. LRMV

The two centrifugal components (B and T) of lilac ring mottle virus were purified by three successive cycles of sucrose density gradient centrifugation. T contains only RNA 3 and 4, while B contains predominantly RNA 1 and 2, but also some RNA 3 and 4. Further cycles of sucrose density gradient centrifugation did not change the patterns. Apparently some RNA 3 and 4 is encapsidated into particles that sediment like B particles. This is consistent with the fact that B alone was infectious and that addition of T resulted in only a small increase of infectivity (Huttinga and Mosch, 1976).

3.3. Infectivity of RNAs

The RNA species of the viruses discussed in this chapter can be separated by sucrose density gradient centrifugation or by electrophoresis on polyacrylamide gels (Section 2.3). The infectivity of each RNA species can then be measured separately or in combination with the other RNA species. First, the role of the major RNAs will be discussed.

The results obtained with the bromo- and cucumoviruses show that the highest infectivity was associated with the combination of RNA 1 plus RNA 2 plus RNA 3; the infectivity of any of the twofold combinations was always less than 10% of that of the threefold combination. Addition of RNA 4 did not enhance the infectivity any further, nor could RNA 4 replace any of the larger RNAs [Lane, 1974a (bromoviruses); Peden and Symons, 1973; Lot et al., 1974 (CMV)]. There is some uncertainty about the genome of BBMV. In this case, only the two largest RNA species were required for infectivity. This could mean either that BBMV does have a bipartite genome or that the three RNA species have not been resolved (Hull, 1972).

For AMV, TSV, the two citrus viruses, and LRMV the infectivity required, besides the three large RNAs, the presence of RNA 4 (Bol et al., 1971; Mohier and Hirth, 1972; Mohier et al., 1974; Van Vloten-Doting, 1975; Gonsalves and Garnsey, 1974, 1975a,b; Huttinga and Mosch, 1976). This finding immediately provokes the question: why four RNAs and only three nucleoprotein components? It seems possible that each of the nucleoproteins always contained small amounts of RNA 4 not detectable by gel electrophoresis. Indeed, it was found that a combination of RNA 1 plus RNA 2 plus RNA 3 with AMV B was highly infectious. However, B particles with degraded RNA were also active in this respect, while the RNA extracted from B preparations lacked this activity (Bol et al., 1971). The only possible conclusion from these experiments was that RNA 4 was functionally equivalent to the coat protein in the onset of infection (Section 3.4).

In RNA preparations from most of these viruses, additional RNA species, the so-called minor RNAs, are also present. Preparations from BMV RNA contained an RNA migrating between RNA 3 and RNA 4 (Lane and Kaesberg, 1971). Philipps (1973) showed that this RNA did not enhance the infectivity, nor could it replace any of the larger RNAs. A similar RNA species was sometimes found in RNA preparations from CMV (Kaper and West, 1972; Marchoux *et al.*, 1973; Lot *et al.*, 1974) and TSV (Clark and Lister, 1971). Since RNA preparations lacking these RNA species were infectious (Lot *et al.*, 1974; Van Vloten-Doting, 1975), this RNA is apparently not essential for infectivity. RNA 5 from CMV was recently shown to be a kind of satellite RNA (Kaper and Waterworth, 1977). CMV RNA 5 has at best about 10% nucleotide sequence homology with CMV RNA 1 + 2 + 3 and none with CMV RNA 4 (Diaz-Ruiz and Kaper, 1977). A minor RNA species migrating somewhat faster than RNA 4 has been found in CLRV (Gonsalves and Garnsey, 1974), while in CVV (Gonsalves and Garnsey, 1975*b*) the amount of this RNA equals that of RNA 4. For infectivity studies with CVV, a mixture of these two RNAs has been used. It is not yet known whether both or only one of these RNAs is active. For AMV, a large number of minor RNA species migrating slower or faster than RNA 4 have been described (Bol and Lak-Kaashoek, 1974). These minor RNAs apparently did not play a role in infectivity.

3.4. Activity of Coat Protein

For the heterocapsidic viruses AMV, TSV, CRLV, CVV, and LRMV, it was found that addition of their own coat protein (instead of RNA 4) to a mixture of RNA 1 plus RNA 2 plus RNA 3 resulted in infectivity (Bol *et al.*, 1971; Mohier and Hirth, 1972; Mohier *et al.*, 1974; Van Vloten-Doting, 1975; Gonsalves and Garnsey, 1975*a,b*; Huttinga and Mosch, 1976). In most cases, the activity of the coat protein preparations was sensitive to heating at 60°C for 5 min, in contrast to the activity of the RNA preparations. Gonsalves and Garnsey (1975*a,b*) subjected the protein preparations to sucrose density gradient centrifugation, and showed that the activity was present in the region of the coat protein. Moreover, the activity could be destroyed by pronase. AMV coat protein was inactive when the -SH groups were blocked (Jaspars and Van Kammen, 1972) or when an *N*-terminal piece of 27 amino acid residues was removed by limited proteolysis (Bol *et al.*, 1974).

Since coat protein from other viruses such as TMV, CMV,

CCMV, or BMV could not activate the genomes of AMV, TSV, CLRV, or CVV (Bol *et al.*, 1971; Van Vloten-Doting, 1975; Gonsalves and Garnsey, 1975c), it is unlikely that the protein activation phenomenon depends on nonspecific protection of the RNAs against the degradative action of plant enzymes at the infection sites. Furthermore, the infectivity of a mixture of RNA and protein from AMV or from CLRV was rapidly lost upon incubation in sap from bean leaves (Bol *et al.*, 1971; Gonsalves and Garnsey, 1975a).

The equivalence of coat protein and RNA 4 can be understood if RNA 4 contains the message for the coat protein. Indeed, it was found that AMV RNA 4 directs *in vitro* the synthesis of coat protein (see Section 5.1). For other heterocapsidic viruses, this has not yet been investigated. In the mixture of RNA 4 and RNA 4a from CVV, RNA 4 is probably the active component since RNA 4a is too small to direct the synthesis of a complete coat protein molecule.

For AMV it was postulated (Bol *et al.*, 1971) that for the initiation of an infection by the three large RNAs a small amount of coat protein is always necessary. This can be provided either as capsid, as low molecular weight coat protein, or by translation of RNA 4 in the cell. This idea is schematically represented for TSV in Fig. 2.

When in 1971 it was found for AMV that the coat protein played a role in the onset of infection, the action of AMV coat protein was thought to be very specific since no other coat protein was active in this regard. Later, the genomes of the two citrus viruses (Gonsalves and Garnsey, 1975a,b) and of TSV (Van Vloten-Doting, 1975) were also found to be dependent for expression on the presence of their coat pro-

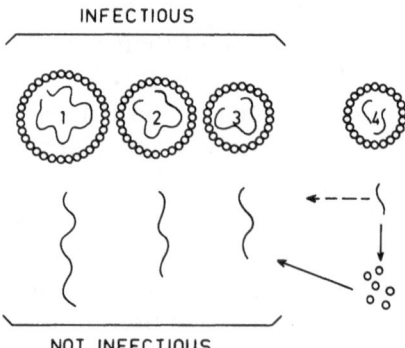

Fig. 2.   Scheme of the requirements for infectivity in a heterocapsidic virus. The mixture of the three large RNAs is not infectious, in contrast to the mixture of the corresponding particles. Infectivity can be induced by adding a small amount of the coat protein or of its messenger, RNA 4. Presumably RNA 4 exerts its action by giving rise to the synthesis of a few coat protein molecules in the cell.

tein. With further experimentation, it was found that the coat proteins from AMV, TSV, and the two citrus viruses were all equally capable of activating their own as well as each other's genome (Van Vloten-Doting, 1975; Gonsalves and Garnsey, 1975c).

The heterologous activation is very remarkable considering the fact that only the two citrus viruses were serologically related, while no serological relationship was observed among AMV, TSV, and the two citrus viruses. Furthermore, the AMV and TSV RNAs do not share nucleotide sequences (Bol et al., 1975), the tryptic peptide maps of AMV and TSV coat proteins are rather different (Van Vloten-Doting, 1975), and the molecular weights reported for these coat proteins are 24,300 (Kraal et al., 1976; Collot et al., 1976) and 29,500 (Ghabrial and Lister, 1974), respectively. TSV RNAs have a high affinity for AMV coat protein since they are able to withdraw subunits from AMV particles (Section 2.2).

The precise function(s) of the coat protein during the initiation of virus multiplication is (are) unknown. We can deduce from the lack of infectivity from the mixture of the three large RNAs that in the absence of coat protein at least RNA 3, which contains the genetic information for the coat protein, is not translated into functional proteins. RNA 3 is not a negative strand, since RNA 4 does not anneal to it (Bol et al., 1975). It is possible that for correct translation the RNA has to be associated with coat protein. To investigate this possibility, the products of AMV RNA-directed translation in a cell-free system from wheat germ were investigated (Section 5.1).

An indication that AMV coat protein in vivo plays a role in the translation process is found in the work of Dingjan-Versteegh and Van Vloten-Doting (1974). They compared the sensitivity of lesion induction on beans by the AMV strains 425 and YSMV to the presence of several antibiotics in the inoculum. Addition of chloramphenicol, which inhibits protein synthesis on organelle ribosomes, did not influence the infectivity of the two AMV strains. Addition of cycloheximide, which is an inhibitor of protein synthesis on cytoplasmic ribosomes, reduced the number of lesions of strain AMV 425 much more than that of strain YSMV. The infectivity of strain YSMV was severely reduced by the simultaneous addition of cycloheximide and chloramphenicol.

An explanation for this could be that the ribosomes of organelles, although normally playing a minor role in the translation of the AMV RNAs, become of primary importance for translation in case the translation by the cytoplasmic ribosomes is blocked by cycloheximide. Apparently AMV 425 does not have this refuge.

By comparing the sensitivity to cycloheximide of inocula consisting of the three large RNAs from YSMV either with coat protein from YSMV or AMV 425 or with RNA 4 from YSMV or AMV 425, it could be shown that the insensitivity to cycloheximide is directly coupled to the presence of YSMV coat protein in the inoculum. This is in accordance with the location of the genetic information for both sensitivity to cycloheximide and the coat protein on RNA 3 (Section 4.1).

The insensitivity to cycloheximide induced by YSMV coat protein can have two explanations: either the YSMV coat protein enables the RNA to pass the chloroplast membrane, or the YSMV coat protein enables the 70 S ribosomes to translate the viral RNAs. In our opinion, the latter explanation seems the more likely, but it has to be confirmed by *in vitro* experiments. Unfortunately, these experiments cannot yet be performed since a cell-free system from plants containing active 70 S ribosomes is not yet available. The experiment has been performed with 70 S ribosomes from *E. coli,* but in this case the translation of AMV 425 RNA 4 was not enhanced by the presence of YSMV coat protein (A. Castel, personal communication).

4. TEST-TUBE EXCHANGE OF GENETIC MATERIAL

4.1. Hybrids

The fact that with most viruses discussed in this chapter the infectivity has been shown to depend on the presence of the three largest RNAs (and in some cases also on protein) suggests that each of these RNAs contains a unique part of the genetic information necessary for the life cycle of the virus. Competitive hybridization studies can show whether the RNAs do share nucleotide sequences (Section 2.2). Translation *in vitro* can give indications about the number and size of the proteins encoded for by the RNAs (Section 5.1). Another way of investigating the relationship between the different RNAs from one virus is to study hybrids constructed from different strains of one virus or even from different viruses.

4.1.1. Isocapsidic Viruses

The only possible way to construct hybrids from strains of isocapsidic viruses is exchange of purified RNA species.

4.1.1a. Bromoviruses

Lane and Kaesberg (1971) obtained BMV isolates with an altered electrophoretic mobility of the nucleoprotein particles. Apparently, the coat protein cistron of these isolates had been mutated. By inoculating heterologous mixtures of the RNAs from the wild type and from one of the mutants, it was found that RNA 3 carries the genetic information for the coat protein.

Bancroft (1972) was able to construct a hybrid virus from RNA 1 and RNA 2 of BMV and RNA 3 of CCMV. The hybrid was serologically indistinguishable from CCMV, indicating that for CCMV as for BMV, the information for the coat protein is located on RNA 3. The compatibility of these CCMV- and BMV-RNAs is rather surprising, since it had earlier been found that the reverse combination was not infectious (Bancroft, 1971). Furthermore, CCMV and BMV, although both classified as bromoviruses, are rather different (Lane, 1974a). *In vitro* particles can be assembled from RNA of BMV and coat protein of CCMV and *vice versa* (Hiebert *et al.*, 1968). The host range of these particles was determined by their RNA. The host range of the BMV-CCMV hybrid was limited to plants that could be infected by both parent viruses, indicating that RNA 3 does more than just provide the coat protein cistron. *In vitro*, RNA 3 was indeed found to direct the synthesis of two proteins (see Section 5.1). The BMV-CCMV hybrid contained only very low amounts of RNA 3 and RNA 4. Since the coat protein is of the CCMV type, at least CCMV RNA 3 must have been present in the plant. The encapsidation of RNA 3 is probably only efficient in the presence of RNA 4. It is conceivable that a product from RNA 1 or RNA 2 is required for the correct assembly of particles or for the regulation of the synthesis of RNA 4 and that this product which is of the BMV type in the hybrid does not efficiently recognize CCMV RNA 3.

Bancroft and Lane (1973) isolated several mutants of BMV and CCMV. The mutations could be assigned to one of the RNAs by means of crosses with wild-type virus RNAs. Since the biochemical basis of symptom expression is unknown and may well be very complex, it is difficult to make comparisons between the results obtained with different viruses about the localization of the information for symptom expression. However, it is striking that none of the symptom mutants of the bromoviruses studied up to now is genetically associated with RNA 1.

Preparations of BMV F (Lane, 1974a), a naturally occurring variant, contain accessory particles in addition to normal particles. The two major classes of the accessory particles contain RNA 3 encapsidated by about 140 coat protein subunits or two molecules of RNA 4 surrounded by about 110 coat protein subunits, respectively. These particles resemble the smaller components from AMV, TSV, and the two citrus viruses (see Section 2.2). A mutation in RNA 2 was responsible for the formation of these smaller particles. This suggests that some factor besides the coat protein specified by RNA 2 is needed for correct assembly of BMV particles *in vivo*.

Bancroft *et al.* (1976) obtained a mutant of CCMV with a perturbed assembly mechanism. The mutant undergoes an abrupt pH induced reversible conformational change at pH values 1.5 lower than in the wild type. A number of amino acid replacements were found in the coat protein. Banding of the mutant in CsCl at pH 5.0 revealed an anomalous dense component. This component contains mainly RNA 4. All these properties were inherited through RNA 3. This indicates that either the formation or the encapsidation of RNA 4 is determined by some property encoded for by RNA 3.

4.1.1b. Cucumoviruses

It was possible to construct hybrids for cucumber mosaic virus by combining RNA species from different strains. The genetic information for the coat protein of CMV was also found to be located on RNA 3 (Marchoux *et al.*, 1974c). From the properties of the hybrids made between strains which cause necrotic lesions of different sizes on *Vigna sinensis* var. Black, it could be concluded that the size of the lesions is determined by RNA 3 (Marchoux *et al.*, 1974a). When hybrids were made between a strain which causes necrotic lesions and a strain which causes chlorotic lesions, it was found that both RNA 2 and RNA 3 influence the type of lesions found. Hybrids containing RNA 2 from the necrotic strain induced necrotic lesions; when RNA 2 from the chlorotic strain was present in the hybrids, chlorotic lesions were found only when RNA 3 was also derived from the chlorotic strain. A new type of symptom was found when the hybrids contained RNA 2 from the chlorotic strain and RNA 3 from the necrotic strain (Marchoux *et al.*, 1974b).

Habili and Francki (1974c) found that RNA 1 and RNA 2 of TAV and RNA 3 of CMV are compatible. TAV, although classified as a cucumovirus, has no detectable serological relationship (Habili and Francki, 1974a) and no significant base sequence homology (Habili and Francki, 1974c) with CMV. The TAV-CMV hybrid has, as expected, the CMV serotype, has base sequences of both TAV and CMV, is, like TAV, unable to infect cucumber, and induces symptoms of the TAV type on a number of host plants (all *Nicotiana*). The reverse combination was not compatible, a similar situation as encountered with BMV and CCMV (Bancroft, 1972). However, Marchoux *et al.* (1975) found that all combinations of their strains of PSV, TAV, and CMV were viable.

4.1.2. Heterocapsidic Viruses

Hybrids of heterocapsidic viruses can be constructed by the exchange of nucleoprotein components as well as by exchange of RNA species.

4.1.2a. AMV

The first report about hybrids between alfalfa mosaic virus strains is by Van Vloten-Doting *et al.* (1968). The experiments were performed on the RNA level, since at that time the infectivity of the nucleoprotein components often declined rapidly. RNA preparations were purified by means of sucrose density centrifugation. The combination of a heavy RNA fraction and a light RNA fraction (which at that time were thought to represent RNA 1 and RNA 4, respectively) was infectious. By combining RNA fractions from different strains, stable hybrids which showed characteristics from both parents could be obtained.

Later, it was found that the AMV genome consists of three RNAs (Bol *et al.*, 1971), while RNA 4, which is required only to start the infection, does not influence the characteristics of the progeny and is apparently not replicated (Bol and Van Vloten-Doting, 1973). By a careful reinvestigation of the hybrids constructed in 1968, it could be shown that the genome of these hybrids consisted of RNA 1 and RNA 2 from one parent and RNA 3 from the other parent (Bol and Van Vloten-Doting, 1973).

In 1969, Majorana and Paul obtained preparations containing mainly components B or Tb and Ta. From leaves inoculated with a mixture of preparations originating from different strains, they could obtain stable single-lesion isolates with a symptom pattern deviating from either parent. It seems plausible that these isolates are true hybrids between the two AMV strains. However, at that time the exact composition of the AMV genome was not yet known and no attention was given to the origin of M in the hybrids. Therefore, it is impossible to draw conclusions from this work about the localization of genetic information on the different components.

Knowing that B, M, and Tb are necessary for infectivity and that each of these components contains mainly one specific RNA, Dingjan-Versteegh *et al.* (1972) inoculated all possible heterologous mixtures of components from two AMV strains. The preparations used were purifed to the stage where the infectivity of the twofold combinations was about or less than 10% of that of the threefold combination. From the leaves inoculated with the heterologous mixtures, ten local lesion isolates were always investigated. When the ten isolates from one particular mixture were not all identical, the minor class was thought to be due either to contamination or to spontaneous mutation, while the characteristics of the major class were thought to belong to the hybrid.

From the results, it could be concluded that RNA 3 carries the genetic information for the coat protein. This RNA also specifies the type of symptoms on tobacco, the ratio of Ta to Tb, and the sensitivity to cycloheximide. RNA 2 determines whether or not the symptoms on bean will become systemic. By constructing hybrids between three AMV strains, it was shown (J. F. Bol, unpublished results) that RNA 3 determines the size of the local lesions on bean, and that the ratio of B to M to Tb is influenced by all three components.

Franck and Hirth (1972) isolated a mutant from AMV-S which could multiply at higher temperatures than AMV-S. From this mutant, three clones were obtained which all multiplied better at 34°C than at 22°C. Hybrids between these mutant clones and AMV-S were constructed (Franck and Hirth, 1976). The factor for thermoresistance was found to be located on RNA 1, while the factor for replication at 22°C was located on RNA 3 of the wild type.

Hartmann *et al.* (1976) isolated three mutants from AMV-S which all differed from the wild type in symptomatology on tobacco, the ratio of nucleoproteins, and the tryptic fingerprints from the coat proteins. The ratio of RNA 4 to 3 increased with increasing temperature in the wild type and in one mutant, in the other two mutants the component composition underwent little change with increasing temperature. All these characters were inherited through RNA 3. This suggests that, as was also seen with CCMV(Section 4.1.1a), the formation or the encapsidation of RNA 4 is specified by RNA 3.

4.1.2b. TSV

Hybrids have also been constructed for tobacco streak virus by combining nucleoprotein preparations from different strains (Fulton, 1970, 1972, 1975). The results are much more difficult to interpret than the results obtained with the viruses discussed before.

Although the preparations used had been purified by four successive cycles of sucrose density gradient centrifugation, the uncombined preparations produced some lesions, and the twofold combinations produced a large number of lesions (compare Section 3.2.2b).

When the TSV hybrids described by Fulton are classified according to their characteristics and not according to the components used to construct the hybrids, all results published up to now fit into a scheme with four linkage groups. When the number of linkage groups is restricted to three, we would have to conclude that in TSV a very high frequency of recombination takes place. In some cases, values up to 50% are found. These values are in line with reassortment of RNA strands rather than with recombination between RNA strands.

Although we do not yet understand the molecular basis of the TSV hybrids, a number of conclusions can be drawn from Fulton's work. The dwarf growth induced by some TSV strains is due to the presence of two determinants; one of these determinants is linked to the determinant of the serotype. The information for local lesion size and local lesion color is, as was also found for CMV and AMV, located on different RNA strands.

4.1.2c. NRSV

Loesch and Fulton (1975) found that the ability of NRSV-S to infect *Vigna sinensis* is determined by genetic information carried in B particles.

4.1.2d. CLRV, CVV, and LRMV

Up to now no hybrids between strains of citrus leaf rugose virus, citrus variegation virus or lilac ring mottle virus have been described.

4.1.2e. Intervirus Hybrids

Although it has been found that heterologous mixtures of RNA and coat protein from AMV, TSV, and the two citrus viruses are all infectious (Section 3.4), the nucleoproteins from the different viruses were found to be incompatible (Van Vloten-Doting, 1975; Gonsalves, personal communication).

For the viruses with tripartite genomes, the study of hybrids has been very successful, since up to now all strains of a given virus and even some combinations of different bromo- and cucumoviruses have been found to be compatible. It is remarkable that in all cases the genetic information for the coat protein is located on RNA 3, the size of local lesions is mostly determined by RNA 3, and chlorotic or necrotic symptoms are often determined by RNA 2.

4.2. Backcross Experiments

The characterization of hybrids showed that the three RNAs, although completely dependent on each other for their replication, retain their own identity as judged by their phenotypic expression. When the RNAs are replicated true to type, it must be possible to reconstruct the parent strains starting from the hybrids.

Bancroft (1972) showed that the RNAs from the BMV-CCMV hybrid, upon recombination with RNAs from BMV and CCMV, yielded strains that were indistinguishable from the parent strains.

Also, in the case of CMV (Marchoux *et al.*, 1974*b*), the genetic information of the RNAs was not detectably altered during replication of the hybrid genome.

For AMV and TSV, similar experiments were performed on the nucleoprotein level. The results obtained with AMV confirm the idea that all RNAs are replicated true to type (Dingjan-Versteegh *et al.*, 1974). The results obtained with TSV (Fulton, 1975) are rather difficult to interpret, which might be due to the ambiguity in the relationship between RNAs and nucleoproteins. Another complicating factor might be that the hybrid clones used for the backcross experiments were not representative for the hybrids to be investigated, because they did not belong to the major class of isolates, and their genotype may well reflect impurities present in the preparations used to construct the hybrids. Nevertheless, Fulton's results (1975) permit the conclusion that also in TSV the RNAs retain their own identity during replication in the presence of RNAs from other strains.

4.3. Thermosensitive Mutants

One way to determine the number of cistrons present in each of the viral RNAs may be by *in vitro* translation of the RNAs (Section 5.1); another way is to determine the number of complementation groups per RNA. The latter approach has been very fruitful in the investigations of phages and animal viruses. A disadvantage of this method is that a rather large number of thermosensitive mutants is required for a reliable estimate of the number of complementation groups per RNA.

For both CCMV and AMV, thermosensitive mutants have been isolated. The mutations were assigned to one of the RNAs (or nucleoproteins) by supplementation tests as described by Bancroft and Lane (1973).

Of the two mutants of CCMV, both induced by nitrous acid treatment, one is located on RNA 1 (Bancroft and Lane, 1973) and one on RNA 3 (Bancroft *et al.*, 1972). The coat protein from the latter mutant had a lower denaturation temperature than the wild-type protein, and in mutant infected leaves kept at 32°C (the nonpermissive temperature) only few virus particles but much free viral RNA was produced.

In tobacco leaves infected with a chlorotic AMV strain, yellow spots are sometimes seen. From these spots stable mutant strains can be isolated. A relatively large proportion (over 25%) of these mutants were found to be thermolabile (Van Vloten-Doting *et al.*, to be published). Apart from complementation studies, these mutants can be helpful in the localization of the replicase and in the investigations about the role of the coat protein.

5. TRANSLATION AND AMINOACYLATION

5.1. *In Vitro* Translation

The genome of viruses with tripartite genomes comprises about 2.5×10^6 daltons of RNA. Of this, only 10% is required for the encoding of the coat protein. The identification of other gene products has been undertaken by attempting to recover purified viral RNA replicases (Section 6).

By investigating the characteristics of hybrids constructed from different strains of viruses, a number of biological properties were found to be determined by the different RNAs (Section 4). However, this does not give insight into the number and size of the proteins encoded for by the viral RNAs. A possible way to study the information present in the viral RNAs is by their translation *in vitro*. Until the beginning of this decade, there were no successful protein-synthesizing systems from plants. Around 1972, it was found that extracts made from wheat embryo gave substantial *in vitro* protein synthesis with a variety of messengers. The products directed by the RNAs from a number of viruses have since been studied in this system. Furthermore, the influence of the cap on the *in vitro* translation was investigated.

5.1.1.   Translation Products of RNA 4

The main product directed by RNA 4 of the bromo- and cucumoviruses and of AMV comigrates with the corresponding coat proteins on SDS polyacrylamide gels (Shih and Kaesberg, 1973; Davies and Kaesberg, 1974; Schwinghamer and Symons, 1975; Van Vloten-Doting *et al.*, 1975; Thang *et al.*, 1975). The electrophoretic patterns of the tryptic peptides from the *in vitro* product of BMV RNA 4 and from BMV coat protein showed substantial similarity in position. However, the ratio of the peaks was not constant, which might be due to the use of a mixture of amino acids with varied specific activity. The products directed by BMV RNA 4 and CMV RNA 4 were both mixed with their corresponding coat protein and subjected to cyanogen bromide cleavage. The electrophoretic patterns of peptides resulting from the *in vitro* product were completely identical to those of the authentic protein (Shih and Kaesberg, 1973; Schwinghamer and Symons, 1975). The translation product of BMV RNA 4 was fully acetylated *in vitro*, as judged from the incorporation of one acetyl group per 11 leucine residues, presumably at the *N*-terminus (Shih and Kaesberg, 1973).

From the main product directed by AMV RNA 4 which comigrates with coat protein, and from a minor product with an apparent molecular weight of 16,000, tryptic peptide maps were made. In both cases, all strong radioactive spots (= *in vitro* products) matched the strong ninhydrin spots (= AMV coat protein). This indicates that both products have all sequences of AMV coat protein. The higher electrophoretic mobility of the minor product must be due to the attachment of a negatively charged molecule. This could be the last tRNA, indicating that termination is the rate-limiting step, which would explain the absence of nascent chains on the gels. The presence of radioactivity on the spot of the first tryptic peptide, with the known sequence of Ac-Ser-Ser-Ser-Gln-Lys (Kraal *et al.*, 1972), shows that the *in vitro* product also has been acetylated (Van Vloten-Doting *et al.*, 1975).

The main product directed by TSV RNA 4 comigrates with TSV coat protein. Further, a small amount of a product which is estimated to be about 2500 daltons heavier is formed. It is not yet known whether this is a precursor or a read-through product of the coat protein (Rutgers, to be published).

The genetic information of the RNA 4 of these various viruses is somewhat larger than required for the coding of the coat protein. For instance, the molecular weight of AMV RNA 4 is 280,000 (Heijtink, 1974). Of this, 85% is required for the coat protein; the remaining information (about 130 bases) is too small for the coding of a second protein. For BMV, it has been found that the last 160 nucleotides at the 3′ terminus were virtually identical in all four RNAs. Apparently this part of the RNA is involved in another process (see Section 2.1 and Section 5.3).

5.1.2. Translation Products of RNA 3

For AMV and isocapsidic viruses it is known from complementation studies (Section 4) that RNA 3 also contains the genetic information for the coat protein. Under the direction of RNA 3 from the bromo- and the cucumoviruses, two main products are formed. One product comigrates on SDS polyacrylamide gels with the corresponding coat protein, while the other has an estimated molecular weight of 35,000 (called 3a protein). The ratio of 3a protein to coat protein is in favor of 3a for BMV (Shih and Kaesberg, 1973) and CMV (Schwinghamer and Symons, 1975), about equal for BBMV, and in favor of coat protein for CCMV (Davies and Kaesberg, 1974). Under the direction of RNA 3 from the two latter viruses, small amounts of products migrating slower than 3a protein were also formed. It cannot be excluded that these products are translated from contaminating RNA 1 or 2. According to Kaesberg (1976) the results obtained with BMV may be interpreted as follows. From RNA 3 only the cistron located near the 5′ terminus of the RNA and coding for the 3a protein is translated. The cistron for coat protein on RNA 3 is closed and the coat protein seen reflects the contamination of the RNA 3 preparation with RNA 4.

Concerning the translation of AMV RNA 3 the results obtained with AMV-S and AMV 425 are contradictory. Translation of AMV-S in a wheat germ extract without spermine gave only a small amount of a 3a-like protein. Addition of spermine resulted in an increase of the amount of 3a-like protein but no coat protein was found (Thang *et al.*, 1976). The translation products of AMV 425 RNA 3 are more heterogeneous: a peak at the position of coat protein, a dominating peak of a 3a-like protein, and a slower-migrating band (Fig. 3B). The ratio of 3a-like protein to coat protein was in favor of coat protein in the absence of spermine and in favor of 3a-like protein in the presence of spermine (Neeleman *et al.,* to be published). The pattern was not significantly influenced by the presence of coat protein during the translation of RNA 3. The formation of coat protein under the direction of RNA 3 is quite surprising, since we know from infectivity studies that *in vivo* coat pro-

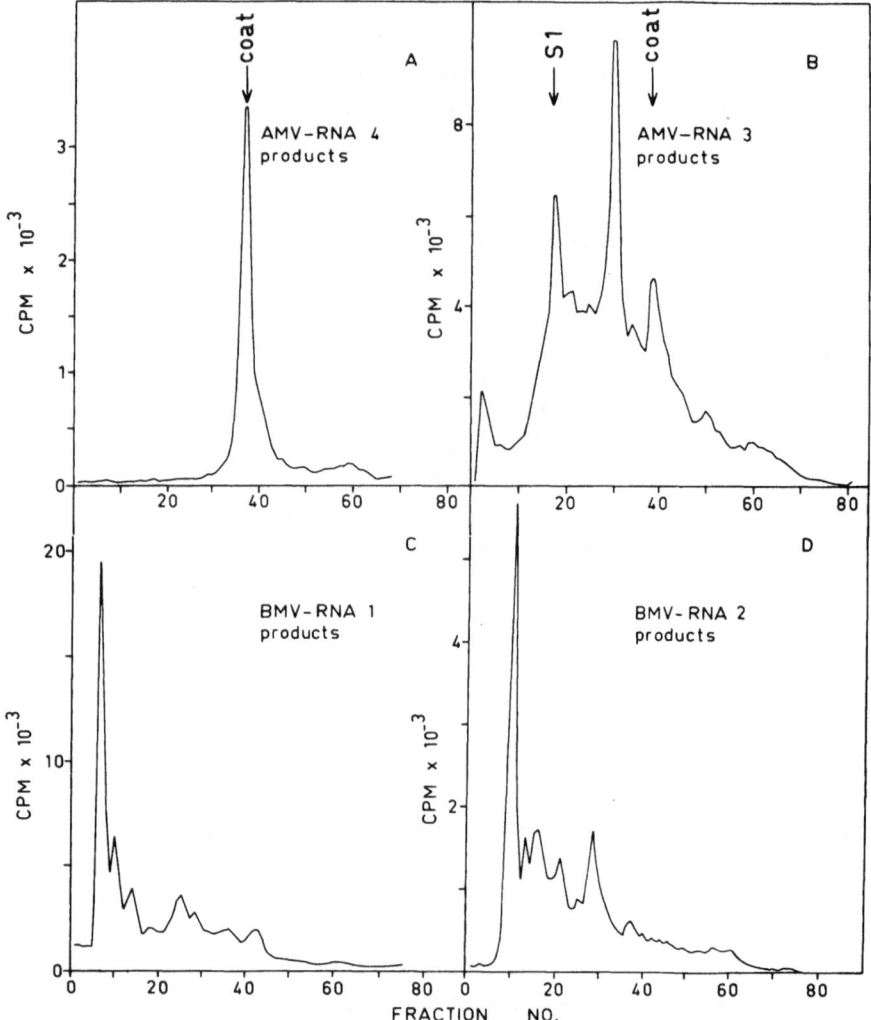

Fig. 3. *In vitro* translation products of AMV RNA 4 (A), AMV RNA 3 (B), BMV RNA 1 (C), and BMV RNA 2 (D). The position of markers in A and B is indicated by arrows. S1 is a ribosomal protein from *Escherichia coli* with a molecular weight of 65,000; the molecular weight of AMV coat protein is 24,300. The molecular weights of the major BMV products are about 100,000. Drawings B and C by courtesy of Dr. D. S. Shih.

tein is required for the formation of coat protein from RNA 3 (Section 3.4). The RNA 3 preparation did not contain any detectable RNA 4. However, it cannot be excluded that during the incubation RNA 3 was processed to an RNA 4-like product. The molecular weight of the largest product, which probably represents the total of genetic information present in RNA 3, is slightly larger than the sum of the molceular weights of 3a and coat protein. The presence of coat protein sequences in this large product and in the material at the coat protein position was demonstrated by the fact that both products could be precipitated by antiserum raised against AMV particles (Van Vloten-Doting, 1976). These results suggest that the large protein is either a precursor of coat protein and 3a protein or a read-through product. Two ribosome binding sites have been found on AMV RNA 3 (Van Vloten-Doting *et al.*, 1977).*

Under the direction of TSV RNA 3, a main product with an estimated molecular weight of 35,000 and some faster migrating material were formed, but no larger products (T. Rutgers, unpublished results). Apparently the formation of a large precursor or readthrough protein is not specific for the coat protein dependent viruses.

Judged from the ratio of incorporated [^{35}S]methionine to incorporated non-sulfur-containing amino acids (phenylalanine, lysine, leucine, isoleucine, and alanine) in coat protein and 3a-like protein, the 3a-like protein of AMV, BMV, and TSV is rather rich in methionine. Comparison of the tryptic peptide maps of the incorporated products (labeled with [^{35}S]methionine) did not reveal corresponding peptides (L. Neeleman and L. Van Vloten-Doting, unpublished results).

5.1.3. Translation Products of RNAs 1 and 2

Since RNAs 1 and 2 of the bromo- and cucumoviruses are rather difficult to separate, a number of *in vitro* studies has been performed with a mixture of these two RNAs. The translation products were very heterogeneous [Shih and Kaesberg, 1973 (BMV); Davies and Kaesberg, 1974 (CCMV); Schwinghamer and Symons, 1975 (CMV); Van Vloten-Doting *et al.*, 1975; Thang *et al.*, 1975 (AMV)]. Assuming that the translation product bands obtained on SDS polyacrylamide gels all

---

* **Note Added in Proof:** Contrary to the results obtained with RNA 3 from AMV 425 by Van Vloten-Doting *et al.* (1977), Gerlinger *et al.* (Gerlinger, P., Mohier, E., Le Meur, M. A., and Hirth, L., 1977, *Nucleic Acid Res.* 4:813) found that RNA 3 from AMV-S could bind only one single ribosome. Furthermore, these authors found that the initiating dipeptides for RNA 3 and RNA 4 were different.

represent complete peptide chains, the total molecular weight of the translation products can be calculated. The observed gene content (in daltons of protein) is much higher than the theoretical maximum, suggesting that the peaks represent either posttranslational cleavage products or incomplete chains. The latter explanation seems the more likely since Shih and Kaesberg (1976) were able to translate RNA 1 as a single major protein of molecular weight 110,000 and RNA 2 as a single major protein of molecular weight 105,000 (Fig. 3C,D). Analysis of *N*-termini and tryptic peptides suggests strongly that the minor bands represent incomplete peptide chains. Furthermore, ribosome binding experiments indicate that the two largest RNAs of both BMV and AMV have only one ribosome binding site (Kaesberg, 1975; Shih and Kaesberg, 1976; Davies, 1976; Van Vloten-Doting *et al.,* 1977).

Since the formation of a protein of a molecular weight of about 100,000 would account for all the coding capacity of RNA 1 or 2, both RNAs seem to be monocistronic.

5.1.4. Translation of RNA Mixtures

Translation of mixtures containing RNA 4 yields in all cases mainly coat protein with small peaks of the slower-migrating products. It has been suggested (BMV: Shih and Kaesberg, 1973; Davies and Kaesberg, 1974; CMV: Schwinghamer and Symons, 1975) that these results reflect the relative accessibility of the ribosome binding sites of the different RNAs. However, this is in contrast to the finding that the optimum number of RNA 4 molecules per incubation volume is about 4 times more than the optimum number of RNA 1 or RNA 2 molecules (Van Vloten-Doting *et al.,* 1975).

5.1.5. Translation in Other Cell-Free Systems

AMV RNA 4 had earlier been used as messenger in the *E. coli* cell-free system. The product formed did have amino acid sequences in common with the authentic coat protein (Van Ravenswaay Claasen *et al.,* 1967). More recently it was shown that RNA 4 directs in the *E. coli* cell-free system the synthesis of a protein of the same size as authentic coat protein. The tryptic peptides of the *in vitro* product are very similar to those of the *in vivo* product with the exception of the *N*-terminal peptide, which is possibly blocked by an *N*-formylmethionine (A. Castel, personal communication). Besides the start with *N*-formylmethionine the protein synthesis on AMV RNA 4 in an *E. coli* cell-free system can also start with *N*-acetylphenylalanine. This initiation takes place probably a few nucleotides prior to the AUG codon (Van Vloten-Doting *et al.*, 1977; A. Castel, to be published).

The RNAs from both AMV and BMV have been translated in a cell-free system from *Bacillus stearothermophilus* (J. W. Davies, personal communication). It is remarkable that the translation of the large AMV RNAs was more efficient at 60°C than at 30°C. This could indicate that at this temperature the secondary structure of the RNAs has been melted. It is tempting to speculate that AMV coat protein has at 30°C a similar effect on the structure of the AMV RNAs.

The BMV RNAs were translated in a cell-free system from mouse L cells and it was found that the major product resembled the authentic coat protein in electrophoretic mobility and in peptide map (Ball *et al.*, 1973).

The AMV RNAs have also been translated in a cell-free system derived from rabbit reticulocytes or from Krebs ascites cells (Mohier *et al.*, 1975). The results obtained with RNA 4 confirm the results obtained with the cell-free system from wheat germ or from *E. coli*. Translation of RNA 3 yields predominantly a 3a-like protein. The peptide map of this protein was shown to be different from that of the coat protein. They also compared the tryptic peptides of the products with molecular weights between 20,000 and 30,000 with those of coat protein and found them to be different (Mohier *et al.*, 1976). However, the autoradiogram will mainly be determined by the dominant product, which in this region was a product of about 30,000. One wonders whether upon longer exposure time, spots corresponding to the other proteins (coat protein?) will appear. Minor slower-migrating bands were also observed, which contained tryptic peptides not found in either 3a-like protein or coat protein. Since RNA 3 in this case had been purified from a total RNA preparation by gel electrophoresis, the possibility exists that these products have been directed by degradation products of RNA 1 or RNA 2 which comigrated with RNA 3. Both RNA 1 and RNA 2 directed the synthesis of a large protein, which could represent the total genetic information present in these RNAs, together with a number of faster migrating products.

5.1.6. Influence of the Cap on the Efficiency of Translation

BMV RNAs from which the terminal m⁷G had been removed could still function as messengers, although much less efficiently than untreated BMV RNAs. The activity of RNA 4 was much more affected than that of RNA 3 (Shih, Dasgupta, and Kaesberg, 1976).

In the presence of the cap analog $m^7G^{5'}p$ the translation of all AMV RNAs was inhibited. However, at high RNA concentration (2.5 $\mu g/100 \mu l$) the amount of inhibition was different for each of the four RNAs. The sensitivity of the translation of different RNAs for $m^7G^{5'}p$ might be inversely related to their affinity for either the ribosomes or the initiation factors. The translation of 3a-like protein and coat protein on RNA 3 were both more sensitive to inhibition by $m^7G^{5'}p$ than the translation of coat protein from RNA 4 (Van Vloten-Doting *et al.*, 1977).

5.2. *In Vivo* Translation

5.2.1. Translation in Protoplasts

For CCMV, extensive studies of protein synthesis in protoplasts have been performed (Sakai *et al.*, 1977). Upon infection of protoplasts previously irradiated with UV light to inhibit host protein synthesis, a number of viral proteins could be detected (Fig. 4). Of the two major peaks, one band apparently corresponds to CCMV coat protein, while peak 2 (estimated molecular weight 36,000) could correspond to

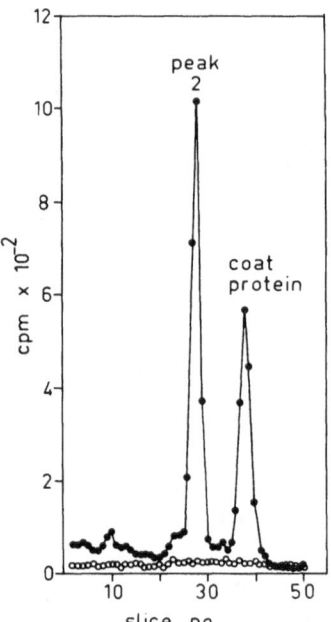

Fig. 4.   Protein synthesis in CCMV-infected proto-plasts. UV-irradiated protoplasts were incubated for 24 h in the presence of actinomycin D with [³H]leucine (●, infected) or [¹⁴C]leucine (○, healthy). Drawing by courtesy of Dr. J. W. Watts.

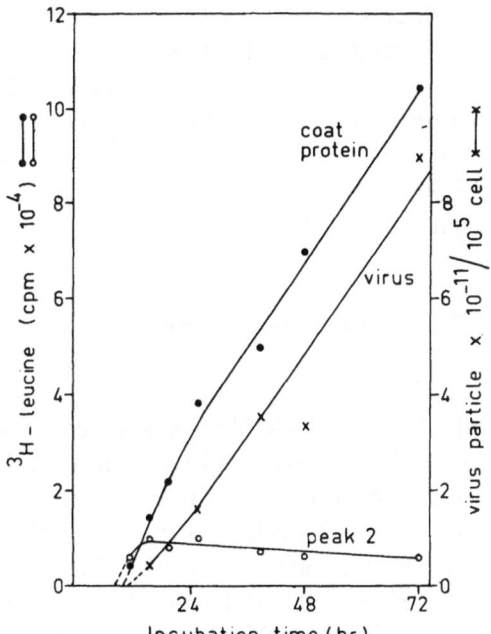

Fig. 5. Time course of synthesis of coat protein, peak 2 protein, and virus in UV-irradiated protoplasts after infection with CCMV. Drawing by courtesy of Dr. J. W. Watts.

the 3a-like product found upon *in vitro* translation of RNA 3 (Section 5.1.2). The two bands with molecular weights of about 100,000 could represent the translation products of RNAs 1 and 2, respectively. The level of translation is apparently regulated, since RNAs 1 and 2 are present in rather large amounts, while only very small bands of the corresponding proteins are found.

The synthesis of coat protein and peak 2 protein was followed in time (Fig. 5). The early appearance of the latter product is in agreement with the suggestion by Hariharasubramanian *et al.* (1973) that a protein of this size is (part of) the replicase.

5.2.2. Translation in Oocytes

The AMV and BMV RNAs have been injected into oocytes of *Xenopus laevis* (G. Marbaix, G. Huez, and T. Rutgers, unpublished results). The products were analyzed on SDS polyacrylamide gels. The following results were obtained with AMV: RNA 4 directs the synthesis of only one protein, which comigrates with authentic coat protein; RNA 3 directs the synthesis of two proteins, coat protein and 3a-like protein, but no larger products are found; upon injection of RNA 1, a product of about 100,000 daltons is formed, while up to now no products directed by RNA 2 have been seen. BMV RNA 1 and 2 each direct the synthesis of a protein with an apparent molecular weight around 100,000 daltons; the product of RNA 1 is slightly larger than that of RNA 2. BMV RNA 3 directs only one product of molecular weight 35,000. The main product directed by BMV RNA 4 appears to be BMV coat protein.

5.2.3. Translation by Polyribosomes Isolated from Infected Tobacco

Bol *et al.* (1976*b*) isolated polyribosomes from tobacco leaves infected with AMV. Six species of viral mRNA were identified: the four AMV RNAs and two additional RNAs with molecular weights of about 600,000. Upon dissociation of the polyribosomes with EDTA, the viral mRNA is released in an mRNP structure. The composition of the mRNP structure is influenced by the isolation procedure. With a low-salt buffer (0.04 M tris–0.06 M KCl), viral coat protein is found to be present in an mRNP structure with a buoyant density of 1.45 g/ml. With a high-salt buffer (0.2 M tris–0.4 M KCl), the buoyant density of the structure is much higher (1.60 g/ml) and no viral coat protein is detectable. This demonstrates that under high salt conditions a considerable amount of protein is dissociated from the mRNP structure or is prevented from association.

Upon addition of a postribosomal supernatant from wheat germ and other requirements for protein synthesis, polyribosomes prepared with high-salt or low-salt buffer are equally efficient in completing nascent peptide chains. In both cases, the only detectable virus-specific polypeptide labeled *in vitro* is viral coat protein.

5.3. Aminoacylation

All four BMV RNAs are known to have a nucleotide sequence terminating in CCA_{OH} (Section 2.1). When it was found that other viral RNAs (TMV and tymoviruses) could accept amino acids, the capacity of BMV RNA to bind amino acids was investigated (Hall *et al.*, 1972). For these experiments, an aminoacyl tRNA-synthesizing system from cotyledons of developing French bean seeds was used. Of all 20 amino acids tested, only tyrosine was bound to BMV RNA. A small binding of phenylalanine was observed; however, this disappeared when the phenylalanine was challenged with tyrosine, while the tyrosine binding was not inhibited by the presence of a large amount of phenylalanine.

The tyrosylation of the BMV RNAs had very similar properties to tyrosyl-tRNA synthesis by cell-free systems from plants: the reaction is enzyme-and-energy-dependent, and the ester bond is rapidly hydrolyzed at alkaline pH.

To determine which component(s) of BMV RNA bind tyrosine, the charged BMV RNA was subjected to sedimentation in a sucrose density gradient at pH 5.0. The UV absorption peaks of the RNA components of authentic BMV RNA, run in a sister tube, coincided with the radioactivity peaks (representing bound tyrosine). An additional peak of radioactivity was observed at the top of the gradient, which was shown to represent tyrosyl-tRNA resulting from endogenous tRNA^{Tyr}, present in the synthetase preparation. From the radioactivity, the UV absorption, and the molecular weights of the BMV RNAs, the extent of aminoacylation of RNAs 1 + 2, RNA 3, and RNA 4 can be calculated. The percentage charging was found to be roughly the same for each RNA (about 58%).

It has been reported (Chen and Hall, 1973) that a small amount of tyrosine could be transferred from tyrosyl-BMV RNA to peptidyl material. However, later experiments indicate that this is not the case and that the earlier results must be attributed to hydrolysis of the BMV RNA tyrosine bond and subsequent binding of the radioactive tyrosine to tRNA^{Tyr} (T. C. Hall, personal communication).

After limited digestion with ribonuclease T_1, a fragment of about 160 nucleotides can be isolated from all four BMV RNAs (Section 2.1). These fragments, which represent the 3′ end of the molecules, are still capable of tyrosine binding (Bastin *et al.* 1976). The tyrosylated 160-nucleotide fragment obtained by partial T_1 digestion was also incapable of transferring its tyrosine to peptidyl material (T. C. Hall, personal communication).

Modification of the 3′ terminus of BMV RNA to a dialdehyde derivative and subsequently to the morpholine derivative resulted in the loss of the ability to accept tyrosine. However, the modified BMV RNA was still capable of functioning as messenger. The pattern of radioactivity obtained for the products of the reaction directed by the dialdehyde derivative was identical to that of the unmodified BMV RNA products, while that of the morpholine derivative showed a different ratio of 3a to coat protein (compare Section 5.1). This could indicate that the structure of BMV RNAs 3 and/or 4 has been altered in such a way that the affinities (or accessibilities) of the ribosomes for the different cistrons have been changed. A possible explanation for these findings could be that not only the ribose residue at the 3′ end of the RNA was attacked but also that of the m⁷G of the cap at the 5′ end. This would mean that the formation of a dialdehyde does not interfere with the function of the cap, but that the formation of a morpholine derivative had a similar effect as the removal of the m⁷G (compare Section 5.1.6). Nevertheless, these results indicate that aminoacylation of BMV RNA is not an obligatory step for translation of this viral RNA (Shih *et al.*, 1974).

Tyrosylated BMV RNA was found to interact with a binary complex of wheat germ elongation factor 1 and [³H]GTP. BMV RNA itself or acetylated aminoacyl BMV RNA did not react with the complex. The interaction seems to be similar to the reaction of EF1 with aminoacyl-tRNAs. However, instead of the formation of a ternary complex, the aminoacylated viral RNA caused a release of GTP from the complex (Bastin and Hall, 1976). The affinity of the acylated viral RNA for EF1 is in favor of the model proposed by Hall and Wepprich (1976) for a role of aminoacylation of viral RNA in transcription.

The RNAs from the other bromoviruses as well as the CMV RNAs were found to be capable of binding tyrosine, provided that plant enzymes were used. Synthetase enzymes of bacteria or yeast were ineffective in the esterification of the bromo- or cucumovirus RNAs. The same enzyme preparations were capable of binding amino acids to TMV or turnip yellow mosaic virus RNAs (Kohl and Hall, 1974). The RNAs from AMV as well as those from TSV could not be charged with any amino acid under the conditions used for the charging of BMV (T. C. Hall, personal communication), not even when coat protein was added to the incubation mixture (unpublished result).

At the moment, the meaning of a tRNA-like 3′ end of viral RNAs is obscure. The present data rule out direct participation of charged viral RNAs as amino acid donors in protein biosynthesis and also the possibility that this 3′ end is obligatory for messenger capacity. The fact that all four BMV RNAs have a (nearly) identical sequence of 160 nucleotides at the 3′ end indicates that this region might be very important. It seems likely that binding of an amino acid, or the tRNA-like structure itself, is involved in the recognition of the replicase.

6. REPLICATION

6.1. Double-Stranded RNAs

It is uncertain whether progeny viral RNA is produced from a double-stranded RNA molecule, but the formation of a complementary strand in infected cells is a prerequisite for RNA replication. Even if double-stranded RNA is a decomposition product resulting from disruption of the replication complex, it is nonetheless characteristic for RNA replication.

In leaves infected with a virus with a tripartite genome, "replicative forms" for each of the parts of the genome are expected. For the bromoviruses (Lane, 1974a; Philipps *et al.*, 1974) and for AMV (Mohier *et al.*, 1974; Bol *et al.*, 1975) this has indeed been found.

There is some ambiguity about the existence of a replicative form corresponding to RNA 4. Lane and Kaesberg (1971), Bastin and Kaesberg (1976), and Bol *et al.* (1975) found a double-stranded RNA molecule with the size expected for the replicative form of RNA 4. Such a molecule was not found by other investigators. It is possible that progeny RNA 4 is transcribed from a strand complementary to RNA 3. RNase treatment of such a complex would yield an apparent double-stranded RNA for RNA 4. The same reasoning could apply to the replicative form corresponding to one of the minor RNA components, which was found in BMV-infected leaves by Lane and Kaesberg (1971) but not in infected protoplasts (Bancroft *et al.*, 1974).

6.2. Replicase

6.2.1. Bromoviruses

In the particulate fraction of BMV-infected barley, an RNA synthetic activity was found which was not present in healthy leaves (Semal and Hamilton, 1968). Semal and Kummert (1971) showed by pulse chase experiments with crude enzyme preparations that the first product labeled is a double-stranded RNA of about 14 S, which is the precursor of single-stranded RNA. The double-stranded RNA remains in the particulate fraction while part of the single-stranded molecules are released in the supernatant (Semal *et al.*, 1974). Since the single-stranded RNA interfered with self-reannealing of double-stranded BMV RNA, its base sequence must be homologous to that of parental viral RNA. When exogenous RNA was added to avoid the degradation of the labeled product by endogenous RNases, the radioactive single-stranded RNAs cosedimented on sucrose density gradients with the BMV RNAs (Kummert and Semal, 1972). Also, on polyacrylamide gels the single-stranded RNAs migrated in the same region as the three largest BMV RNAs (Kummert and Semal, 1974). The double-stranded RNA had the expected gel electrophoretic mobilities (Kummert, 1974).

In the particulate fraction from broad bean infected with BBMV, an enzyme activity is present which is very similar to the one found in BMV-infected barley (Romero and Jacquemin, 1971). The RNA produced during a short pulse was shown by reannealing experiments to have sequences homologous to parental viral RNA (Jacquemin, 1972). By polyacrylamide gel electrophoresis, Jacquemin and Lopez (1974) could show that the product made in the first 2 min had the properties of replicative forms of the large BBMV RNAs. Upon heating, radioactive RNAs of the size of the BBMV genome were produced.

The BMV RNA replicase can be released from the membrane and the template by the use of a nonionic detergent (Triton X100) in the presence of a reducing agent (Hadidi and Fraenkel-Conrat, 1973). The addition of template stimulates the soluble enzyme about fivefold. BMV RNA is the most efficient template, followed by CCMV RNA. Other viral RNAs, including BBMV RNA, are less efficient. The replicase activity is dependent on the presence of all four triphosphates. Optimal activity is found at pH 8.0 and 32 mM Mg^{2+}. In a sucrose density gradient, the enzyme activity sediments with about 6 S. However, in this purified form the enzyme loses its activity in a few hours at 0°C. All four BMV RNAs can stimulate the activity of the soluble RNA polymerase. The main product formed is about 0.5×10^6 daltons. A small amount of material of about 1.5×10^6 daltons is also found. These two products could correspond to replicative forms for RNA 4 and RNA 3, respectively. Products corresponding to replicative forms of RNA 1 and RNA 2 were not found (Hadidi, 1974). From the fact that an unfractionated BMV RNA preparation, which had been heated until all three RNAs had been degraded and only a peak of RNA 4 remained, still retained 40% of its original template activity it was concluded that RNA 4 is the most active component (Hadidi *et al.*, 1973). In fractions which contain the BMV replicase, a protein of about 34,500 daltons is found. A protein comparable in size is synthesized early after infection in leaves (Hariharasubramanian *et al.*, 1973), as well as in protoplasts (Section 5.2.1) and is translated *in vitro* from BMV RNA 3 (Section 5.1.2).

6.2.2.   CMV

In leaf homogenates from CMV-infected cucumbers, three virus-induced RNA polymerase activities have been found, one in the supernatant (Gilliland and Symons, 1968; May *et al.*, 1969) and two in the particulate fraction. Only one of the two latter activities was independent of added RNA (May *et al.*, 1970). The bound replicase could be solubilized by a high concentration of MgSO$_4$. The properties of the solubilized enzymes were very similar to the properties of the enzyme of the supernatant. Clark *et al.* (1974) purified the supernatant enzyme by a polymer partition system followed by a DEAE Sephadex and a phosphocellulose column. From healthy leaves, only a negligible RNA replicase activity was obtained by the same purification procedure. The preparation obtained from infected leaves contained, besides an RNA-dependent polymerase activity, a poly(C)-dependent activity. The two activities eluted at different salt concentrations from a DNA agarose column. The purified enzyme was unstable at 0°C and at −15°C, but it could be stored in liquid nitrogen without loss of activity. The purified enzyme was not specific for CMV RNA as it copied also three other RNAs (*E. coli* ribosomal RNA, TMV RNA, and yeast RNA) tested. This could indicate that the enzyme obtained is an incomplete form and that the subunit(s) determining the specificity has been lost. The authors speculate about the possibility that the poly(C)-dependent activity represents also an incomplete form of the real enzyme. At the moment, there is only circumstantial evidence (Peden *et al.*, 1972) that this enzyme is involved in the *in vivo* replication of viral RNA, either as isolated or as part of a more complex enzyme structure.

6.2.3. AMV

In the particulate fraction of AMV-infected broad beans (Weening and Bol, 1975) as well as of AMV-infected tobacco leaves (Semal, 1969; Weening, 1975), a membrane-bound enzyme–template complex has been found. A complicating factor in these experiments is the presence of an actinomycin D-insensitive RNA synthetic activity in healthy leaves. However, the product made by the particulate fraction of healthy leaves was RNase sensitive and sedimented with about 4 S, while the product made by the particulate fraction from infected leaves was RNase resistant and sedimented with about 15 S. Furthermore, it contained base sequences from AMV RNA since it could be displaced by AMV RNA in reannealing experiments.

Attempts have been made to solubilize the virus-induced enzyme from tobacco by treatment with nonionic detergents. RNA polymerase activity was indeed found in the supernatant after treatment with Lubrol. However, the detergent released a similar RNA polymerase activity from healthy leaves. Both enzymes could be stimulated by a variety of RNAs. About half of the product was RNase resistant.

Optimum pH for both enzymes was around 7.5. Both enzymes were dependent on a rather high concentration of Mg^{2+}. These results suggest that the two enzymes are identical and that the virus-induced enzyme or the virus-induced subunit(s) had remained in the particulate fraction (Bol *et al.*, 1976*a*). The virus-induced enzyme could be solubilized by extracting the pellet with a buffer devoid of magnesium. Similar treatment of healthy material did not yield any activity. The activity was not dependent upon addition of RNA. Apparently, the enzyme was still associated with template. However, added AMV RNA could also function as template (Clerx-van Haaster *et al.*, to be published).

6.2.4. Comparison of the Time of Appearance of the Replicase

When we look at the time of appearance of infection-related RNA polymerase activity, we find a striking difference between different hosts infected with the same or with different viruses.

In broad bean infected with BBMV, a peak of replicase was found 4 days after infection in the third verticil (Romero and Jacquemin, 1971). Upon infection of the same host with AMV, the activity was maximal in the same leaves 9 days after infection. In BMV-infected barley, a peak of replicase was found 3 days after infection by Semal and Kummert (1970) and 6 days after infection by Hadidi and Fraenkel-Conrat (1973).

In all these cases, the level of replicase activity rose rather sharply and decreased at the time that the virus started to accumulate.

A rather different situation is found in CMV-infected cucumbers; here, the replicase activity could be detected 2 days after infection and its level increased until about 10 days after infection and remained high for at least another week (May *et al.*, 1970). A similar situation seems to exist in AMV-infected tobacco, where the polymerase activity increases from 2 to 6 days after infection (Weening, 1975) while symptoms often already appear 3 days after infection.

7. DISCUSSION

Research on the plant viruses with tripartite genomes leaves us with a number of interesting questions to which there is as yet no answer. The first question is, of course: why do viruses have their genetic information in several molecules? Multipartite genomes have been found now in a considerable number of plant and animal RNA viruses (for a review on plant viruses with multipartite genomes, see Jaspars, 1974), but not in DNA viruses. Since recombination mechanisms for RNA are probably very scarce, it may be an advantage for RNA viruses to have their genetic information in freely exchangeable parts. On the other hand, the multipartite genome may be an adaptation of RNA viruses to the translation machinery of the eukaryotic cell, which does not seem to favor translation of large polycistronic messengers (see Chapter 4). In any case, there must be an important biological advantage compensating for the drawback which a plant virus with a tripartite genome has in infecting cells with three particles instead of one.

Another question concerns the origin of tripartite genomes. Did they develop from a common ancestor with a nonfragmented genome, and how could this genome become fragmented without losing its infectivity? The striking similarity of their RNA patterns and the fact that their coat protein gene is always located on the same RNA strand strongly suggest that the tripartite genomes do have a common ancestor. However, no sequence homology was found between the RNAs of AMV on the one hand and those of TSV, BMV, CCMV, and CMV on the other hand (Bol *et al.*, 1975). Even with the two cucumoviruses CMV and TAV, no homologous RNA sequences could be detected (Habili and Francki, 1974c).

Van Vloten-Doting (1968) has suggested that multipartite genomes developed as complexes of mutually dependent deletion mutants derived from a single genome or from different genomes. In case the mutants were derived from the same genome, an explanation can be given for the fact that a replicase recognizes different RNA molecules, for it is obvious that the recognition site was conserved in all molecules.

The role of the coat protein in the activation of the genomes of the heterocapsidic viruses is still enigmatic. A regulatory function in translation is conceivable. Such a function, although in a negative sense, has been found for the coat protein of RNA phages (Weissmann *et al.*, 1973). A function of the coat protein in posttranslational cleavage of large primary viral translation products is also possible. Lawrence and Thach (1975) have found that one of the coat proteins of encephalomyocarditis virus has proteolytic activity. At the moment we favor the idea that the coat protein is somehow involved in the replication process. This idea is stimulated by the finding that the sites with high affinity for the coat protein are located near the 3′ end of AMV RNA 4 (Section 2.2). If the 3′-terminal parts of all four AMV RNAs are similar, as was found for the BMV RNAs (Sections 2.1 and 5.3), this could point to a function of the coat protein in the 3D-structure of the replicase recognition site. Furthermore one of the main differences between the heterocapsidic viruses and isocapsidic viruses is the fact that the latter can all accept an amino acid at their 3′ terminus. This phenomenon is also thought to be related to the replication process (Section 5.3). This raises another intriguing question, namely, whether there is any functional relationship between coat protein independency of tripartite genomes and their amino acid acceptor function. It is the feeling of the authors of this chapter that the answers to the questions raised above will not only give more insight into the life cycle of eukaryote RNA viruses but also into the secrets of the eukaryotic cell itself.

ACKNOWLEDGMENTS

We wish to thank Drs. J. W. Davies, R. W. Fulton, D. Gonsalves, T. C. Hall, P. Kaesberg, R. M. Lister, L. Pinck, D. S. Shih, and J. W. Watts for sending us manuscripts or information prior to publication.

The authors' work on AMV and TSV was sponsored in part by the Netherlands Foundation for Chemical Research (S.O.N.), with financial aid from the Netherlands Organisation for the Advancement of Pure Research (Z.W.O.).

8. REFERENCES

Adams, J. M., and Cory, S., 1975, Modified nucleosides and bizarre 5′ termini in mouse myeloma mRNA, *Nature* (*London*) **255**:28.

Ball, L. A., Minson, A. C., and Shih, D. S., 1973, Synthesis of plant virus coat proteins in an animal cell-free system, *Nature New Biol.* **246**:206.

Bancroft, J. B., 1970, The self-assembly of spherical plant viruses, *Adv. Virus Res.* **16**:99.

Bancroft, J. B., 1971, The significance of the multicomponent nature of cowpea chlorotic mottle virus RNA, *Virology* **45**:830.

Bancroft, J. B., 1972, A virus made from parts of the genomes of brome mosaic and cowpea chlorotic mottle viruses, *J. Gen. Virol.* **14**:223.

Bancroft, J. B., and Flack, I. H., 1972, The behaviour of cowpea chlorotic mottle virus in CsCl, *J. Gen. Virol.* **15**:247.

Bancroft, J. B., and Lane, L. C., 1973, Genetic analysis of cowpea chlorotic mottle and brome mosaic viruses, *J. Gen. Virol.* **19**:381.

Bancroft, J. B., Rees, M. W., Dawson, J. R. O., McLean, G. D., and Short, M. N., 1972, Some properties of a temperature-sensitive mutant of cowpea chlorotic mottle virus, *J. Gen. Virol.* **16**:69.

Bancroft, J. B., Motoyoshi, F., Watts, J. W., and Dawson, J. R. O., 1974, Cowpea chlorotic mottle and brome mosaic viruses in tobacco protoplasts, in: *Modification of the Information Content of Plant Cells* (R. Markham, D. R. Davies, D. A. Hopwood, and R. W. Horne, eds.), p. 133, North-Holland, Amsterdam.

Bancroft, J. B., McDonald, J. G., and Rees, M. W., 1976, A mutant of cowpea chlorotic mottle virus with a perturbed assembly mechanism, *Virology* **75**:293.

Basit, A. A., and Francki, R. I. B., 1970, Some properties of rose mosaic virus from South Australia, *Aust. J. Biol. Sci.* **23**:1197.

Bastin, M., and Hall, T. C., 1976, Interaction of elongation factor 1 with aminoacylated brome mosaic virus and tRNAs, *J. Virol.* **20**:117.

Bastin, M., and Kaesberg, P., 1976, A possible replicative form of brome mosaic virus RNA 4, *Virology* **72**:536.

Bastin, M., Dasgupta, R., Hall, T. C., and Kaesberg, P., 1976, Similarity in structure and function of the 3′ terminal region of the four brome mosaic viral RNAs, *J. Mol. Biol.* **103**:737.

Boatman, S., and Kaper, J. M., 1976, Molecular organization and stabilizing forces of simple RNA viruses. IV. Selective interference with protein–RNA interactions by use of sodium dodecyl sulfate, *Virology* **70**:1.

Bockstahler, L. E., and Kaesberg, P., 1961, Bromegrass mosaic virus: a virus containing an unusually small ribonucleic acid, *Nature (London)* **190**:192.

Bockstahler, L. E., and Kaesberg, P., 1965, Infectivity studies of bromegrass mosaic virus RNA, *Virology* **27**:418.

Bol, J. F., and Kruseman, J., 1969, The reversible dissociation of alfalfa mosaic virus, *Virology* **37**:485.

Bol, J. F., and Lak-Kaashoek, M., 1974, Composition of alfalfa mosaic virus nucleoproteins, *Virology* **60**:476.

Bol, J. F., and Van Vloten-Doting, L., 1973, Function of top component *a* RNA in the initiation of infection by alfalfa mosaic virus, *Virology* **51**:102.

Bol, J. F., and Veldstra, H., 1969, Degradation of alfalfa mosaic virus by pancreatic ribonuclease, *Virology* **37**:74.

Bol, J. F., Van Vloten-Doting, L., and Jaspars, E. M. J., 1971, A functional equivalence of top component *a* RNA and coat protein in the initiation of infection by alfalfa mosaic virus, *Virology* **46**:73.

Bol, J. F., Kraal, B., and Brederode, F. T., 1974, Limited proteolysis of alfalfa mosaic virus. Influence on the structural and biological function of the coat protein, *Virology* **58**:101.

Bol, J. F., Brederode, F. T., Janze, G. C., and Rauh, D. K., 1975, Studies on sequence homology between the RNAs of alfalfa mosaic virus, *Virology* **65**:1.

Bol, J. F., Clerx-van Haaster, C. M., and Weening, C. J., 1976a, Host and virus specific RNA polymerases in alfalfa mosaic virus infected tobacco, *Ann. Microbiol. (Inst. Pasteur)* **127A**:183.

Bol, J. F., Bakhuizen, C. E. G. C., and Rutgers, T., 1976b, Composition and biosynthetic activity of polyribosomes associated with alfalfa mosaic virus infections, *Virology* **75**:1.

Bruening, G., and Agrawal, H. O., 1967, Infectivity of a mixture of cowpea mosaic virus ribonucleoprotein components, *Virology* **32**:306.

Chen, J. M., and Hall, T. C., 1973, Comparison of tyrosyl transfer ribonucleic acid and brome mosaic virus tyrosyl ribonucleic acid as amino acid donors in protein synthesis, *Biochemistry* **12**:4570.

Clark, G. L., Peden, K. W. C., and Symons, R. H., 1974, Cucumber mosaic virus-induced RNA polymerase: Partial purification and properties of the template-free enzyme, *Virology* **62**:434.

Clark, M. F., and Lister, R. M., 1971, Preparations and some properties of the nucleic acid of tobacco streak virus, *Virology* **45**:61.

Collot, D., Peter, R., Das, B., Wolff, B., and Duranton, H., 1976, Primary structure of alfalfa mosaic virus coat protein (strain S), *Virology* **74**:236.

Corbett, M. K., and Grant, T. J., 1967, Purification of citrus variegation virus, *Phytopathology* **57**:137.

Dasgupta, R., Shih, D. S., Saris, C., and Kaesberg, P., 1975, Nucleotide sequence of a viral RNA fragment that binds to eukaryotic ribosomes, *Nature (London)* **256**:624.

Dasgupta, R., Harada, F., and Kaesberg, P., 1976, Blocked 5′ termini in brome mosaic virus RNA, *J. Virol.* **18**:260.

Davies, J. W., 1976, The multipartite genome of brome mosaic virus: Aspects of *in vitro* translation and RNA structure, *Ann. Microbiol. (Inst. Pasteur)* **127A**:131.

Davies, J. W., and Kaesberg, P., 1974, Translation of virus mRNA: Protein synthesis directed by several virus RNAs in a cell-free extract from wheat germ, *J. Gen. Virol.* **25**:11.

De Sequeira, O. A., 1967, Purification and serology of an apple mosaic virus, *Virology* **31**:314.

Desjardins, P. R., and Steere, R. L., 1969, Separation of top and bottom components of alfalfa mosaic virus by combined differential and density gradient centrifugation, *Arch. Gesamte. Virusforsch.* **26**:127.

Diaz-Ruiz, J. R., and Kaper, J. M., 1977, Cucumber mosaic virus-associated RNA 5. III. Little nucleotide sequence homology between Carna 5 and helper RNA, *Virology*, (in press).

Dingjan-Versteegh, A., and Van Vloten-Doting, L., 1974, The effect of inhibitors of protein biosynthesis on the infectivity of alfalfa mosaic virus: Role of coat protein, *Virology* **58**:136.

Dingjan-Versteegh, A., Van Vloten-Doting, L., and Jaspars, E. M. J., 1972, Alfalfa mosaic virus hybrids constructed by exchanging nucleoprotein components, *Virology* **49**:716.

Dingjan-Versteegh, A., Van Vloten-Doting, L., and Jaspars, E. M. J., 1974, Confirmation of the constitution of alfalfa mosaic virus hybrid genomes by backcross experiments, *Virology* **59**:328.

Finch, J. T., Klug, A., and Van Regenmortel, M. H. V., 1967, The structure of cucumber mosaic virus, *J. Mol. Biol.* **24**:303.

Fraenkel-Conrat, H., and Fowlks, E., 1972, Variability at the 5′ ends of two plant viruses, *Biochemistry* **11**:1733.

Franck, A., and Hirth, L., 1972, Isolement et propriétés d'une souche thermophile du virus de la mosaïque de la luzerne, *C. R. Acad. Sci. Ser. D* **274**:745.

Franck, A., and Hirth, L., 1976, Temperature-resistant strains of alfalfa mosaic virus, *Virology* **70**:238.

Francki, R. I. B., 1968, Inactivation of cucumber mosaic virus (Q strain) nucleoprotein by pancreatic ribonuclease, *Virology* **34**:694.

Fulton, R. W., 1962, The effect of dilution on necrotic ringspot virus infectivity and the enhancement by non-infective virus, *Virology* **18**:477.

Fulton, R. W., 1967, Purification and some properties of tobacco streak and Tulare apple mosaic viruses, *Virology* **32**:153.

Fulton, R. W., 1968, Relationships among the ringspot viruses of *Prunus, Dtsch. Akad. Landwirtschaftwiss. Berl. Tagungsber.* **97**:123.

Fulton, R. W., 1970, The role of particle heterogeneity in infection by tobacco streak virus, *Virology* **41**:288.

Fulton, R. W., 1972, Inheritance and recombination of strain-specific characters in tobacco streak virus, *Virology* **50**:810.

Fulton, R. W., 1974, The biological activity of heterogeneous particle types of plant viruses, in: *Viruses, Evolution and Cancer* (E. Kurstak and K. Maramorosch, eds.), p. 723, Academic Press, New York.

Fulton, R. W., 1975, The role of top particles in recombination of some characters of tobacco streak virus, *Virology* **67**:188.

Furuichi, Y., Morgan, M., Shatkin, A. J., Jelinek, W., Saldit-Georgieff, M., and Darnell, J. E., 1975, Methylated, blocked 5′ termini in HeLa cell mRNA, *Proc. Natl. Acad. Sci. USA* **72**:1904.

Garnsey, S. M., 1975, Purification and properties of citrus leaf rugose virus, *Phytopathology* **65**:50.

Ghabrial, S. A., and Lister, R. M., 1974, Chemical and physiochemical properties of two strains of tobacco streak virus, *Virology* **57**:1.

Gilliland, J. M., and Symons, R. H., 1968, Properties of a plant virus-induced RNA polymerase in cucumbers infected with cucumber mosaic virus, *Virology* **36**:232.

Glitz, D. G., and Eichler, D., 1971, Nucleotides at the 5′ linked ends of bromegrass mosaic virus RNA and its fragments, *Biochim. Biophys. Acta* **238**:224.

Gonsalves, D., and Garnsey, S. M., 1974, Infectivity of the multiple nucleoprotein and RNA components of citrus leaf rugose virus, *Virology* **61**:343.

Gonsalves, D., and Garnsey, S. M., 1975a, Functional equivalence of an RNA component and coat protein for infectivity of citrus leaf rugose virus, *Virology* **64**:23.

Gonsalves, D., and Garnsey, S. M., 1975b, Nucleic acid components of citrus variegation virus and their activation by coat protein, *Virology* **67**:311.

Gonsalves, D., and Garnsey, S. M., 1975c, Infectivity of heterologous RNA-protein mixtures from alfalfa mosaic, citrus leaf rugose, citrus variegation, and tobacco streak viruses, *Virology* **67**:319.

Habili, N., and Francki, R. I. B., 1974a, Comparative studies on tomato aspermy and cucumber mosaic viruses. I. Physical and chemical properties, *Virology* **57**:392.

Habili, N., and Francki, R. I. B., 1974b, Comparative studies on tomato aspermy and cucumber mosaic viruses. II. Virus stability, *Virology* **60**:29.

Habili, N., and Francki, R. I. B., 1974c, Comparative studies on tomato aspermy and cucumber mosaic viruses. III. Further studies on relationship and construction of a virus from parts of the two viral genomes, *Virology* **61**:443.

Hadidi, A., 1974, The nature of the products of brome mosaic virus RNA polymerase, *Virology* **58**:536.

Hadidi, A., and Fraenkel-Conrat, H., 1973, Characterization and specificity of soluble RNA polymerase of brome mosaic virus, *Virology* **52**:363.

Hadidi, A., Hariharasubramanian, V., and Fraenkel-Conrat, H., 1973, Template activity of brome mosaic virus-RNA components with soluble brome mosaic virus RNA polymerase, *Intervirology* **1**:201.

Hall, T. C., and Wepprich, 1976, Functional possibilities for aminoacylation of viral RNA in transcription and translation, *Ann. Microbiol. (Inst. Pasteur)* **127A**:143.

Hall, T. C., Shih, D. S., and Kaesberg, P., 1972, Enzyme-mediated binding of tyrosine to brome-mosaic-virus ribonucleic acid, *Biochem. J.* **129**:969.

Hariharasubramanian, V., Hadidi, A., Singer, B., and Fraenkel-Conrat, H., 1973, Possible identification of a protein in brome mosaic virus infected barley as a component of viral RNA polymerase, *Virology* **54**:190.

Harrison, B. D., Murant, A. F., and Mayo, M. A., 1972, Evidence for two functional RNA species in raspberry ringspot virus, *J. Gen. Virol.* **16**:339.

Hartmann, D., Mohier, E., Leroy, C., and Hirth, L., 1976, Genetic analysis of alfalfa mosaic virus mutants, *Virology* **74**:470.

Heijtink, R. A., 1974, Fysisch-chemische karakterisering van nucleoproteïnen en nucleinezuurmoleculen van alfalfa mosaic virus, Ph.D. Thesis, University of Leiden.

Heijtink, R. A., and Jaspars, E. M. J., 1974, RNA contents of abnormally long particles of certain strains of alfalfa mosaic virus, *Virology* **59**:371.

Heijtink, R. A., and Jaspars, E. M. J., 1976, Characterization of two morphologically distinct top component *a* particles from alfalfa mosaic virus, *Virology* **69**:75.

Hiebert, E., Bancroft, J. B., and Bracker, C. E., 1968, The assembly *in vitro* of some small spherical viruses, hybrid viruses, and other nucleoproteins, *Virology* **34**:492.

Hill, J. H., and Shepherd, R. J., 1972, Molecular weights of plant virus coat proteins by polyacrylamide gel electrophoresis, *Virology* **47**:817.

Hull, R., 1969, Alfalfa mosaic virus, *Adv. Virus Res.* **15**:365.

Hull, R., 1970*a*, Studies on alfalfa mosaic virus. IV. An unusual strain, *Virology* **42**:283.

Hull, R., 1970*b*, Studies on alfalfa mosaic virus. III. Reversible dissociation and reconstitution studies. *Virology* **40**:34.

Hull, R., 1972, The multicomponent nature of broad bean mottle virus and its nucleic acid, *J. Gen. Virol.* **17**:111.

Hull, R., 1976, The behaviour of salt-labile plant viruses in gradients of cesium sulphate, *Virology* **75**:18.

Huttinga, H., and Mosch, W. H. M., 1976, Lilac Ring Mottle Virus: a coat protein-dependent virus with a tripartite genome, *Acta Horti.* **59**:113.

Jacquemin, J. M., 1972, *In vitro* product of an RNA polymerase induced in broad bean by infection with broad bean mottle virus, *Virology* **49**:379.

Jacquemin, J. M., and Lopez, M., 1974, RNAs labelled *in vitro* by polymerase from leaves infected with broad bean mottle virus, *Intervirology* **4**:45.

Jaspars, E. M. J., 1974, Plant viruses with a multipartite genome, *Adv. Virus Res.* **19**:37.

Jaspars, E. M. J., and Van Kammen, A., 1972, Analysis of the genome constitution of cowpea mosaic and alfalfa mosaic viruses, *Proc. 8th FEBS Meet. Amsterdam* **27**:121.

Jones, A. T., and Mayo, M. A., 1973, Purification and properties of elm mottle virus, *Ann. Appl. Biol.* **75**:347.

Jones, A. T., and Mayo, M. A., 1975, Further properties of black raspberry latent virus and evidence for its relationship to tobacco streak virus, *Ann. Appl. Biol.* **79**:297.

Kado, I. C., 1972, Mechanical and biological inoculation principles, in: *Principles and Techniques in Plant Virology* (C. I. Kado and H. O. Agrawal, eds.), p. 3, Van Nostrand Reinhold, New York.

Kaesberg, P., 1975, The RNAs of brome mosaic virus and their translation in cell-free extracts derived from wheat embryo, *INSERM (Colloque)* **47**:205.

Kaesberg, P., 1976, Translation and structure of the RNAs of brome mosaic virus, in: *Animal Virology,* Proceedings of the Fourth ICN–UCLA Symposium on Molecular and Cellular Biology (D. Baltimore, A. S. Huang, and C. F. Fox, eds.) p. 555, Academic Press, New York and London.

Kaper, J. M., 1972, Experimental analysis of the stabilizing interactions of simple RNA viruses: A systematic approach, *Proc. 8th FEBS Meet. Amsterdam, 1972* **27**:19.

Kaper, J. M., 1973, Arrangement and identification of simple isometric viruses according to their dominating stabilizing interactions, *Virology* **55**:299.

Kaper, J. M., and Geelen, J. L. M. C., 1971, Studies on the stabilizing forces of simple RNA viruses. II. Stability, dissociation and reassembly of cucumber mosaic virus, *J. Mol. Biol.* **56**:277.

Kaper, J. M., and Re, G. C., 1974, Redetermination of the RNA content and the limiting RNA size of three strains of cucumber mosaic virus, *Virology* **60**:308.

Kaper, J. M., and Waterworth, H. E., 1973, Comparison of molecular weights of single-stranded viral RNAs by two emperical methods, *Virology* **51**:183.

Kaper, J. M., and Waterworth, H. E., 1977, Cucumber mosaic virus associated RNA 5: causal agent for tomato necrosis, *Science*, (in press).

Kaper, J. M., and West, C. K., 1972, Polyacrylamide gel separation and molecular weight determination of the components of cucumber mosaic virus RNA, *Prep. Biochem.* **2**:251.

Keith, J., and Fraenkel-Conrat, H., 1975, Tobacco mosaic virus RNA carries 5'-terminal triphosphorylated guanosine blocked by 5'-linked 7-methylguanosine, *FEBS Lett.* **57**:31.

Kohl, R. J., and Hall, T. C., 1974, Aminoacylation of RNA from several viruses: Amino acid specificity and differential activity of plant, yeast and bacterial synthetases, *J. Gen. Virol.* **25**:257.

Kraal, B., De Graaf, J. M., Bakker, T. A., Van Beynum, G. M. A., Goedhart, M., and Bosch, L., 1972, Structural studies on the coat protein of alfalfa mosaic virus, *Eur. J. Biochem.* **28**:20.

Kraal, B., Van Beynum, G. M. A., De Graaf, J. M., Castel, A., and Bosch, L., 1976, The primary structure of the coat protein of alfalfa mosaic virus (strain 425), *Virology* **74**:232.

Kruseman, J., Kraal, B., Jaspars, E. M. J., Bol, J. F., Brederode, F. T., and Veldstra, H., 1971, Molecular weight of the coat protein of alfalfa mosaic virus, *Biochemistry* **10**:447.

Kummert, J., 1974, *In vitro* pulse-labeling of the replicative forms of bromegrass mosaic virus RNA, *Virology* **57**:314.

Kummert, J., and Semal, J., 1972, Properties of single-stranded RNA synthesized by a crude RNA polymerase fraction from barley leaves infected with brome mosaic virus, *J. Gen. Virol.* **16**:11.

Kummert, J., and Semal, J., 1974, Polyacrylamide gel electrophoresis of the RNA products labeled *in vitro* by extracts of leaves infected with bromegrass mosaic virus, *Virology* **60**:390.

Lane, L. C., 1974a, The bromoviruses, *Adv. Virus Res.* **19**:151.

Lane, L. C., 1974b, The components of barley stripe mosaic and related viruses, *Virology* **58**:323.

Lane, L. C., and Kaesberg, P., 1971, Multiple genetic components in bromegrass mosaic virus, *Nature (London) New Biol.* **232**:40.

Lawrence, C., and Thach, R. E., 1975, Identification of a viral protein involved in posttranslational maturation of the encephalomyocarditis virus capsid precursor, *J. Virol.* **15**:918.

Lebeurier, G., Wurtz, M., and Hirth, L., 1969a, Dissociation et réassociation de la protéine et du RNA du virus de la mosaique de la luzerne, *C. R. Acad. Sci. Ser. D* **268**:1897.

Lebeurier, G., Wurtz, M., and Hirth, L., 1969b, Auto assemblage de RNA extraits de trois types de virus différents et des sous unités protéique du virus de la mosaïque de la luzerne, *C. R. Acad. Sci. Ser. D* **268**:2002.

Lister, R. M., and Saksena, K. N., 1976, Some properties of Tulare apple mosaic virus and ILAR viruses suggesting grouping with tobacco streak virus, *Virology* **70**:440.

Lister, R. M., Ghabrial, S. A., and Saksena, K. N., 1972, Evidence that particle size heterogeneity is the cause of centrifugal heterogeneity in tobacco streak virus, *Virology* **49**:290.

Loesch, L. S., and Fulton, R. W., 1975, *Prunus* necrotic ringspot virus as a multicomponent system, *Virology* **68**:71.

Lot, H., and Kaper, J. M., 1973, Comparison of the buoyant density heterogeneity of cucumber mosaic virus and brome mosaic virus, *Virology* **54**:540.

Lot, H., and Kaper, J. M., 1976*a*, Physical and chemical differences of three strains of cucumber mosaic virus and peanut stunt virus, *Virology* **74**:209.

Lot, H., and Kaper, J. M. 1976*b*, Further studies on the RNA component distribution among the nucleoproteins of cucumber mosaic virus, *Virology* **74**:223.

Lot, H., Marchoux, G., Marrou, J., Kaper, J. M., West, C. K., Van Vloten-Doting, L., and Hull, R., 1974, Evidence for three functional RNA species in several strains of cucumber mosaic virus, *J. Gen. Virol.* **22**:81.

Majorana, G., and Paul, H. L., 1969, The production of new types of symptoms by mixtures of different components of two strains of alfalfa mosaic virus, *Virology* **38**:145.

Marchoux, G., Douine, L., Lot, H., and Esvan, C., 1973, Identification et estimation du poids moléculaire des acides ribonucléïques du virus de la mosaïque du concombre (VMC souche D), *C. R. Acad. Sci. Ser. D* **277**:1409.

Marchoux, G., Marrou, J., Douine, L., Lot, H., Quiot, J.-B., and Clement, M., 1974*a*, Complémentation entre souches du virus de la mosaïque du concombre. Localisation d'un gène sur l'ARN-3, *C. R. Acad. Sci. Ser. D* **278**:889.

Marchoux, G., Marrou, J., and Quiot, J.-B., 1974*b*, Complémentation entre ARN de différentes souches du virus de la mosaïque du concombre. Mise en évidence d'une interaction entre deux ARN pour déterminer un type de symptôme, *C. R. Acad. Sci. Ser. D* **279**:1943.

Marchoux, G., Devergne, J.-C., Marrou, J., Douine, L., and Lot, H., 1974*c*, Complémentation entre ARN de différentes souches du virus de la mosaïque du concombre. Localisation sur l'ARN-3, de plusieurs propriétés, dont certaines liées à la nature de la capside, *C. R. Acad. Sci. Ser. D* **279**:2165.

Marchoux, G., Devergne, J.-C., and Douine, L., 1975, Cucumovirus: Studies on construction of pseudo recombinants from parts of their RNA genomes, in: *Third International Congress of Virology* (H. S. Bedson, R. Najéra, L. Valenciano, and P. Wildy, eds.), p. 90.

May, J. T., Gilliland, J. M., and Symons, R. H., 1969, Plant virus-induced RNA polymerase: Properties of the enzyme partly purified from cucumber cotyledons infected with cucumber mosaic virus, *Virology* **39**:54.

May, J. T., Gilliland, J. M., and Symons, R. H., 1970, Properties of a plant virus-induced RNA polymerase in particulate fractions of cucumbers infected with cucumber mosaic virus, *Virology* **41**:653.

Mellema, J. E., 1975, A model for the capsid structure of alfalfa mosaic virus, *J. Mol. Biol.* **94**:643.

Mellema, J. E., and Van den Berg, H. J. N., 1974, The quaternary structure of alfalfa mosaic virus, *J. Supramol. Struct.* **2**:17.

Mink, G. I. 1975, Inactivation of peanut stunt virus by pancreatic ribonuclease, *Virology* **63**:466.

Mink, G. I., Silbernagel, M. J., and Saksena, K. N., 1969, Host range, purification, and properties of the western strain of peanut stunt virus, *Phytopathology* **59**:1625.

Moed, J. R., 1966, Onderzoekingen over alfalfa mosaic virus: Ontmantelingsvraagstuk, Ph.D. thesis, University of Leiden.

Mohier, E., and Hirth, L., 1972, Etude des fonctions complémentaires des acides ribonucléiques du virus de la mosaïque de la luzerne, *C. R. Acad. Sci. Ser. D* **274**:337.

Mohier, E., Pinck, L., and Hirth, L., 1974, Replication of alfalfa mosaic virus RNAs, *Virology* **58**:9.

Mohier, E., Hirth, L., Le Meur, M.-A., and Gerlinger, P., 1975, Translation of alfalfa mosaic virus RNA's in mammalian cell-free systems, *Virology* **68**:349.

Mohier, E., Hirth, L., Le Meur, M.-A., and Gerlinger, P., 1976, Analysis of alfalfa mosaic virus 17 S RNA translational products, *Virology* **71**:615.

Peden, K. W. C., and Symons, R. H., 1973, Cucumber mosaic virus contains a functional divided genome, *Virology* **53**:487.

Peden, K. W. C., May, J. T., and Symons, R. H., 1972, A comparison of two plant virus-induced RNA polymerases, *Virology* **47**:498.

Pfeiffer, P., and Hirth, L., 1975, The effect of conformatinal changes in brome mosaic virus upon its sensitivity to trypsin, chymotrypsin and ribonuclease, *FEBS Letters* **56**:144.

Philipps, G., 1973, Réplication des RNAs d'un virus à composants multiples. Le virus de la mosaïque du brome, Ph.D. thesis, University of Strasbourg.

Philipps, G., Gigot, C., and Hirth, L., 1974, Replicative forms and viral RNA synthesis in leaves infected with brome mosaic virus, *Virology* **60**:370.

Pinck, L., 1975, The 5'-end groups of alfalfa mosaic virus RNAs are $m^7G^{5'}ppp^{5'}Gp$, *FEBS Lett.* **59**:24.

Pinck, L., and Fauquet, C., 1975, Analysis of the pancreatic-ribonuclease-digestion products of alfalfa-mosaic-virus ribonucleic acid, *Eur. J. Biochem.* **57**:441.

Price, W. C., 1964, Strains, mutation, acquired immunity and interference, in: *Plant Virology* (M. K. Corbett and H. D. Sisler, eds.), p. 93, University of Florida Press, Gainesville.

Romero, J., and Jacquemin, J. M., 1971, Relation between virus-induced RNA polymerase activity and the synthesis of broad bean mottle virus in broad bean, *Virology* **45**:813.

Sakai, F., Watts, J. W., Dawson, J. R. O., and Bancroft, J. B., 1977, Synthesis of proteins in tobacco protoplasts infected with cowpea chlorotic mottle virus, *J. Gen. Virol.* **34**:285.

Schwinghamer, M. W., and Symons, R. H., 1975, Fractionation of cucumber mosaic virus RNA and its translation in a wheat embryo cell-free system, *Virology* **63**:252.

Semal, J., 1969, Synthesis of ribonucleic acid in cell-free extracts of broad bean leaves infected with broad bean mottle virus, *Phytopathology* **59**:881.

Semal, J., and Hamilton, R. I., 1968, RNA synthesis in cell-free extracts of barley leaves infected with bromegrass mosaic virus, *Virology* **36**:293.

Semal, J., and Kummert, J., 1970, Virus-induced RNA polymerase and synthesis of bromegrass mosaic virus in barley, *J. Gen. Virol.* **7**:173.

Semal, J., and Kummert, J., 1971, Sequential synthesis of double-stranded and single-stranded RNA by cell-free extracts of leaves infected with bromegrass mosaic virus, *Virology* **36**:293.

Semal, J., Kummert, J., and Dekegel, D., 1974, Localization of viral RNA polymerase activity and its products in extracts of barley leaves infected with bromegrass mosaic virus, *Phytopathology* **64**:446.

Shih, D. S., and Kaesberg, P., 1973, Translation of brome mosaic viral ribonucleic acid in a cell-free system derived from wheat embryo, *Proc. Natl. Acad. Sci. USA* **70**:1799.

Shih, D. S., and Kaesberg, P., 1976, Translation of the RNAs of brome mosaic virus: the monocistronic nature of RNA 1 and RNA 2, *J. Mol. Biol.* **103**:77.

Shih, D. S., Lane, L. C., and Kaesberg, P., 1972, Origin of the small component of brome mosaic virus RNA, *J. Mol. Biol.* **64**:353.

Shih, D. S., Kaesberg, P., and Hall, T. C., 1974, Messenger and amino-acylation functions of brome mosaic virus RNA after chemical modification of 3′ terminus, *Nature (London)* **249**:353.

Shih, D. S., Davies, J. W., and Kaesberg, P., 1975, The *in vitro* synthesis of viral protein and its regulation, *Proc. First Int. Congr. Int. Assoc. Microsc. Soc.* **3**:83.

Shih, D. S., Dasgupta, R., and Kaesberg, P., 1976, 7-Methylguanosine and efficiency of RNA translation, *J. Virol.* **19**:637.

Stace-Smith, R., and Tremaine, J. H., 1973, Biophysical and biochemical properties of tomato aspermy virus, *Virology* **51**:401.

Symons, R. H., 1975, Cucumber mosaic virus RNA contains 7-methylguanosine at the 5′ terminus of all four RNA species, *Mol. Biol. Rep.* **2**:277.

Symons, R. H., 1976, Studies on the replication of cucumber mosaic virus, *Ann. Microbiol. (Inst. Pasteur)* **127A**:161.

Thang, M. N., Dondon, L., Thang, D. C., Mohier, E., Hirth, L., Le Meur, M.-A., and Gerlinger, P., 1975, Translation of alfalfa mosaic virus RNAs in plant cell and mammalian cell extracts, *INSERM (Colloque)* **47**:225.

Thang, M. N., Dondon, L., and Mohier, E., 1976, Translation of alfalfa mosaic virus RNA. Effect of polyamines, *FEBS Lett.* **61**:85.

Van Beynum, G. M. A., 1975, The primary structure of the coat protein of alfalfa mosaic virus, Ph.D. thesis, University of Leiden.

Van Beynum, G. M. A., Kraal, B., De Graaf, J. M., and Bosch, L., 1975, Structural studies on the coat protein of alfalfa mosaic virus. Isolation and characterization of the tryptic peptides and alignment of the cyanogen -bromide fragments, *Eur. J. Biochem.* **52**:23.

Van Beynum, G. M. A., De Graaf, J. M., Castel, A., Kraal, B., and Bosch, L., 1977, Structural studies on the coat protein of alfalfa mosaic virus, *Eur. J. Biochem.* **72**:63.

Van Boxsel, J. A. M., 1976, High-affinity sites for coat protein on alfalfa mosaic virus RNA, Ph.D. Thesis, University of Leiden.

Van Der Meer, F. A., Huttinga, H., and Maat, D. Z., 1976, Lilac ring mottle virus: isolation from lilac, some properties, and relation to lilac ringspot disease, *Neth. J. Plant Path.* **82**:67.

Van Ravenswaay Claasen, J. C., Van Leeuwen, A. B. J., Duijts, G. A. H., and Bosch, L., 1967, *In vitro* translation of alfalfa mosaic virus RNA, *J. Mol. Biol.* **23**:535.

Van Regenmortel, M. H. V., 1967, Biochemical and biophysical properties of cucumber mosaic virus, *Virology* **31**:391.

Van Regenmortel, M. H. V., Hendry, D. A., and Baltz, T., 1972, A reexamination of the molecular size of cucumber mosaic virus and its coat protein, *Virology* **49**:647.

Van Vloten-Doting, L., 1968, Verdeling van de genetische informatie over de natuurlijke componenten van een plantevirus: Alfalfa mosaic virus, Ph.D. thesis, University of Leiden.

Van Vloten-Doting, L., 1975, Coat protein is required for infectivity of tobacco streak virus: Biological equivalence of the coat proteins of tobacco streak and alfalfa mosaic viruses, *Virology* **65**:215.

Van Vloten-Doting, L., 1976, Similarities and differences between viruses with a tripartite genome, *Ann. Microbiol. (Inst. Pasteur)* **127A**:119.

Van Vloten-Doting, L., and Jaspars, E. M. J., 1967, Enhancement of infectivity by combination of two ribonucleic acid components from alfalfa mosaic virus, *Virology* **33**:684.

Van Vloten-Doting, L., and Jaspars, E. M. J., 1972, The uncoating of alfalfa mosaic virus by its own RNA, *Virology* **48**:699.

Van Vloten-Doting, L., Kruseman, J., and Jaspars, E. M. J., 1968, The biological function and mutual dependence of bottom component and top component *a* of alfalfa mosaic virus, *Virology* **34**:728.

Van Vloten-Doting, L., Dingjan-Versteegh, A., and Jaspars, E. M. J., 1970, Three nucleoprotein components of alfalfa mosaic virus necessary for infectivity, *Virology* **40**:419.

Van Vloten-Doting, L., Rutgers, T., Neeleman, L., and Bosch, L., 1975, *In vitro* translation of the RNAs of alfalfa mosaic virus, *INSERM (Colloque)* **47**:233.

Van Vloten-Doting, L., Bol, J. F., Neeleman, L., Rutgers, T., Van Dalen, D., Castel, A., Bosch, L., Marbaix, G., Huez, G., Hubert, E., and Cleuter, Y., 1977, in: *NATO Advanced Studies on Nucleic Acids and Protein Synthesis in Plants* (L. Bogorad and J. H. Weil, eds.), p. 387, Plenum Press, New York.

Verhagen, W., 1973, Structuurveranderingen van alfalfa mosaic virus in zwak alkalisch milieu, Ph.D. thesis, University of Leiden.

Verhagen, W., and Bol, J. F., 1972, Evidence for a pH-induced structural change of alfalfa mosaic virus, *Virology* **50**:431.

Verhagen, W., Van Boxsel, J. A. M., Bol, J. F., Van Vloten-Doting, L., and Jaspars, E. M. J., 1976, RNA-protein interactions in alfalfa mosaic virus, *Ann. Microbiol. (Inst. Pasteur)* **127A**:165.

Weening, C. J., 1975, Synthese van alfalfa mosaic virus RNA *in vitro*, Ph.D. Thesis, University of Leiden.

Weening, C. J., and Bol, J. F., 1975, Viral RNA replication in extracts of alfalfa mosaic virus-infected *Vicia faba*, *Virology* **63**:77.

Weissmann, C., Billeter, M. A., Goodman, H. M., Hindley, J., and Weber, H., 1973, Structure and function of phage RNA. *Annu. Rev. Biochem.* **42**:303.

CHAPTER 2

Plant Covirus Systems: Two-Component Systems

George Bruening
Department of Biochemistry and Biophysics
University of California
Davis, California 95616

1. INTRODUCTION

The central concept concerning the viruses described in this chapter is that they have in common the following characteristic: the minimum genetic entity which can be derived from the virus, and which can induce an infection in which virions are formed, is two pieces of RNA. The two pieces of RNA, which can be considered to be the two chromosomes composing the genome of the virus, are (for the plant viruses described here) found in distinguishable ribonucleoprotein particles. That is, the genome is distributed in two kinds of virions. The notion of the extracellular phase of a virus life cycle being represented by "virions" rather than "virion" is generally alien to bacterial, animal, and fungal virology. However, probably nearly half of the recognized groups of plant viruses have virions rather than a virion. What advantage does such an arrangement give a plant virus? Why do such viruses find a niche which apparently has not been occupied by a monochromosomal, monovirion virus? *A priori*, the potential disadvantage of having to bring at least two particles or RNA molecules into a cell, rather than one, is most obvious. A potential advantage which comes to mind is a possibly more ready interchange of genetic information (chromosomes) when more than one (closely related) virus strain is replicating in the same cell, or even when more than one strain is being transmitted by the same vector. (Genetic recombination has not been convicingly demonstrated for any RNA plant virus.) Also, having the genome divided among smaller particles rather than in one large particle may facilitate movement of the virus in the plant or in the vector. It is possible that independent chromosomes can replicate in different cellular compartments (Harrison *et al.*, 1976) and separately become structurally and functionally optimized for replication and service as template in different compartments. Since smaller RNAs seem to be more readily translated in cell-free protein-synthesizing systems, and a similar situation may hold *in vivo*, smaller virion RNAs may allow more ready translation early in infection. Perhaps the apparent disadvantage of requiring more than one particle to enter a cell in order to infect it is not a disadvantage for plant viruses spread by vectors. Perhaps in almost all transmissions (vector or "mechanical") many virions are involved, and requiring that the virions be of two kinds rather than one has little effect on the probability of achieving infection. That infectivity dilution curves of the single-hit type frequently have been observed for viruses with more than one virion as well as for single-virion viruses is possible support for this idea. These are speculations; at the present time, the remarkable phenomenon, the existence of covirus systems, is without thoroughly supported causal explanation.

If the two pieces of RNA which are associated with the two components of the two-component viruses are independent "chromosomes," then two chromosomes of different type from two virus strains (if the strains are sufficiently similar in their detailed mode of replication) ought to be infective. The new virus so formed ought to have properties which are a hybrid of the properties of the parent strains. For the sake of simplicity, such artificially formed virus strains will be referred to here as "hybrid viruses." However, it must be recognized that these viruses are not recombinants in the usual sense since no breaking and rejoining of nucleic acid strands is considered to have occurred. The term "pseudo-recombinant" has been used (e.g., Gibbs and Harrison, 1976) to describe the hybrid viruses which are the subject of this chapter, and that term also has merit because it is more specific and tends to avoid the connotation of "recombinant" which "hybrid" has.

Most of this chapter is concerned with the three groups of two-component virus systems which have been most intensely studied: tobraviruses, comoviruses, and nepoviruses. In addition, pea enation mosaic virus, barley stripe mosaic virus, soil-borne wheat mosaic virus, and Nodamura virus and an insect virus are discussed briefly. The tobraviruses, barley stripe mosaic virus, and soil-borne wheat mosaic virus have rod-shaped virions of helical symmetry. The others have polyhedral (or "isometric") particles, apparently of icosahedral symmetry. The names "tobravirus" and "comovirus" are derived from the names of the type members, *tobacco rattle virus* (TRV) and *cowpea mosaic virus* (CPMV), respectively. "Nepovirus" is derived from *nematode-borne, polyhedral virus* (Harrison *et al.*, 1971; Cadman, 1963). The tobraviruses were formerly referred to as "netuviruses" (for *nematode-borne, tubular viruses*).

2. TOBRAVIRUSES

The members of the tobravirus group are unique among known covirus systems because the largest of the two or more virion RNA molecules can be propagated in susceptible plants independently of the other virion RNAs. However, no capsid protein is formed under these circumstances. A complete and well-illustrated summary of the early work on the genetic and other properties of this group was prepared by Lister (1969).

Tobraviruses can be spread by nematodes (*Trichodorus* species), and the virus has been shown to be very persistent in the nematode (reviewed by Taylor, 1972; Cooper and Harrison, 1973), with one report of persistence for more than 2 years (van Hoof, 1970). Tobraviruses have been shown to be seed-borne in a few instances (Lister and Murant, 1967; Kitajima and Costa, 1969). They are easily transmitted by mechanical inoculation. *Nicotiana clevelandii* often has been utilized as a host for obtaining chemically useful amounts of virus, but various tobaccos, other solanaceous plants, legumes, and other species have been useful for increasing, distinguishing, or assaying the various strains. Kubo *et al.* (1975) have demonstrated replication of TRV in tobacco protoplasts.

2.1. Serotypes and Particle Dimensions; Separation of Virions

Many isolates of TRV have been obtained. Three serotypes have been distinguished (Harrison and Woods, 1966). TRV strains BEL, BLU, PMK, PRN, and SP from the United Kingdom, A and HSN from Japan (Miki and Okada, 1970), B and C from California (Semancik and Kajiyama, 1967), and VH from the Netherlands can be considered members of serotype I. TRV GER (Sänger, 1968) from Germany may also be serotype I. FLA, ORE, and SAL from the United States were assigned to serotype II, and CAM and Z (Ghabrial and Lister, 1973*b*) from Brazil were assigned to serotype III. The pea early browning viruses (PEBV) have many characteristics in common with the tobacco rattle viruses and must be considered members of the tobravirus group. Several PEBVs have been isolated, and some of these have been distinguished by serological reaction, host range, and transmission by specific nematodes (Gibbs and Harrison, 1964; Harrison, 1966). Weak serological relationships to TRV strains have been demonstrated in some, but not all, cases (Maat, 1963; Gibbs and Harrison, 1964; Allen, 1967; Cooper and Mayo, 1972).

From two to four distinct modal lengths are found in TRV and PEBV preparations by electron microscopy, and these correspond to two to four zones analyzed by centrifugation (Harrison and Woods, 1966; Semancik, 1966*b*). Rods of the longest class are from 180 to 200 nm in length, depending on the particular TRV strain. The PEBV long rods are about 210 nm in length. Where more than one class of shorter rods is present, all but one of them usually, but not always, have been minor components. For the purposes of this chapter, the long rods will be designated L rods and the predominant (or only) shorter rods will be designated S rods. The lengths of the S rods and minor components vary from 45 to 115 nm, depending on the virus strain. Serotype and S-rod length are not correlated (Harrison and Woods, 1966).

Estimates of particle outside diameter range from 20 or 21 nm (cylindrically averaged diameter from X-ray diffraction or electron microscopic image of hexagonally packed rods) to 25 nm (maximum diameter from X-ray diffraction or electron microscopic image of isolated particles) (Nixon and Harrison, 1959; Finch, 1965; Offord, 1966; Tollin and Wilson, 1971; Cooper and Mayo, 1972). A canal of about 4–5 nm diameter is concentric with the long axis of the rods and appears flared at one end of the particle (Harrison and Woods, 1966; Cooper and Mayo, 1972). The flared end may be due to a tilted orientation of protein subunits within the helix. Concentric, cylindrical regions of elevated density have been observed at radii of 4 and 8 nm, the latter perhaps due to RNA phosphate residues (Offord, 1966; Tollin and Wilson, 1971). In all structural features other than length, the S rods and L rods cannot be distinguished.

Separation of L and S rods is essential to many genetic studies of TRV. Separations have been accomplished on the basis of sedimentation coefficient on sucrose density gradients (e.g., Semancik, 1966*b*) and on the basis of solubility in polyethylene glycol solutions (Clark and Lister, 1971; Huttinga, 1973). Complete separation of L and S rods is difficult to achieve, probably because of the aggregation of S rods to form entities with properties similar to those of L rods. Separation of S-rod RNA and L-rod RNA, rather than the virions, avoids this difficulty.

2.2. Particle Structural Homologies

Particles of all three TRV serotypes appear to form a homologous series in which the sedimentation coefficient can be predicted from particle length by assuming that the frictional coefficient of the particle is proportional to the calculated frictional coefficient for a prolate ellipsoid of the same major axis length and volume (Harrison and Klug, 1966). The existence of such a homologous series implies that particles of the different strains have the same diameter, partial specific volume, and mass per unit length (or that these properties vary with strain and particle length in some mutually compensating manner). A pea early browning virus isolate had a smaller sedimentation coefficient than would have been predicted from its length, implying a smaller mass per unit length for PEBV than for TRV. PEBV rods appear 6–8% narrower than TRV rods in the electron microscope (Harrison and Woods, 1966; Cooper and Mayo, 1972). L rods have sedimentation coefficients of about 300 S.

Cooper and Mayo (1972) found the L rods of TRV CAM to migrate 1.16 times more rapidly than the S rods during free-boundary or sucrose density gradient electrophoresis. The inadequacy of present theory of electrophoretic mobility makes it difficult to predict a relationship between particle length and electrophoretic mobility with the certainty possible in predicting relationships between length and sedimentation coefficient. However, the force in an electrophoretic field on cylindrical particles of the same diameter and formal ionic charge per unit length might be expected to increase more with increasing particle length than the frictional forces retarding migration (Tanford, 1961). Thus higher electrophoretic mobility for L rods cannot be taken as unequivocal evidence for a greater charge per unit length on L rods than on S rods.

X-ray diffraction patterns of TRV are consistent with helical symmetry (Finch, 1965; Tollin and Wilson, 1971). Therefore, there ought to be a single kind of polypeptide in any particle (Crick and Watson,

1956), or equimolar amounts if more than one kind is present. Some analyses of TRV protein by polyacrylamide gel electrophoresis, with or without detergent, have revealed a single zone (Ghabrial and Lister, 1973a; Cooper and Mayo, 1972; Lesnaw and Reichmann, 1970; Miki and Okada, 1970) for a given TRV strain. Minor zones have been found (Semancik, 1970). These may be due to limited proteolysis of the virions (Mayo and Cooper, 1973; Mayo et al., 1974b), which removes a few amino acids from the carboxyl terminus (unpublished results of Mayo and Robinson, cited by Mayo et al., 1976). However, the presence of contaminating strains is difficult to rule out (Cooper and Mayo, 1972). The similar amino acid composition of protein from L and S rods (Miki and Okada, 1970) and similar serological reactivity (Lister and Bracker, 1969), together with the genetic evidence reviewed below, show that L and S rods have the same protein subunits. In cross-absorption tests (Cooper and Mayo, 1972), antiserum absorbed with S rods still reacted very weakly with L rods, although no reaction could be detected in the reciprocal experiment. This result may have been due to the higher valency of L rods rather than to any antigenic difference between the L rods and S rods. However, the sensitivities of the methods used in published reports do not allow the possibility to be excluded that a minor protein (e.g., one molecule per virion) is associated with one of the two kinds of virions.

2.3. Protein and RNA Molecular Weights

Both amino acid analyses and polyacrylamide gel electrophoresis in the presence of sodium dodecylsulfate provide estimates of the capsid protein molecular weight. Valid estimates by gel electrophoresis require homologous properties for the complexes of sodium dodecylsulfate with the standard and with the viral polypeptides. However, capsid polypeptides of different TRV strains migrated at different rates (Ghabrial and Lister, 1973a), although they would be expected to have the same molecular weight (because of the implied approximately constant mass per unit length of TRV particles based on their sedimentation behavior). Estimates for TRV capsid polypeptide molecular weights from electrophoretic mobility at single gel concentrations range from ~20,000 to ~38,000 (Lesnaw and Reichmann, 1970; Miki and Okada, 1970; Cooper and Mayo, 1972; Ghabrial and Lister, 1973a). It is possible that TRV capsid proteins, like certain other proteins (Makino et al, 1975; Robinson and Tanford, 1975), interact with detergents in a way that is different from the interactions exhibited by typical water-soluble proteins. The detergent–protein complex of a TRV protein might be more asymmetrical or it may have a lower SDS-to-protein ratio than the corresponding complexes with "standard" proteins. In gels of 1% agarose, the SDS–protein complexes should not be retarded in their electrophoretic mobility by the gel matrix, and mobilities should be equal for complexes of similar surface charge density. Mayo and Robinson (1975) found that TRV CAM protein migrated more slowly than bovine serum albumin or tobacco mosaic virus proteins in 1% agarose (all as SDS complexes), implying that less SDS was bound by the TRV protein–SDS complex. They compared the retardation of electrophoretic mobilities (rather than the absolute mobilities) of TRV CAM protein and standard proteins by increasing concentrations of polyacrylamide in SDS-impregnated gels, and by interpolation, obtained a molecular weight of 23,000 $\pm$ 2800 for the TRV protein. However, the retardation with increasing gel concentration seems to vary with the TRV strain (Ghabrial and Lister, 1973a; Mayo et al., 1974b), implying that the proteins from the different strains may vary in symmetry. Unpublished results of Mayo and Robinson (cited by Mayo et al., 1976) indicate that the mobility is less dependent on gel concentration after removal of a few amino acids from the carboxyl terminus.

Molecular weight estimates from amino acid analyses depend not only on the reliability of the analysis but also on how the data are weighted when computations are made (Gibbs and McIntyre, 1970). The range of molecular weights calculated from amino acid analysis of capsid protein from several strains of TRV is 19,000–24,000 (Offord, 1966; Semancik, 1966b, 1970; Miki and Okada, 1970; Gibbs and McIntyre, 1970; Ghabrial and Lister, 1973a). Mayo and Robinson (1975) have reevaluated the published amino acid composition data by the procedure of Gibbs and McIntyre and have concluded that a number of molecular weight values in the range of 18,000 to a little over 24,000 are equally probable. They also estimated a molecular weight of 21,700 $\pm$ 700 for TRV PRN protein by sedimentation equilibrium in guanidine hydrochloride and concluded from the various estimates that the molecular weight of TRV proteins is in the range of 22,000 $\pm$ 2000.

The molecular weight of the capsid protein can also be estimated from properties of the virions. Evidence from X-ray diffraction and analysis of electron microscopic images favors $25\frac{1}{3}$ as the number of protein subunits per turn of the TRV helix. From the helix pitch ($\sim$2.55 nm), the estimated mass per unit length of the TRV helix ($2.54 \times 10^5/$

nm, derived from sedimentation data and particle dimensions), and the percentage of protein in the virion (~95%), the protein mass per capsomer is calculated to be ~24,000. An integral number of nucleotide residues would be expected to be associated with each protein subunit in the helix. If one takes an average nucleotide residue weight of 320 and a 19:1 ratio of protein to RNA, the protein subunit molecular weight ought to be an integral multiple of 6000. Four nucleotide residues per capsomer and $25\frac{1}{3}$ capsomers per turn of the helix would result in $101\frac{1}{3}$ nucleotide residues per turn. The currently accepted structure for tobacco mosaic virus has 49 nucleotide residues per turn, the phosphodiester chain disposed at a distance of 4 nm from the helix axis and a helix pitch of 2.3 nm. Thus the region of elevated electron density at 8 nm from the helix axis of TRV could accommodate the phosphodiester chain of TRV RNA at approximately the same density of nucleotide residues along the RNA helix as is found in TMV (~0.52 nm from phosphorus atom to phosphorus atom). Wilson *et al.* (1975) have presented a model for RNA conformation in TRV rods. In summary, current information on the virion structure is consistent with a capsid polypeptide molecular weight of ~24,000, one polypeptide per capsomer (Tollin and Wilson, 1971; Offord, 1966; Harrison and Klug, 1966; Finch, 1965; Nixon and Harrison, 1959; Harrison and Nixon, 1959). However, this estimate depends on the precision to which such quantities as particle dimensions, percentage of RNA in the virions, and partial specific volume are known. An experimentally determined value of the last quantity has not been published. The molecular weight of a TRV capsid protein will be known, probably, only when an amino acid sequence has been determined.

The molecular weights of TRV RNAs have been estimated by comparing their electrophoretic mobilities to those of ribosomal RNAs in polyacrylamide gels. The results are consistent with those discussed in the previous paragraph. For eight published values of particle length and the corresponding RNA molecular weights (Harrison and Woods, 1966; Cooper and Mayo, 1972; Morris and Semancik, 1973a; Huttinga, 1973; Reijnders *et al.*, 1974) (four TRV strains), the average mass of RNA per unit particle length and the standard deviation is 12,750 ± 180 nm^{-1}. The same quantity, derived from virion mass per unit length (Harrison and Klug, 1966) and the percentage of RNA in the virions (or from the redundant information of helix pitch, number of nucleotide residues per turn, and nucleotide residue weight), can be calculated to be 12,700 nm^{-1}. Therefore, 190 nm of L rods, for example, can be expected to contain RNA of molecular weight ~2.4×10^6.

2.4. Virion Reconstitution Experiments*

TRV protein has been isolated by treating virions with acetic acid or formic acid (Semancik and Reynolds, 1969), urea plus acetic acid (Miki and Okada, 1970), or 1.5 M $CaCl_2$ (Ghabrial and Lister, 1973a). RNA can be recovered by phenol extraction (e.g., Darby and Minson, 1972) or by protease digestion of the capsid protein (Cooper and Mayo, 1972). The first report on the reconstitution of TRV from isolated TRV protein and RNA is that of Semancik and Reynolds (1969). Aggregation of the protein (in the absence of RNA) has also been studied by Fritsch *et al.* (1973) and by Morris and Semancik (1973b). The two groups used protein from TRVs of two different serotypes (CAM, serotype III, and C, serotype I). Both report the formation of ~35 S protein aggregates (possibly double disks composed of about 50 monomers of capsid protein) at pH values close to or above neutrality. At low pH, the degree of aggregation decreases, and material sedimenting at less than 10 S was observed. At ionic strength 0.1, approximately equal amounts of 36 S and < 10 S material were found at 2°C and pH 4.5–5.3 for CAM protein (Fritsch *et al.*, 1973), and at 11°C and approximately pH 5.4 for C protein (Morris and Semancik, 1973b). Since the behavior of the CAM protein was nearly temperature-independent over the range 0–20°C, the TRV proteins from the two strains apparently show a very similar pH dependence of aggregation. However, at pH 8, the < 10 S aggregates of TRV-C protein accounted for 10–20% of the total, whereas only a trace of < 10 S protein was present in CAM protein preparations at pH 8. Both proteins aggregated more readily at low ionic strength.

In contrast to the results reported for protein aggregation, summaries of the conditions found to be optimal for reconstitution of CAM virions (0.5 ionic strength phosphate buffer, pH 4.7, 20 h at 1°C; Abou Haidar *et al.*, 1973) and to be optimal for reconstitution of C virions (0.25 M glycine buffer, pH 8.0, 12 h at 4–10°C; Morris and Semancik, 1973b) appear to be very different. However, these conditions may represent the separate optima for two different steps in the reconstitution, and the reconstitution of CAM virions and that of C virions may be very similar processes. Abou Haidar *et al.* (1973) attempted to reconstitute CAM at pH 8 under a variety of conditions which were the same as or similar to those reported by Semancik and Reynolds (1969), i.e., RNA plus protein dialyzed against 0.25 M glycine buffer, pH 8,

---

* See chapter by L. Hirth in Vol. 6 for a detailed discussion of this topic.

9°C for 48 h, then against 0.1 M phosphate buffer, pH 7.0. (The secondary dialysis, at pH 7.0, has been utilized by Semancik and Reynolds, 1969, and by Morris and Semancik, 1973b, in order to disrupt any C-strain protein aggregates which were not associated with RNA.) No long CAM nucleoprotein rods were formed at pH 8. Electron microscopic images of complexes formed after only a few minutes at pH 8 indicate that the protein was associated with only one end of any RNA molecule. However, the encapsidation process failed to proceed further. Since at pH 8 and low ionic strength the 36 S aggregate is the only form of the CAM protein detectable in other than trace amounts (Fritsch et al., 1973), the presumed reconstitution initiation complex observed in the electron microscope may be formed most readily from the 36 S aggregate. Further extension of the encapsidation may require protein in a less aggregated form, as has been postulated for the reconstitution of tobacco mosaic virus (reviewed by Casjens and King, 1975). Isolated protein of TRV C does exist to an extent of 10–20% as < 10 S aggregates at pH 8.

   Successful reconstitution of CAM virions (to 5–10% of the specific infectivity of native CAM nucleoprotein) was accomplished by mixing at 1°C RNA in pH 8 buffer plus protein in water and then adding pH 4.7 sodium phosphate to a final ionic strength of 0.5 (Abou Haidar et al., 1973). Thus the RNA–protein mixture was exposed first and briefly to a condition favoring the 36 S aggregate and second to a condition under which the 36 S aggregate is marginally stable and less extensive protein aggregates are favored. Successful reconstitution of C virions (60% recovery of input RNA as nucleoprotein) was accomplished by dialysis of RNA plus protein against a low ionic strength pH 8 buffer (a condition under which the 36 S aggregate predominates but the < 10 S protein concentration is significant) and then against 0.1 M phosphate buffer, pH 7.0 (a condition under which aggregates of C protein dissociate). For both CAM and C reconstitution, the yield of nucleoprotein particles having length of the corresponding L rod appears to be low. This may be the result of a facile initiation of nucleoprotein rods but a subsequent slow growth of the coated region which allows nucleases to act on the RNA.

2.5. Conversion of Unstable TRV to Stable TRV

   Early experiments (Köhler, 1956) on the transmission of TRV isolates gave indications of an unusual kind of apparent genetic instability. Most infections spread well into young leaves of tobacco, and the sap from such leaves is highly infectious. Other infections spread slowly, never becoming fully systemic. Sap derived from plants with the latter type of infection is weakly infectious, and the infectivity it does possess declines rapidly in extracts. Sänger and Brandenburg (1961) and Cadman (1962) contributed to our current understanding of the unstable form of TRV with the discovery that the infectivity in sap could be stabilized by phenol extraction, the infectivity remaining in the aqueous phase. This and other observations (such as the absence of virus antigen in the sap) led to the conclusion that the infectious entity of the unstable form of the virus is RNA not protected by capsid protein. Inoculation of a local lesion host with the stable form induces lesions of two kinds (Fig. 1), those which upon transfer yield a stable infection and those which yield an unstable infection. [In a few cases the two kinds of lesions can be distinguished by appearance (Lister, 1967), but in most cases they cannot; however, freezing of the excised lesion for a period of days usually causes "unstable" infectivity to

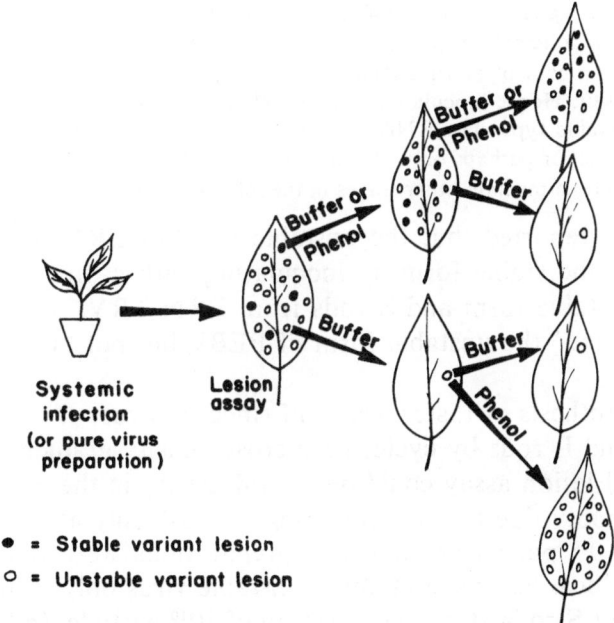

Fig. 1. Derivation of "stable" and "unstable" variants of a tobravirus. Stable variants, containing viral nucleoprotein, are readily transferred in buffer extracts, whereas "unstable" variants, being RNA devoid of protective viral protein, are not. Both are readily transferred using phenol extraction. For simplicity, the two kinds of lesion produced are represented as looking different, although this is usually not the case. From Lister (1969) with permission of the Federation of American Societies for Experimental Biology.

disappear, whereas "stable" infectivity is preserved.] Unstable infections do not revert to the stable form (Cadman and Harrison, 1959); stable infections give rise to both forms, the unstable form being favored by dilution of the inoculum.

Harrison and Nixon (1959) showed by local lesion assay of fractions from sucrose density gradients on which TRV had been centrifuged that most of the infectivity was associated with the L rods. Lister (1966) repeated this experiment and extended it in a way which allowed the phenomena of unstable TRV and two principal TRV rod lengths to be related. Subculturing of the local lesions derived from the sucrose gradient fractions revealed that those resulting from inoculation of the L-rod fractions were almost entirely of the unstable type, whereas those derived from the S-rod region, or the region of overlap of S rods and L rods, were predominantly of the stable type. Lister (1966) interpreted the infectivity observed in both the S-rod and overlap regions of the gradient as being derived from mixtures of L and S rods, and suggested that

> . . . the simplest explanation of this system would be that the RNA of "long" particles of the TRV type is deficient in the information required for some stage of the process leading to the enrobement of viral RNA with virus protein; possibly the coding of the virus protein itself. Hence inocula containing only long particles give rise to infections only of the unstable type. The RNA of "short" particles, on the other hand, though containing at least, or perhaps only, the information lacking in that of the "long" particles, is inadequate to mediate other stages in the infection cycle.

Lister (1966) reported that the unstable form of PRN TRV could be converted to the stable form by inoculating with a mixture of phenol-extracted unstable form and S rods from PRN TRV. S rods of PEBV could "stabilize" the unstable form of PEBV but not "unstable" PRN TRV.

The hypothesis of Lister was confirmed by Frost *et al.* (1967), who purified S and L rods by cycles of sucrose density gradient centrifugation. A local lesion assay could detect infectivity in the S-rod preparation (presumably due to contaminating L rods) only at concentrations of $\geq 5 \times 10^{10}$ particles/ml. L-rod preparations were infectious, but gave rise to local lesions containing unstable virus only. From a mixed inoculation of S rods at a concentration of 10^{10} particles/ml and L rods at 2×10^8 particles/ml, half of the lesions were of the stable type. The proportion of stable infections increased monotonically with increasing S-rod concentration. S-rod RNA, but not ultraviolet-irradiated S rods, could induce stable infections, implying that the RNA is the active agent. Frost *et al.* (1967) also observed that stabilization was achieved by homologous but not by heterologous S-rod and L-rod mixtures (and not by the corresponding mixtures of RNAs) and pointed out that this implies that RNA of the S rods must be dependent on aid from the L rods (e.g., a specific RNA polymerase) because neither short nor long particles accumulate after the heterologous mixed inoculations.

The ability of the L-rod RNA to replicate independently of the S-rod RNA in a defective type of infection (no capsid protein formed), the inability of the S-rod RNA to replicate independently, and the ability of S-rod RNA to convert the defective L-RNA infection to one in which both L and S virions are produced has been well documented in later publications (e.g., Lister, 1968; Semancik and Kajiyama, 1968; Sänger, 1968, 1969).

2.6. Infectivity as a Function of Virion Concentration

Local lesion counts have been shown to vary as the first power of the L-rod concentration in the inoculum (also containing S rods) over a more than hundredfold range for two strains of TRV (Frost *et al.*, 1967; Sänger, 1968). Frost *et al.* reported that for the CAM strain of TRV the number of lesions on *Chenopodium amaranticolor* remained the same, within experimental error, with increasing S-rod concentration (over a 25-fold range) at constant L-rod concentration. In contrast to the above results, Morris and Semancik (1973*a*) observed a decline in the number of local lesions formed on leaves of cucumber or cowpea plants as the concentration of S rods, added to a constant concentration of L-rod RNA, was increased. (The L-rod RNA was actually phenol-extracted sap from plants inoculated with CAM L rods, so the L-RNA concentration is not known; at low S-rod concentrations, the local lesion counts increased with increasing S-rod concentration; S-rod concentration was varied over a thousandfold range.) *Nicotiana clevelandii* was inoculated with the same mixtures (L-rod RNA concentration constant); the amount of virions (nucleoprotein) recovered increased with increasing low concentrations of S rods but declined when a sufficient amount of S rods was supplied. S rods from a serotype II strain did not stimulate or inhibit, within experimental error, local lesion formation by the (serotype III) CAM L-rod RNA. It is not known whether this phenomenon of homologous interference of S rods with local lesion formation depends on the species of local lesion host used (*Chenopodium* by Frost *et al.* vs. cucumber, etc., by Morris and Semancik), on whether L-rod RNA or L rods are in the inoculum, or on using a sufficient range of S-rod concentrations.

Sänger (1968) analyzed not only the total number of lesions as a

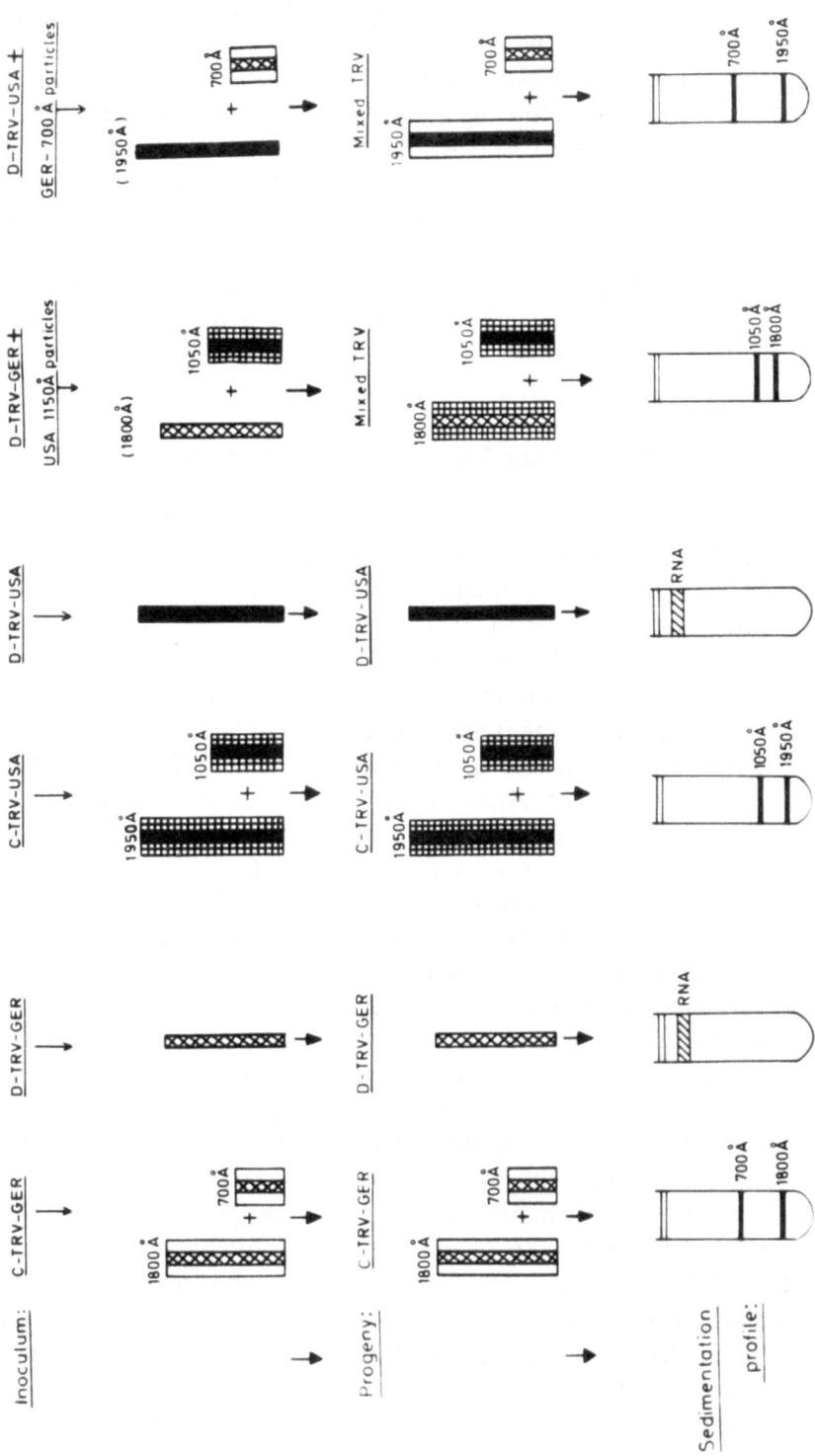

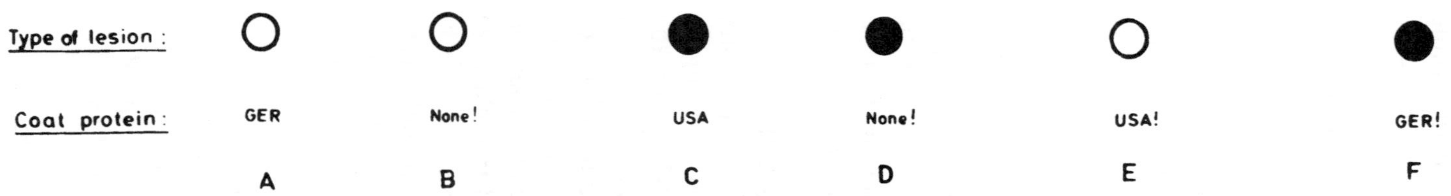

Type of lesion :	○	○	●	●	○	●
Coat protein :	GER	None!	USA	None!	USA!	GER!
	A	B	C	D	E	F

Fig. 2. Complementation of two unstable TRV isolates with the heterologous short particles. The genetic markers of the two systems (particle size, lesion morphology, and coat protein specificity) are represented diagramatically. D-TRV inoculum (for defective TRV) was prepared by homogenizing tissue infected with unstable TRV in the presence of bentonite, a ribonuclease inhibitor, and clarifying it by centrifugation. Infectivity in such preparations is associated with an RNA (and upon inoculation gives rise to an RNA) which sediments at the rate of L-rod RNA, as indicated in parts B and D. A C-TRV (for complete TRV) inoculum is a virion preparation consisting of L rods and S rods. When inoculated on tobacco, TRV USA induced fully necrotic spots and TRV GER induced necrotic rings, as indicated, regardless of whether the infection was of the stable or the unstable type. Diagrams E and F present results obtained after inoculation of heterologous mixtures of unstable TRV and S rods. They are consistent with local lesion type being specified by the source of L-rod RNA and the capsid protein (serological reaction) being specific by the source of S rods. From Sänger (1969) with permission of Springer-Verlag and H. L. Sänger.

function of TRV concentration (S and L rods at a constant ratio) but also the proportion of them which represented infections of the stable type. As has been stated above, the total number of lesions varied as the first power of the inoculum concentration. The *proportion* of local lesions of the stable type varied as the second power of the inoculum concentration. This is an unexpected result since it means that the absolute number of stable-type lesions varied as the third power of the inoculum concentration. A simple extension of the most simple infection hypothesis (a minimum of one S-rod RNA molecule plus one L-rod RNA molecule initiating a stable infection) would predict a second power dependence (e.g., Fulton, 1962).

2.7. TRV Hybrids

The hypothesis of Lister (1966) holds that S-rod RNA and L-rod RNA encode different genetic information. Therefore, it might be possible to derive a hybrid virus by combining the S rods and the L rods from two different TRV strains. Such hybrids have been recognized by the phenotypic markers of rod length (not a genetic marker in the usual sense), type of capsid protein (usually recognized serologically), symptoms on infected plants, and temperature sensitivity. Experiments with hybrid TRV have been thoroughly reviewed by Jaspars (1974) and Gibbs and Harrison (1976), and the subject will be considered only briefly here. Semancik and Kajiyama (1968) inoculated cucumbers with the nine possible combinations of purified S rods and L rods derived from the serotype I isolates B, C, and PRN. At the inoculum concentrations used, the S rods produced no lesions, and only 0–10% of the lesions from the L-rod inocula were of the stable type. The three isolates have L rods of the same length, have S rods of different lengths (80–115 nm), and are serologically very similar or identical; B and C seem to have the same capsid protein (Semancik, 1970). From 35 to 95% of the lesions from the mixed inocula were of the stable type, with no noticeable trend in the percentages of stable type in favor of either homologous or heterologous mixtures. The lengths of the S rods in the stable infections, as estimated from the sedimentation coefficients, were determined by the source of S rods in the mixed inocula and were independent of the source of L rods. These results support very strongly the concept of S-rod RNA having independent genetic information not derived from the L-rod RNA.

Hybrids which can be recognized by capsid protein as the

phenotypic marker are inherently difficult to construct. This is because it is precisely those pairs of strains that are serologically most distinct which are least likely to form a stable infection when inoculated as heterologous mixtures of S rods and L rods (or the corresponding RNAs). Sänger (1968, 1969) found only two out of 20 heterologous inocula derived from the RNAs of five serologically distinct TRV strains to produce stable infections. These were the two reciprocal S and L combinations of strains GER and USA (Fig. 2). The lengths of both the L rods and S rods of these strains are different, and the rod lengths of the hybrid TRVs were determined by the sources of the corresponding RNAs of the original mixed inocula. As expected, the type of capsid protein (serological reaction) of the hybrid was determined by the source of S-rod RNA in the inoculum. All S rods known to be capable of stabilizing a TRV infection of the unstable type have RNAs larger than the minimum size (molecular weight approximately 240,000) required to code for capsid protein, so it is reasonable to conclude that a "factor" contributed by the S-rod RNA to the induction of a stable infection is the structural gene for the capsid protein.

Symptoms induced in the host are markers which vary in reliability and reproducibility from system to system. However, it has been possible to demonstrate that, in different systems, symptoms are controlled by the S-rod RNA, the L-rod RNA, or by the combination. Sänger (1969) found the morphology of local lesions induced on tobacco by five TRV strains to be determined solely by infectious L-rod RNA and not to be influenced by the presence of S rods. Lister and Bracker (1969) found the symptoms characterized as mild, severe, and yellow (as well as the S-rod lengths) for three isolates of TRV ORE to be determined in mixed inoculations by the source of S rods. Ghabrial and Lister (1973b) inoculated a mixture of S rods of the TRV ORE (serotype II) isolate which produced yellow symptoms (designated TRV Y) plus L rods of TRV Z (serotype III). A virus was recovered which has an amino acid composition and two-dimensional tryptic peptide map characteristic of Y capsid protein but the symptoms of Z-TRV on *Petunia*. However, symptoms on *N. clevelandii* were most like those of Y-TRV, indicating that symptoms induced by a single virus may be dependent on both S-rod and L-rod RNAs. The hybrid produced about one-tenth the amount of virions as did either of the parental strains and one-eighth the total amount of antigen as Y-TRV. A stable form of the reciprocal hybrid (S rods of Z plus L rods of Y) was not recovered.

Robinson (1973a) induced mutants of TRV CAM with 1.0 M NaNO$_2$ at pH 6 for 40 h at room temperature. The solution was diluted, CAM S rods were added, and *Chenopodium* plants were inoculated with the mixture. Local lesions were excised, frozen, and thawed (to eliminate unstable TRV) and transferred to pairs of *Chenopodium* plants. One member of each pair was held at 20°C, the other at 30°C. Putative temperature-sensitive mutants were selected as the local lesion isolates producing few lesions at 30°C. Wild-type CAM on *Chenopodium* at 30°C produced 49% of the lesions produced at 20°C, whereas mutants N8 and N10 produced 0% and 3%, respectively. The virions of the mutants were no more heat-sensitive than the wild-type virions, and, suprisingly, N10 replication was not temperature-sensitive in *Nicotiana clevelandii* (Robinson, 1973*b*). As expected because of the procedure used to recover the mutants (S rods added before the selection step), the temperature sensitivity of hybrids of wild type and mutant was dependent on the source of L rods, and the mutations are presumed to be in the L-rod RNA. The mutants and wild-type CAM could not be distinguished when all were propagated at 20°C.

2.8. *In Vitro* Protein Synthesis

Protein synthesis in a cell-free system to which viral RNA is added potentially provides a system for unequivocally demonstrating the presence of a gene on the viral RNA. Ball *et al.* (1973) utilized extracts of mouse L cells which had been preincubated to consume L-cell messenger RNA and thereby reduce the level of endogenous (no added messenger RNA) amino acid incorporation. The L-rod RNA or S-rod RNA of CAM TRV at 50 μg/ml stimulated incorporation to a level only about double the endogenous level. [^{35}S]Methionine-labeled incubation mixtures, both endogenous and S-rod RNA-stimulated, were analyzed by polyacrylamide gel electrophoresis. A prominent zone corresponding in mobility to TRV capsid protein was observed for the latter analysis but not for the former. No further test (e.g., peptide analysis) was made of identity of the material in this zone, nor was any analysis presented of the products from incubations to which L-rod RNA had been added. The low amount of incorporation relative to the endogenous level does not encourage further use of the L-cell system stimulated by TRV RNAs.

Cell-free protein-synthesizing systems derived from wheat germ can be prepared so that the endogenous incorporation is very low. What incorporation there is, is spread among several sizes of polypeptides so that, generally, only few and faint zones can be seen after analysis by gel electrophoresis. Mayo *et al.* (1976) found that TRV CAM S-rod RNA stimulated the incorporation of about 40 mol of [^{35}S]methionine per mole of RNA added to a wheat germ system. L-rod RNA of the same virus was only about one-sixteenth as effective; however, L RNA of TRV PRN seemed to be a more effective messenger RNA than the S-RNA of PRN. The incorporation level was comparable to that for tobacco mosaic virus RNA in the same system (i.e., a few percent of the added radioactive amino acid was incorporated). The major portion of the product directed by TRV CAM S-RNA comigrated with authentic TRV CAM capsid protein during electrophoresis in gels of two different concentrations. No product was recognized which could account for the S-RNA sequences not devoted to the capsid protein gene. Antiserum to CAM precipitated 30% of the S-RNA product, but it precipitated only 2% or less of the radioactivity incorporated in incubation mixtures to which CAM L-RNA, PRN S-RNA, or tobacco mosaic virus RNA had been added. Under the proper conditions of pH and ionic strength, the CAM S-RNA product formed 36 S aggregates as expected for capsid protein (see Section 2.4). The *in vitro* product apparently represented TRV CAM capsid protein completed to, or nearly to, the normal carboxyl terminus since the anomalous electrophoretic behavior associated with CAM capsid protein with an intact carboxyl terminus (see Section 2.3) was also exhibited by the *in vitro* product. CAM L-RNA stimulated incorporation into a spectrum of polypeptides with apparent molecular weights extending to about 100,000. When S-RNA and L-RNA were incubated together in the wheat germ extract, only the S-RNA product (capsid protein) was observed. Fritsch *et al.* (1976) have extended this work and have found polypeptides of apparent molecular weights greater than 170,000 in reactions mixtures to which spermidine (0.9 mM) and either CAM or PRN L-rod RNA had been added. PRN S-rod RNA stimulated the synthesis not only of a polypeptide which comigrated with PRN capsid protein (apparent weight 29,000) but also of several other zones, one with an apparent molecular weight (32,000) larger than that of the capsid protein. (See Chapter 4 for further discussion.)

2.9. Nucleotide Sequence Relationships

Minson and Darby (1973a) and Darby and Minson (1973) utilized RNA-RNA hybridization, both competition hybridization and direct hybridization, to show that nucleotide sequences in TRV CAM L-rod RNA correspond to a small but significant fraction of the sequences in S-rod RNA. Materials for the competition hybridization experiments were melted double-stranded RNA from TRV-infected tissue, ^{3}H-labeled S-rod RNA, and varying amounts of unlabeled L-rod RNA. The amounts of radioactivity which were found to be ribonuclease resistant after annealing decreased hyperbolically with increasing concentrations of L-rod RNA, as expected for a direct competition of the L-rod RNA with the ^{3}H-labeled S-rod RNA for complementary nucleotide sequences of the melted double-stranded RNA. The decrease in ribonuclease-resistant radioactivity, extrapolated to infinite concentration of L-rod RNA and expressed as a fraction of the resistant radioactivity found in the absence of added L-rod RNA, was 0.27. High-molecular-weight, single-stranded RNA isolated from tissue infected with unstable TRV (containing about 0.2% L-rod RNA but presumably free of S-rod RNA) competed to the extent of 0.29; S-rod RNA competed completely (extrapolated fraction of 1.0), and RNA from uninfected tissue did not compete detectably. Thus, on the average, approximately $(0.28)(2070)$ ~600 nucleotide residues of the S-rod RNA must correspond to some degree with sequences in L-rod RNA. The correspondence need not be exact since complete displacement of the S-rod RNA by the excess L-rod RNA, or labilization of a double-stranded region involving the S-rod RNA because it was close to a double-stranded region involving the L-rod RNA, would result in a decrease in ribonuclease-resistant radioactivity.

Materials for the direct hybridization experiments of Darby and Minson (1973) were ^{3}H-labeled S-rod RNA, ^{3}H-labeled L-rod RNA, and double-stranded RNA isolated from tissue infected with defective TRV. The fraction of either S-rod or L-rod RNA made ribonuclease resistant increased hyperbolically with increasing concentrations of melted double-stranded RNA in the annealing reaction, as expected for direct hybridization of the radioactive RNA with nucleotide sequences in the complementary strand derived from the double-stranded RNA. The extrapolated values (to infinite concentration of double-stranded RNA) were 0.80–0.85 of the ^{3}H-labeled L-rod RNA made ribonuclease resistant and 0.21 of the ^{3}H-labeled S-rod RNA. Possible explanations for the L-rod RNA values being less than 1.0 are the presence of L-rod RNA in the double-stranded RNA preparation and the partial susceptibility of double-stranded RNA to the ribonuclease concentrations used in the digestion step. If these factors affect the hybrids with S-rod RNA and those with L-rod RNA equally, then the calculated fraction of S-rod RNA sequences for which corresponding sequences in L-rod RNA exist is 0.25–0.26, comparable to the numbers derived from competition hybridization experiments. The melting temperatures of RNA hybrids were compared by heating them to various temperatures, cooling quickly, and digesting with ribonuclease to determine the fraction of radioactivity made ribonuclease-sensitive. Two homologous hybrids (radioactive S-rod RNA annealed to melted TRV double-stranded RNA and radioactive L-rod RNA annealed to double-stranded RNA from tissue infected with unstable TRV) melted 7°C higher than the heterologous hybrid formed by annealing radioactive S-rod RNA to the melted double-stranded RNA of unstable TRV. This observation provides evidence that the two strands of the heterologous hybrid were not fully complementary. The annealing conditions (70°C and 0.3 M NaCl-0.03 M sodium citrate) were such that nearly complementary as well as exactly complementary nucleotide sequences could be expected to hybridize. TRV RNAs have been labeled with [125]I (Shoulder *et al.*, 1974), and it may be possible to carry out more sensitive assays with this high-specific-activity [^{125}I]RNA.

Since the length ratio of CAM S rods to L rods is 52/197, unlabeled S-rod RNA ought to compete with labeled L-rod RNA in a hybridization reaction with melted double-stranded RNA to the extent of $(52/197)(0.28) = 0.07$. Minson and Darby (1973*a*) were unable to detect competition by S-rod RNA against ^{3}H-labeled L-rod RNA when both were annealed with melted double-stranded RNA from a stable TRV infection. Whether a competition to 7% would be undetectable or whether some other phenomenon (e.g., titration of the competing S-rod RNA by complementary RNA from the melted double-stranded RNA) explains the lack of competition by S-rod RNA remains to be determined. No similar competition experiment, using double-stranded RNA from unstable TRV rather than from stable TRV, has been presented. Darby and Minson (1973) reported that unpublished RNA-RNA hybridization experiments by them and D. J. Robinson showed no detectable sequence homology among TRV strains CAM, Y, and PRN (serotypes III, II, and I, respectively).

The significance of the partial and inexact sequence homology of L-rod RNA sequences with sequences in S-rod RNA is not known. Similarities almost certainly exist in the two RNAs with regard to recognition sites for RNA replicase enzyme(s), ribosomes, and capsid protein. However, if the current concepts of the structure and replication of RNA bacteriophages (Zinder, 1975) can be applied to TRV, the observed extent of sequence homology far exceeds the requirements for recognition.

Minson and Darby (1973*b*) have determined that the 3'-terminal sequence of both RNAs is -GpCpCpC-OH. Polyadenylate sequences could not be detected in the RNAs of TRV B and TRV C by hybridization with [^{3}H]polyuridylate (Semancik, 1974).

2.10. Events in TRV Replication

Our knowledge of the molecular biology of the replication of TRV and the other viruses discussed in this chapter is in a primitive state. Both L-rod RNA and mixed TRV RNAs are infective. They stimulate polypeptide synthesis in cell-free amino acid incorporating systems, and S-rod RNA can direct the synthesis of capsid protein *in vitro*. Therefore, the viral RNAs and not their complementary strands probably function as messengers *in vivo*. Tissue infected with stable-form TRV contains RNAs which are complementary to the L-rod and S-rod RNAs. Undoubtedly the complementary RNAs are involved in viral RNA synthesis, but neither the sizes of the complementary RNAs nor the enzyme or enzymes which synthesize them have been characterized.

Harrison and Crockatt (1971) compared the effects of various antibiotics on the replication of CAM TRV in *N. clevelandii* leaf disks floated on solutions of those antibiotics beginning 4–5 h after inoculation of the intact leaf. The amont of stable TRV infectivity which was recovered from the disks after incubation for 3–4 days was not reduced by chloramphenicol (100 μg/ml), actinomycin D (25 μg/ml), or rifampicin (100 μg/ml), which are generally considered to inhibit protein synthesis on 70 S ribosomes, DNA-dependent RNA synthesis, and DNA-dependent RNA polymerase of prokaryotes, respectively. However, cycloheximide (an inhibitor of protein synthesis on 80 S ribosomes) at 2 μg/ml reduced the accumulated stable TRV infectivity by thirtyfold. Cycloheximide at 0.4 μg/ml had a retarding effect on the virus increase, reducing it tenfold at 1 day after inoculation but only 10% at 4 days. Stable TRV accumulated only to the detection limit (corresponding to a several hundredfold reduction) for stable TRV when the disks were incubated in 10 μg/ml cycloheximide, but accumulation of unstable TRV (in the one experiment presented) was inhibited only approximately thirtyfold under these conditions. If, as this result implies, RNA synthesis was inhibited less than protein synthesis, it is consistent with the expected mode of action of cycloheximide. Synthesis of both stable and unstable TRV was prevented if 10 μg/ml cycloheximide was infiltrated into leaves 17 h prior to inoculation. The stronger effect of cycloheximide on viral RNA synthesis when it was applied prior to inoculation and the retarding effect of a low concentration (0.4 μg/ml) of the inhibitor on the rate of virus synthesis imply a dependence of viral RNA synthesis on the synthesis of protein(s) (on 80 S ribsomes) early in infection. Unfortunately, no test was reported of the effects of the other antibiotics at times earlier than 4 h postinoculation.

Robinson (1974) compared the number of lesions on *Chenopodium amaranticolor* 5 days postinoculation for leaves that had been UV irradiated at various times before and after inoculation. Irradiation just prior to inoculation reduced lesion counts by 30%; irradiation just after inoculation reduced them 95%. Irradiation at various times after inoculation caused succeedingly less drastic reductions until, at about 24 h after inoculation, the lesion counts approached those of unirradiated controls. A reduction of about 50% was seen for irradiation at about 5 h postinoculation. The time dependence of the irradiation sensitivity of local lesion development could have a number of causes. The stability of a nascent lesion could be increased by an increase in the number of infective units in it, by the synthesis or interposition of structures capable of shielding against the radiation, or by a stimulation of RNA repair systems. Robinson (1974) found that the temperature-sensitive mutant N8 (see Section 2.7) failed at 30°C to induce ultraviolet-resistant local lesions (tested for by incubation of the plants at 20°C after irradiation). This implies that the step in the induction of local lesions which is blocked at 30°C is the same as or precedes the step(s) which allows lesion development to become ultraviolet-resistant.

The distinctive shape of TRV particles makes it possible by electron microscopy to identify sites of virion accumulation. Harrison and Roberts (1968) observed in TRV CAM-infected *N. clevelandii* parallel arrays of particles with the dimensions of L rods and abutting the surfaces of mitochondria, rod long axis perpendicular to the surface of the mitochondrion. Even in the situations in which two mitochondria were close enough to allow contact at both ends of the viruslike rods, only one end of the rod seemed to be attached to the mitochondrion surface (polar attachment). The mitochondrial surface membrane did not appear to be pierced. Particles with the dimensions of S rods were seen in the cytoplasm but not abutting mitochondria. Kitajima and Costa (1969) obtained similar results with various isolates of pepper ringspot virus (serologically related to Brazilian strains of TRV) in several host species, except that these authors had greater difficulty identifying S-rod-like particles in the cytoplasm. Even meristematic tissue had the arrays of rods apparently attached to mitochondria. De Zoeten (1966) found parallel arrays of rods in tobacco inoculated with a California strain of TRV, but no evidence of attachment to mitochondria. The phenomenon may be strain specific. The lack of inhibition of TRV CAM by chloramphenicol administered 4–5 h after inoculation implies that mitochondrial protein synthesis at late times after inoculation is not required for virus replication and that attachment of L rods to mitochondria probably is not indicative of their protein being synthesized in them.

Tobacco mesophyll protoplasts inoculated with TRV CAM were studied by Harrison *et al.* (1976); they assayed infective RNA, infective nucleoprotein, the relative amounts of short and long particles, and the binding of fluorescent antibodies (antiserum raised against virions). Infective RNA was detected at 7 h and approached a maximum at 12 h. Fluorescent antibody staining and infective nucleoprotein were observed at 9 h after inoculation and increased up to about 40 h. The kinetics of L-rod and S-rod synthesis were distinct, with half the final amount of L rods appearing at 22 h but half the final yield of S rods occurring at 30 h. (Semancik and Kajiyama, 1967, had found the ratio of S rods to L rods of TRVs B and C to decline rather than increase with time after inoculation of intact plants.) L rods were closely associated with mitochondria at all times. In other experiments, the S and L rods were inoculated at different times. The amounts of infectious nucleoprotein were reduced as the time of inoculation of the S rods was varied from being simultaneous with the long rod to being up to 8 h before or 4 h after the long rods. However, the proportions of the protoplasts which were stained by fluorescent antibody remained approximately constant over the stated range of inoculation intervals. This result testifies to the degree of stability and independence exhibited by the two TRV RNAs. This protoplast system obviously has great potential for further elucidation of the events in TRV replication (see Chapter 5).

2.11. Possible Significance of Other TRV Components

Some TRV isolates have more than one major class of rods shorter than the L rods (180–200 nm). The possible biological significance of the multiple classes has not been extensively investigated. A TRV isolated from pepper had rods of lengths 50, 85, 115, and 190 nm, but was resolved by local lesion transfer into two viruses: TRV B with particles of 50, 115, and 190 nm lengths and TRV C with particles of 50, 85, and 190 nm lengths (Semancik, 1966*b*). The capsid proteins of B and C are apparently identical. The 85- and 115-nm S rods, but not the 50-nm rods, were able to convert the unstable infections of these viruses to the stable form (Semancik and Kajiyama, 1968). These S rods must have the same or a very similar capsid protein gene.

Therefore, some instances of multiple length classes probably are due to the TRV being a mixture of strains. Harrison and Woods (1966) found the number of length classes of rods to vary during serial passage of several TRVs.

However, a mixture of strains is not a likely explanation for the persistence in both TRV B and TRV C of the 50-nm rods which were not necessary to initiate a TRV stable infection, yet were recovered from tissue inoculated with a mixture of the L and S rods (Semancik and Kajiyama, 1968). The 50-nm rods may contain RNA molecules with their entire nucleotide sequence derived from the RNA of the L rod or S rod. Such encapsidated derivative RNAs have been observed for a cowpea strain of tobacco mosaic virus (Morris, 1974; Whitfeld and Higgins, 1976; Higgins et al., 1976; Bruening et al., 1976). The RNA in a 50-nm TRV rod could be expected to be capable of specifying a polypeptide of molecular weight > 60,000.

3. COMOVIRUSES

Two ribonucleoprotein particles of viruses from the comovirus group, or their RNA molecules, are required to initiate an infection. No independent propagation of either of the ribonucleoprotein components or their RNAs has been demonstrated (e.g., see Kassanis et al., 1973). Two unusual features of the these isometric virions which have been observed for several members of the group and which serve to distinguish them from other known plant viruses are the presence in the capsid of two major kinds of proteins and the presence in the RNAs of polyadenylate sequences. (However, see comments on broad bean wilt virus group, Section 3.1.) Various properties of comoviruses have been reviewed by van Kammen (1972), Brown and Hull (1973), and Jaspars (1974).

Chewing insects (beetles, grasshoppers, weevils) have been shown to be capable of transmitting various comoviruses (see review by Walters, 1969; Whitney and Gilmer, 1974; Gerhardson and Petersson, 1974; Fulton et al., 1975; Cockbain et al., 1975). Beetles retain and continue to transmit the virus over a period of days (Walters, 1969). Several viruses in the group are seed transmitted (see review by Shepherd, 1972; Moghal and Francki, 1974; Nelson and Knuhtsen, 1973a; Haque and Persad, 1975). Most are legume viruses; most have a host range limited to a few species; all can be mechanically transmitted. Various *Chenopodium* species are useful as local lesion hosts. Cowpea mosaic virus growth in protoplasts has been demonstrated (Beier and

Bruening, 1975; Hibi *et al.*, 1975). The RNA of cowpea mosaic virus also infects cowpea protoplasts (Beier and Bruening, 1976).

3.1. Members of the Comovirus Group

The comovirus group was formerly referred to as the squash mosaic virus group, after the first member to be demonstrated to have two ribonucleoprotein components and to be characterized biophysically (Rice *et al.*, 1955; Mazzone *et al.*, 1962). The SB (Agrawal, 1964) isolate of CPMV is now considered to be the type member of the comovirus group (Harrison *et al.*, 1971). Members of the group include the following:

Broad bean stain virus	BBSV
Broad bean true mosaic virus	BBTMV
(or Echtes Ackerbohnemosaik-Virus)	(EAMV)
Bean pod mottle virus	BPMV
Bean rugose mosaic virus	BRMV
Cowpea mosaic virus	CPMV
Desmodium virus	
Pea green mottle virus	PGMV
Quail pea mosaic virus	QPMV
Radish mosaic virus	RaMV
Red clover mottle virus	RCMV
Squash mosaic virus	SqMV

Many serological relationships have been reported between viruses considered to be in this group. A selection of these relationships is presented in Table 1. No attempt is made in the table to distinguish the degrees of serological cross-reaction. Some of the cross reactions shown have titers which are 1/100th or less of the homologous titers. In many cases, the investigators have been unable to show serological relationships between specific pairs of viruses listed in the table. By serological criteria, the members of the comovirus group are generally distantly related. Among those viruses labeled as CPMVs, SB and Nigerian (of the "yellow" subgroup), on one hand, and VU and Trinidad (of the "severe" subgroup), on the other, are no more closely related serologically than some other comoviruses which are named according to different hosts (Swaans and van Kammen, 1973). However, two subgroups of SqMV were found to be closely related (Nelson and Knuhtsen, 1973*b*), as are BPMV, type, and BPMV, J-10 (Moore and Scott, 1971).

TABLE 1

Selected Reports of Serological Relationships between Comoviruses[a]

Virus	a	b	c	d	e	f	g	h	i	j	k	l
BBSV				xo								
BBTMV (EAMV)			o				ox					
BPMV, type	xo		x		x	x	o	ooo		o	o	
BPMV, J-10		x						xoo			o	
BRMV									x			
CPMV, Arkansas	ooo		x			x	x	x		o	o	x
CPMV, Trinidad	oxo	ooooo										o
CPMV-VU		ooxoo								o		o
CPMV-SB		oxo	o				xo					o
CPMV, Nigerian	x	xoo	o						o			
Desmodium virus					o							
PGMV (F1)			ox	oo			o					
QPMV											x	
RaMV, type		o						oo				
RaMV-HZ								xo				
RaMV-KV								x				
RCMV		x		x	ooo		o					
SqMV			x	ox	x		o	x				

[a] x, Antiserum reacting with virus, o.

[b] a, Shepherd (1963); b, Agrawal and Maat (1964); c, Campbell (1964); d, Valenta and Gressnerova (1966); e, Gibbs *et al.* (1968); f, Lee and Walters (1970); g, R. J. Shepherd (personal communication); h, Moore and Scott (1971); i, Stefanac and Mamula (1971) and Kassanis *et al.* (1973); j, Gaméz (1972); k, Moore (1973); l, Siler, Scott, and Bruening (unpublished observations).

Broad bean wilt virus (BBWV), nasturtium ringspot virus, petunia ringspot virus, and parsley virus 3 (PV3) are serologically very similar (Frowd and Tombinson, 1972; Sahambi *et al.*, 1973; Doel, 1975). However, no serological relationship of these to the comoviruses has been demonstrated (e.g., Taylor *et al.*, 1968), and at least some are transmitted by aphids rather than by chewing insects. The capsid proteins of BBWV comigrate with CPMV capsid proteins in gel electrophoresis, as do the larger RNAs. A possible requirement has been indicated for two kinds of nucleoproteins in order to initiate infections (Doel, 1975). If BBWV or the related viruses can be shown to have polyadenylate sequences in the RNAs, they probably should be considered to be comoviruses regardless of whether or not serological relationships or common vectors can be demonstrated.

The serological reactivity of CPMV has been utilized in solid phase radioimmune assay (Ball, 1973) and in serologically-specific electron microscopy (Beier and Shepherd, to be published).

3.2. Chemical Composition of the Centrifugal Components

Rice *et al.* (1955) found that carefully isolated preparations of SqMV were composed of not one but three centifugal components. Sedimentation coefficients of 56 S, 88 S, and 111 S (later revised to 57 S, 95 S, and 118 S, Mazzone *et al.*, 1962) were determined with the Svedberg oil turbine ultracentrifuge. These were designated as the top, middle, and bottom components, respectively. The top component seemed to have less RNA than the middle or bottom component and showed no infectivity except at the highest concentration available. However, means for efficiently separating the components were not available and no local lesion host was available, so no firm conclusion could be made about component infectivities or the presence of RNA in the top component. A local lesion host has been discovered recently (Lastra *et al.*, 1975).

The sedimentation patterns for various comoviruses are similar to those observed by Rice *et al.* (1955) except for variations in the relative amounts of the components. For many of these viruses, top component is absent. Bruening and Agrawal (1967) measured the sedimentation coefficients of the type member CPMV-SB at a concentration of about 100 μg/ml (using an analytical ultracentrifuge equipped with ultraviolet absorption optics). Values of $s_{20,w}$ = 97.5 $\pm$ 1.5 S (15 determinations) and 119 $\pm$ 3 S (17 determinations) were obtained for the middle (M) and bottom (B) components, respectively (the uncertainties listed are standard deviations). The sedimentation coefficient of the top (T) component was reported to be 60.2 $\pm$ 1 S (5 determinations). The concentration of virus was low enough so that extrapolation to zero concentration was unnecessary. Almost all sedimentation coefficients reported for comovirus particles fall in the ranges 118 $\pm$ 8 S for B, 98 $\pm$ 7 S for M, and 58 $\pm$ 4 S for T. The observed ranges of the ratios of sedimentation coefficeints are 2.02 $\pm$ 0.05 for B/T and 1.65 $\pm$ 0.03 for M/T (Mazzone *et al.*, 1962; Bancroft, 1962; Paul, 1963; Bruening and Agrawal, 1967; van Kammen, 1967; Moghal and Francki, 1974; Sahambi *et al.*, 1973; Blevings and Stace-Smith, 1976). The fact that the ranges of observed ratios of sedimentation coefficients are proportionately smaller than the ranges of observed sedimentation coefficients implies that the magnitudes of the latter ranges may be due in part to systematic errors such as improper measurement of the temperature of centrifugation. The formula of Reichmann (1965) may be used to calcuate an RNA content of 34% for B and 25% for M from the sedimentation ratios given above. (The formula is applicable only if the top component is indeed devoid of RNA. El Manna and Bruening (unpublished observations) found that T was not labeled above the background level with [^{32}P]phosphate *in vivo* under conditions in which B was labeled to 5000 cpm/μg.) These percentages of RNA content are within a few percent of the values derived from chemical analyses (Mazzone *et al.*, 1962). Doel (1975) observed cosedimentation of components from viruses of the BBWV group with those of Nigerian CPMV.

Wu and Bruening (1971) demonstrated that the capsids of CPMV-SB are composed principally of two kinds of polypeptides. The polypeptides were isolated by treating virions with a mixture of LiCl and guanidinium chloride which precipitated RNA but maintained the protein in solution. The larger (L) and smaller (S) polypeptides had apparent molecular weights of 42,000 and 22,000, respectively, according to their electrophoretic mobilities on SDS polyacrylamide gel and amino acid compositions. (The limitations of these two methods have been discussed in Section 2.3.) The insolubility and strong tendency to aggregate (especially for the L polypeptide) shown by the CPMV capsid proteins represent major technical difficulties in working with them. However, it was found that in 5 M urea at room temperature both polypeptides are soluble to a few mg/ml. The L polypeptides were present as aggregates under these conditions, but the S polypeptide apparently was dispersed. Because of this specific aggregation, it was possible to separate L and S polypeptides by chromatography on Sephadex G200 in 5 M urea, the L polypeptide aggregates eluting at the void volume. Two-dimensional analyses of the tryptic peptides and amino acid analysis were consistent with the two polypeptides having distinct amino acid sequences. (Amino acid analyses of BBTMV proteins are also distinct; Blevings and Stace-Smith, 1976.) The relative amounts of amino groups, absorbency at 280 nm, staining intensity in the gels, and ^{35}S-label of the two polypeptides, as well as the amino acid composition of L and S as compared to the unfractionated capsid proteins, were all consistent with an approximately 1:1 molar ratio of L and S in components T, M, and B of CPMV. Wu and Bruening (1971) postulated that the CPMV capsid is composed of 60 copies each of L and S. Geelen *et al.* (1972) confirmed the existence of the two capsid polypeptides. The corresponding molecular weights determined by them were 44,000 and 22,000 for underivatized polypeptides and 49,000 and 25,000 for carboxymethylated proteins. A particle weight for T, estimated by light scattering, was found to be approximately consistent with 60 copies of each kind of polypeptide in the capsid (see also Section 3.3, below).

Pairs of capsid proteins with electrophoretic mobilities similar to those of CPMV have been observed for BBTMV, BPMV, RaMV, RCMV, and SqMV (Wu and Bruening, 1971; J. Carpenter, as reported by Kassanis *et al.*, 1973; Blevings and Stace-Smith, 1976; Oxefelt, 1976). The corresponding molecular weights of L and S calculated in these experiments are 37,500 and 20,000 for BBTMV (Blevings and Stace-Smith, 1976) and 40,000 and 18,000 for RCMV (Oxefelt, 1976). However, RCMV proteins comigrated with CPMV-SB proteins in electrophoresis. CPMV-SB and SqMV polypeptides appeared to have very similar electrophoretic mobilities (Wu and Bruening, 1971). Molecular weights of 42,000 and 26,000 were calculated for polypeptides from viruses of the BBWV group and these could not be resolved from polypeptides of Nigerian CPMV in coelectrophoresis experiments.

In order to recover CPMV RNA in good yield, phenol extraction must be performed at a slightly alkaline pH (El Manna and Bruening, 1973) or with organic solvent added to the phenol (Reijnders *et al.*, 1974; Zabel *et al.*, 1974). Reijnders *et al.* (1974) have reviewed the reported molecular weights of CPMV RNAs. The range for M-component RNA is $1.37 - 1.45 \times 10^6$ and for B-component RNA is $2.02-2.5 \times 10^6$. These values were all derived by comparing electrophoretic mobilities or sedimentation rates of the CPMV RNAs with other RNAs used as standards. The CPMV RNA molecular weights were derived by interpolation. No absolute method for determining the molecular weights has been applied to CPMV RNAs or proteins. Therefore, one cannot expect to reconcile exactly, at this time, the molecular weights of the macromolecular virion components with the percentages of RNA in the virions or the particle weights. Mazzone *et al.* (1962) determined the particle weights of SqMV components by the theoretically sound method of sedimentation and diffusion, including experimental determination of the partial specific volumes. The results were particle weights of 4.5×10^6 for T, 6.1×10^6 for M, and 6.9×10^6 for B. A value of 4.6×10^6 for top component of Nigerian CPMV was estimated by light scattering (Geelen *et al.*, 1972).

Mazzone *et al.* (1962) found that the B component of SqMV did not behave as a homogeneous material when analyzed by RbCl density gradient centrifugation. Two zones had 118 S (i.e., bottom component) material in them. One had a buoyant density only slightly greater than that of M, whereas the other was found, at equilibrium, near the bottom of the centrifuge tube. Bruening (1969) found a similar situation for CPMV-SB. The two forms of the bottom component were designated B_U (for B-upper) and B_L (for B-lower). The densities of the components (in g/ml) in CsCl gradients buffered at pH ~5.8 were estimated to be T, 1.297; M, 1.402; B_U, 1.422; and B_L, 1.470. Either B_U or B_L could serve with M to initiate infections (Bruening, 1969), and the RNAs of B_U and B_L were found to be equivalent in apparent molecular weight and in terminal nucleotide sequences (El Manna and Bruening, 1973). As was found with SqMV, the difference in density between B_U and B_L was greater than the difference between M and B_U. Component B_L was present in lesser amounts than B_U in most CPMV preparations (Bruening, 1969). A high-density form of bottom component may be present in BPMV preparations (see Fig. 6 of Bancroft, 1962). White *et al.* (1973) found four zones in the density range expected for middle and bottom components when RaMV-KV and RaMV-HZ were analyzed on CsCl gradients. No assignment of middle or bottom components to specific density zones was made. Only two zones were seen in RbBr gradients (buffered with phosphate at pH ~7) containing RaMV-HZ. RaMV-KV similarly gave two major zones and, in addition, a spectrum of minor zones considered to represent virion aggregates containing more than one kind of component. The minor zones were and would be expected to be intermediate in density.

Van Kammen and van Griensven (1970) observed, for Nigerian CPMV, component buoyant densities in CsCl gradients (phosphate buffered at pH ~7) similar to those reported by Bruening (1969). They considered B_U to be "an artifact of CsCl gradient centrifugation" simply because the buoyant densities of the series T, M, B_L bear a more linear relationship to the RNA contents of the particles than do the densities of the series T, M, B_U. This contention has little basis. That is, the buoyant densities of B_U and B_L almost certainly depend on the amounts of CsCl bound, but it is not necessarily artifactitious if B_U binds less than B_L. Van Kammen and van Griensven (1970) reported that B_U and B_L separately recovered from CsCl gradients each gave rise to both B_U and B_L when centrifuged again under similar conditions. No data were presented, and it is not clear whether the zone seen in the second centrifugation was "manufactured" in the process of centrifugation or was a contaminant due to insufficient resolution in the first centrifugation.

Wood (1971) found that CPMV-VU components M and B had densities, in CsCl gradients buffered at pH ~6.5, of 1.386 ± 0.004 and 1.395 ± 0.002 g/ml, respectively; these values are more reminiscent of M and B_U of CPMV-SB than they are of M and B_L. At pH ~8.5, the CPMV-VU components had buoyant densities of 1.404 ± 0.003 and 1.443 ± 0.002 g/ml, similar to the densities of CPMV-SB components

M and B_L, although the densities of CPMV-SB components M and B_L at pH 8.5 have not been reported. The VU components were recovered from the pH 8.5 gradients and were analyzed on pH ~6.5 gradients. The buoyant densities were 1.394 and 1.436. That is, the process of centrifugation in a CsCl gradient at pH 8.5 increased the buoyant densities by 0.008 g/ml for component M and 0.041 g/ml for B. It seems as if a $B_U \rightarrow B_L$ conversion had been accomplished, although this was not claimed by the author. He regarded the "increased density observed [after centrifugation] at alkaline pH values, especially with the bottom component particles, [as] an artifact of CsCl centrifugation . . . resulting in different amounts of cesium binding and/or hydration." The implication is that B_L (and the slightly higher density form of M) may be artifacts.

The chemical basis of the apparent $B_U \rightarrow B_L$ conversion is probably loss of polyamines from the particles; however, this has not been firmly established. El Manna (1968) identified (by gas–liquid chromatography and other techniques) the polyamine spermidine as a constituent of the M and B components of CPMV-SB. Subsequently, putrescine and spermine were found to be minor constituents. CPMV-SB component B_U was converted to a particle with the buoyant density (and unchanged electrophoresis and sedimentation) properties of B_L by dialysis against 3 M KCl–0.05 M Tricine, pH 8.6. The spermidine content of the particles was reduced from about 100 nmol/mg of virion protein to about 20 in this *in vitro* $B_U \rightarrow B_L$ conversion (Bruening, unpublished results). A reasonable hypothesis is that polyamines in the B_U particle bind to the RNA, blocking sites which otherwise would be able to associate with cesium ions. Exposure of B_U to solutions of high ionic strength (CsCl or KCl) at a sufficiently alkaline pH apparently allows the polyamine(s) to diffuse out of the particle, exposing more sites for association with cesium ions and thereby increasing the buoyant density.

Partridge *et al.* (1974) discovered that CPMV, but not BPMV, capsid protein (unfractionated) contains covalently bound sugars (principally glucosamine, glucose, and galactosamine). The total amount of all sugars found is almost 2 g per 100 g of protein. The authors postulate that the carbohydrate may be involved in seed transmission of the virus since, of the five viruses they studied, only CPMV and barley stripe mosaic virus (see Section 5) have been demonstrated to be seed transmissible and only those two were found to have covalently bound carbohydrate.

3.3. Virion Electrophoretic Forms

Bancroft (1962) found that BPMV, which had been transferred serially through well-separated local lesions and then increased in soybeans, was nevertheless heterogeneous when analyzed by free-boundary electrophoresis in 0.1 ionic strength phosphate-buffered NaCl solution, pH 7. Two symmetrical zones representing approximately equal masses of nucleoprotein were consistently seen. The two materials were resolved by hanging-curtain electrophoresis. When these were separately inoculated, both gave rise to both electrophoretic forms. The separated electrophoretic forms each had the M and B components represented in similar amounts; thus the electrophoretic forms could not be identified with centrifugal forms, and possible differences in virion surface charge due to RNA content cannot explain the mobility differences. Agrawal (1964) observed similarly paired, symmetrical boundaries for the SB and Nigerian isolates of CPMV (in 0.1 M phosphate buffer, pH 7.0) and less dramatic electrophoretic heterogeneity for two other CPMVs. BBTMV also has fast and slow electrophoretic forms (Blevings and Stace-Smith, 1976). SqMV was found to have a single electrophoretic form (Rice et al., 1955).

Component T, as well as M and B, of Nigerian CPMV (and M and B of BPMV) were found to have two forms when analyzed by polyacrylamide gel electrophoresis at pH 9.5 (Semancik, 1966a). The two electrophoretic forms of various comoviruses have been separated on a preparative scale (in addition to hanging-curtain electrophoresis) by cellulose acetate strip electrophoresis, free-boundary electrophoresis, sucrose density gradient electrophoresis, centrifugation through inverse gradients of polyethylene glycol, and isoelectric precipitation (Semancik, 1966a; Niblett and Semancik, 1969; Clark and Lister, 1971; Blevings and Stace-Smith, 1976; Siler et al., 1976), in order of increasing capacity of the separation methods.

Siler et al. (1976) confirmed that CPMV-SB has two electrophoretic forms at both pH 7 and pH 9.3. However, four zones were observed for analyses on polyacrylamide gels at pH 7.5 and 8.2. These four zones, in order of increasing mobility, were shown to contain slow form of component T, slow form of components M and B, fast form of component T, and fast form of components M and B. The hydrogen ion titration curve of T deviated from the curve for M and B (all components were electrophoretic fast form) within the pH range 7.2–8.8, but the curves coincided outside that range (Siler and Bruening, to be published). The electrophoresis and titration experiments indicate that the empty capsids and the nucleoproteins of the fast electrophoretic form have similar numbers of ionizable groups. However, a subset of the ionizable groups of component T must be less acidic than the counterpart subset in M and B. The difference in electrophoretic mobility at pH 7.5 and 8.2 cannot be a direct effect of the charge on the RNA because of the limited pH range over which the difference is seen and because the zones for T and for M plus B were equally sharp, giving no hint of different electrophoretic mobilities of M and B even though they contain different amounts of RNA. There may be a valid analogy in comparing T and M plus B of CPMV on one hand and, on the other, aggregates of tobacco mosaic virus protein and tobacco mosaic virus ribonucleoprotein, which have different titration curves (reviewed by Durham and Klug, 1971). The RNA may indirectly alter protein ionization constants in both systems by inducing conformation changes. Component T of BBTMV was observed only if a mercaptan was present during purification and storage (Blevings and Stace-Smith, 1976) indicating a qualitative difference between T and M plus B for this virus as well.

Geelen *et al.* (1972) first recognized that the molecular weight of the S polypeptide is larger by about 2500–3000 in the slow form than it is in the fast electrophoretic form of CPMV ($\sim$25,000 vs. $\sim$22,000). Similarly, Blevings and Stace-Smith (1976) demonstrated that BBTMV slow-form virions had an S polypeptide of molecular weight $\sim$24,500 vs. the $\sim$20,000 observed for the fast form. Oxefelt (1976) observed forms of RCMV S polypeptide with apparent molecular weights of 20,200 and 18,300. It may be true in general for the comoviruses that the slow and fast electrophoretic forms differ in the molecular weights of the S polypeptide, implying that the *in vivo* conversion of forms is mediated by proteases.

The first reported investigation (Niblett and Semancik, 1969) of the chemical differences between the slow and fast forms was hindered both in experimental design and in interpretation because the existence of two kinds of polypeptides in the capsid was not known at that time. Digestion of BPMV fast electrophoretic form with trypsin converted it to particles with the same electrophoretic mobility as the slow form. The implication is that the slow form will be found to have an S polypeptide of lower molecular weight than that of the fast form, contrary to the results with CPMV and BBTMV. Chymotrypsin and a mixture of carboxypeptidase A and carboxypeptidase B did not cause a change in the mobility of BPMV fast or slow forms. Amino acid analysis of BPMV fast and slow electrophoretic forms revealed a lower glutamic acid content for the latter. Therefore, it is possible that the trypsin released an acidic peptide which was responsible for the higher anionic mobility of BPMV fast form. Blevings and Stace-Smith (1976) could find no statistically significant difference between that amino acid composition of proteins from the slow and fast electrophoretic forms of BBTMV.

Chymotrypsin or a mixture of carboxypeptidases A and B converted CPMV-SB slow electrophoretic form to particles migrating as the fast form (Niblett and Semancik, 1969). Trypsin converted the slow form to a form migrating at a rate intermediate between those of the slow and fast forms. Therefore, it is possible that digestion by chymotrypsin released a basic polypeptide which was responsible for the lower anionic mobility of the CPMV slow form. Leucine was detected as the predominant carboxyl-terminal amino acid of both the fast form and the form with the same mobility that was enzymatically produced from slow form. Leucine was not detected as a carboxyl-terminal amino acid of the slow form. These results imply possible identity of the *in vivo* and *in vitro* fast electrophoretic forms. However, no peptide maps or other information is available to more firmly establish this point. A more detailed interpretation of the carboxypeptidase digestions and amino acid analyses reported by Niblett and Semancik (1969) is not possible because the contributions of the two capsid proteins cannot be distinguished. A hypothesis supported by their results is that a carboxyl-terminal region of the S polypeptide which is present in the slow form of CPMV is missing in the fast form, exposing a carboxyl-terminal leucine residue. The mobility of Nigerian CPMV slow form was increased by incubation with trypsin (Geelen *et al.*, 1973) and that of BBTMV slow form by treatment with chymotrypsin or carboxypeptidases (Blevings and Stace-Smith, 1976). However, in neither case did the mobility of the treated slow form increase enough to equal that of the corresponding fast form.

The relative amounts of slow and fast electrophoretic forms vary in the course of an infection. The fast form of BPMV predominates early in infection and the slow form predominates late in infection (Gillaspie and Bancroft, 1965; Semancik, 1966a), whereas for CPMV-SB (Niblett and Semancik, 1969) and BBTMV (Blevings and Stace-Smith, 1976) it is the fast form which predominates late in infection. At 80 h after they had been inoculated with CPMV, plants were fed [^{32}P]phosphate. In the period 130–170 h postinoculation, the specific radioactivity of the fast form increased more than did that of the slow form. In experiments with unlabeled, CPMV-infected plants, the ratio of fast form to slow form increased more than sixfold in the period 9–14 days postinoculation, whereas the total amount of virions increased only about 30%. Therefore, both in "young" infections, in which the virus concentration is increasing rapidly, and in older infections the fast form of CPMV seems to be derived from the slow form, presumably by proteolysis (Niblett and Semancik, 1969). When primary leaves of cowpeas of various ages were inoculated with CPMV-SB and then harvested 3 days after inoculation, the ratio of fast form to slow form in the recovered virus increased steadily with the age of the plants at inoculation (Lee *et al.*, 1975*a*). Apparently, aging of the plant can contribute to the increased conversion of slow to fast form in infections held for long periods. Obviously, *in vivo* proteolysis is a possible explanation for the *in vivo* interconversions of the electrophoretic forms of BPMV and BBTMV.

Incubation of purified Nigerian CPMV increased the slow form mobility but did not make it equal to that of the fast form. The most highly purified CPMV preparations showed the least tendency to change slow-form mobility, supporting the notion that the conversion is induced by protease(s) contaminating the virus preparation. However, no published experiment rules out the possibility that the virion has intrinsic protease activity as has been found for encephalomyocarditis virus (Lawrence and Thach, 1975). The electrophoretic components of BBTMV also showed altered behavior during storage of virus preparations at 4°C. The mobility of the slow form generally increased 30–40%, whereas the fast-form mobility increased only slightly over a 3-week period. Different preparations "stabilized" (no longer showed mobility changes with continued incubation) at different relative mobilities of the slow, as compared to the fast, electrophoretic form. Preparations recovered after a precipitation by polyethylene glycol and stored for 3–4 weeks at 4°C had in the slow-form particles an S polypeptide of apparent molecular weight 21,500 rather than the 24,500 observed in the freshly isolated slow-form virions. However, the authors were not able to detect other differences in polypeptide apparent molecular weights which would correlate with the observed changes in mobilities of the virions as a function of the time of storage. Changes which are not proteolytic in origin may contribute to the alterations in electrophoretic mobility of BBTMV particles.

Proteolytic activities which modify the mobility of CPMV slow form have been found in infected and uninfected tissue. When slow-form Nigerian CPMV was incubated with centrifuged sap from infected cowpeas, the mobility of the particles increased to approach, but not equal, the mobility of fast form (Geelen *et al.*, 1973). Lee *et al.* (1975*a*) partially purified (by centrifugation, a heat step, and precipitation by ammonium sulfate) an activity which converted slow form to fast form (rather than to a form of intermediate mobility). Equal amounts were recovered from uninoculated or CPMV-SB-inoculated cowpeas. However, upon chromatography on Sephadex G100, quantitatively distinct profiles were obtained for the preparations from healthy and infected tissue. Similar profiles were not obtained when the assays were performed with several synthetic substrates. That is, the enzymatic activity(ies) seemed specific for slow-to-fast conversion. Plant tissues and conditions of plant culture which promoted only inefficient conversion of slow form to fast form *in vivo* also yielded only small amounts of the enzymatic activity. Since it is not known whether the partially purified protease activity(ies) resides *in vivo* in a compartment to which virions are exposed, it is difficult to know whether the activity is responsible for slow-to-fast conversion *in vivo*. *In vivo* conversion may be under genetic control of the virus (see Section 3.6).

Niblett and Semancik (1969, 1970) found the specific infectivity (local lesions per A_{260} unit) of fast-form CPMV-SB to be higher than that of slow form for CPMV isolated 7–35 days after inoculation. The infectivity of isolated viral RNA declined over this same period of time after inoculation, and the heterogeneity of the RNA (judged by sucrose density gradient centrifugation), while significant at 9 days, increased at the longer times. RNA from 11-day slow form was less heterogeneous than RNA from 11-day fast form. Niblett and Semancik concluded that the modifications resulting in the fast-form capsid caused the fast form to have enhanced infectivity in spite of the more extensively degraded RNA those capsids contained. More recently, Lee *et al.* (1975*a*) have isolated virions from an 8-day infection utilizing two procedures. The slow and fast forms of CPMV-SB were immediately separated by sucrose density gradient electrophoresis and inoculated for local lesions assay. For virus isolated by either procedure, the fast form had a specific infectivity about twice that of slow form. When the unfractionated virions were treated with the protease activity recovered from cowpea tissue (see previous paragraph), their specific infectivity increased.

Geelen *et al.* (1973) observed that slow-form and fast-form Nigerian CPMV isolated form cowpeas 5 days after inoculation were equally infectious, contrary to the results described in the previous paragraph. The RNAs recovered from the two forms were also equally infectious and similar in distribution of mobilities on gels. Slow form which had been sufficiently purified could be incubated ("aged") in 0.1 M sodium phosphate–10 mM mercaptoethanol, pH 7.0, at 25°C for 18 h without altering the electrophoretic mobility. However, this treatment reduced the infectivity to a range of 24–30% of the value for slow form maintained at 0°C; fast-form infectivity was reduced to a range of 79–86% of the value for fast form held at 0°C. A subsequent incubation with trypsin increased the mobility of the slow form and returned its infectivity to control (virus held at 0°C) levels. The infectivity of freshly prepared slow form was not increased by incubation with trypsin, nor was the electrophoretic mobility or infectivity of the fast form. Different specific infectivities of the electrophoretic forms of CPMV-SB and Nigerian CPMV in different laboratories may mean that the two strains are really different in this regard, or that there are differences in experimental approach which are not obvious (Lee *et al.*, 1975*a*).

We are left without a satisfactory explanation for the recovery of infectivity of aged slow form of Nigerian CPMV upon incubation with trypsin (or chymotrypsin) *in vitro* or of what value, if any, *in vivo* conversion of electrophoretic forms is to the virus. Equally mysterious is the apparent synchrony with which the transition from slow to intermediate migrating forms occurs *in vitro* (e.g., Fig. 6 of Geelen *et al.*, 1973). Instead of forming a broad distribution of migrating species, the transitions seem to occur as discrete steps with a narrow distribution of migrating species at each stage.

3.4. Capsid Structure

Virus particles in a matrix of stain suspended across holes in the carbon film provide electron microscopic images of sufficient quality for detailed analysis. Crowther *et al.* (1974) used uranyl acetate at pH 4.2 to stain the slow electrophoretic form of a Nigerian strain of CPMV (a mixture of the centrifugal forms). Digital versions of densitometric tracings from images of single particles were converted to two-dimensional Fourier transforms by computerized calculations. The best estimate was made of the orientation of the original particle, i.e., the orientation of axes of symmetry characteristic of an icosahedron, and of the degree to which finer details could be determined from the image. Because unique orientations were obtained from analysis of the images showing the finer details, the CPMV particles can be considered to have icosahedral symmetry (five-, three-, and twofold symmetry axes) to a resolution of as little as 2.5–3 nm. From a few two-dimensional transforms, a three-dimensional transform was constructed. Fourier inversion of the three-dimensional transform gave a three-dimensional image of the regions from which stain had been excluded, i.e., a three-dimensional image of the capsid. Thus these calculations allow an averaged, three-dimensional image to be derived from several two-dimensional images.

Crowther *et al.* state that "The reconstruction shows the capsid to have a rather smooth but modulated surface, a structure not easily described in terms of an arrangement of capsomers." Because "knobs" project more strongly at the fivefold symmetry axes of the reconstruction (to a radius of about 12 nm) than at the threefold axes (to a radius of about 10.5 nm), they propose that the L polypeptides are arranged as pentamers at the 12 fivefold positions (for a total of 60 copies). The S polypeptides would then be disposed as trimers at the 20 threefold positions. The stain-excluded volume corresponding to the fivefold and threefold positions is consistent with a 2:1 volume ratio of L polypeptide to S polypeptide. Figure 3 compares a model of this struc-

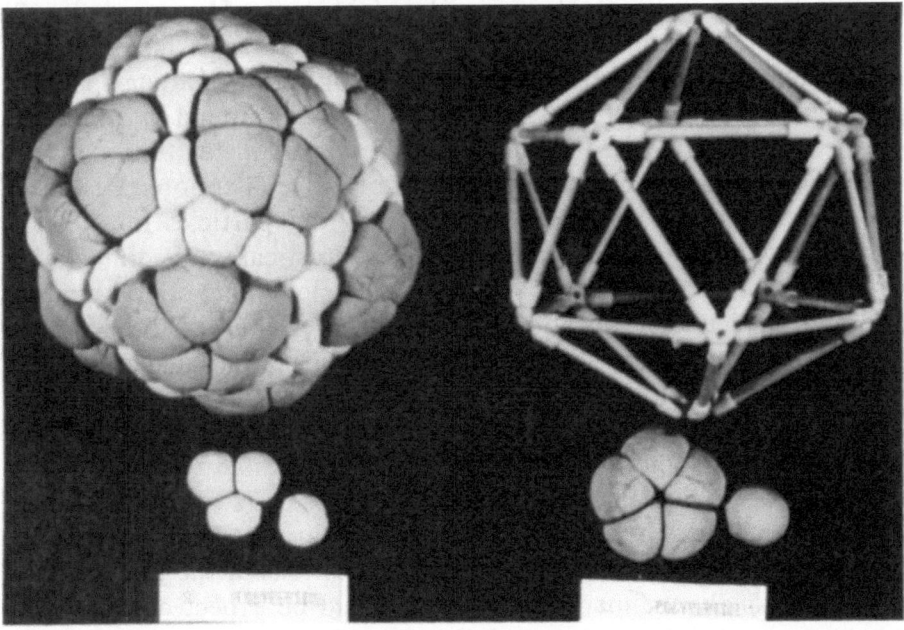

Fig. 3. Capsid structure of cowpea mosaic virus. The capsid is composed of 60 copies each of two different polypeptides, S and L. They are arranged, according to the electron microscopic image reconstructions of Crowther *et al.* (1974), in 12 pentamers of L polypeptide at the vertices of a regular icosahedron and 20 trimers at the faces. A stick model of an icosahedron is shown on the right in approximately the same orientation as the capsid model on the left.

ture and a stick model of an icosahedral surface lattice. The particle dimensions (circularly averaged diameter of ~20 nm) and the mass of protein in the capsid are consistent with all polypeptides being exposed at the surface. Crowther *et al.* point out that the S polypeptides probably are on the surface since they are modified in the slow-to-fast conversion of electrophoretic forms. The volume of S polypeptides would not be sufficient to cover an isometric shell of L polypeptides unless the S polypeptides assumed a very unusual, nonglobular conformation, so the L polypeptides probably are also exposed. The images of particles of the fast electrophoretic form could not be distinguished from those of the slow form.

The only report of any difference in the dimensions of the centrifugal components of a comovirus is that of Juretić and Fulton (1974). The T, M, and B components of the HZ strain of RadMV could not be distinguished by immunodiffusion tests using antiserum prepared against unfractionated virus. Therefore, the components would be expected to have very similar surfaces. Electron microscopic images showed many particles with hexagonal outlines, as expected for an icosahedron viewed down a threefold axis. However, the B-component particle images had average diameters of 28 nm vs. 24 nm for the other components. No photograph of an unfractionated virion preparation was presented. (Crowther *et al.*, (1974) found that particles on the carbon film were about 30% larger in diameter than particles suspended in stain over holes in the carbon film. Therefore, it is possible that the conditions used to prepare CPMV particles for electron microscopy affect the observed diameter drastically.) Sedimentation coefficients of RaMV-HZ T, M, and B in a low ionic strength buffer and at a particle concentration of several mg/ml were 54 S, 83 S, and 98 S, respectively (Juretić and Fulton, 1974). The low value of 98 S for component B (by comparison with the values observed for other comoviruses) makes it tempting to conclude that the B particles have an unusual conformation. However, it is not possible to assume from this observation that the B-component particles are swelled in solution. The asymmetrical shapes of the sedimenting boundaries indicate interactions between particles under the conditions of the analysis, and the most rapidly sedimenting particles would be expected to be most severely retarded (Johnston and Ogston, 1946) by such interactions. More extensive hydrodynamic measurements will be required to determine whether the RdMV-HZ B component has a larger diameter in solution than the T and M components.

Semancik and Bancroft (1965) found that the middle component of BPMV could be destroyed by emulsification with chloroform at pH 9.5, whereas bottom component was stable under these conditions.

In summary, eight kinds of comovirus particles have been distinguished: the slow and fast electrophoretic forms of T, M, B_U, and B_L. These have not been distinguished serologically (Bruening and Agrawal, 1967; Valenta and Marcinka, 1968; Juretić and Fulton, 1974). All reports which deal with the capsid structure, except that of Juretić and Fulton (1974), imply that the capsids of all these particles are of the same size and general structure. There are probably 60 copies of each of two kinds of polypeptides. The slow-to-fast (or fast-to-slow, depending on the virus) conversion is probably mainly a proteolytic reaction. The molecular weights of the polypeptides are known only approximately. The L polypeptide has a molecular weight of about 43,000 in both electrophoretic forms. The capsids of the slow and fast forms do differ in the molecular weight of the S polypeptide, it being about 24,000 before the proteolytic step and about 21,000 after, according to analyses by electrophoresis in polyacrylamide gels permeated with SDS. Component T, for both the slow and the fast electrophoretic forms of CPMV, has some ionizable groups which differ in dissociation constant from the corresponding groups in M, B_U, and B_L. CPMV has covalently bound sugar residues in the capsid protein. B_U and B_L apparently do not differ from M in capsid structure but differ from each other in buoyant density on CsCl density gradients, probably because of different polyamine contents.

3.5. Infectivity of the Components

The existence of defective tobravirus infections from which only one of the two chromosomes of the virus, the L-rod RNA, can be recovered makes it possible to determine unequivocally that the RNA is infectious. Every comovirus infection which has been examined has yielded both M and B particles (e.g., Bruening and Agrawal, 1967). However, it is not possible to determine unequivocally that M or M-RNA alone, or B or B-RNA alone, is not infectious, because that conclusion must be drawn from negative results: no observed infection after inoculation of the purified component or component RNA. The conclusion that both M-RNA and B-RNA are required to initiate an infection rests on the observation that the infectivity of the individual components declines (but the infectivity of the binary mixture remains approximately constant) as the preparations of those components (or their RNAs) are subjected to succeeding steps of fractionation designed to discard traces of the other component. It is convenient to consider an infectivity–activation ratio: the number of lesions produced by inoculating M plus B, divided by the sum of the two numbers of lesions obtained by inoculating the preparations of M and B separately (when mixed inocula have the same concentrations of M and B particles as the individual inocula; or, when the M inoculum and B inoculum are simply mixed in equal proportions, the same ratio is multiplied by 2 to approximately compensate for the dilution effect of mixing the inocula). Wood and Bancroft (1965) separated by sucrose density gradient centrifugation the M and B components of CPMV and BPMV. Activation ratios of 2.2–18 were obtained for BPMV and 4–10 for CPMV. The B-component preparations all were at least a fewfold more infectious than the M-component preparations, so it was not possible for these authors to discard the notion that the B component is infectious.

Bruening and Agrawal (1967) observed activation ratios of 8–17 for CPMV-SB components separated by two cycles of zone sucrose density gradient centrifugation and mixed in 1:1 particle ratios. The M and B preparations were analyzed by analytical centrifugation and were shown to be at least 97% and 99% pure, respectively (the limitations of the analysis). The infectivity of M plus B mixed in various ratios gave an inverted "U"-shaped curve. Similar data are plotted in Fig. 4 (Siler and Bruening, unpublished results). The steepness of these curves at the extreme values of the particle ratios indicates that even if the pure components are not in fact infective, a component preparation will be infective if contaminated by even a trace of the other component. When the mixing curve of Bruening and Agrawal (1967) (a mixing curve for the component RNAs had a similar appearance) was extrapolated to zero percentage of component B, the extrapolated value for the infectivity was zero. This implies that M is not infectious. The corresponding extrapolation to 100% B was more ambiguous and could be interpreted as either zero or nonzero infectivity. From the shape of the curves and the apparent intercepts, the authors concluded that it is likely that "Most infections are initiated by a group of M and B particles rather than by a single B particle or B plus M particle pair." This statement is at variance with current ideas only in that it concedes (because of the ambiguous intercept) that an infection could be initiated by a B particle. It does appear that most infections are initiated by groups of M and B particles, although no evidence excludes the possi-

Fig. 4. Infectivity of cowpea mosaic virus as a function of the proportions of components M and B in the inoculum. The total component concentration was held constant for each curve and was 6×10^9, 12×10^9, and 18×10^9 particles/ml for the lower, middle, and upper curves, respectively. At these concentrations, both the B (i.e., 0% M) and the M (i.e., 100% M) preparations did not produce lesions on the host (*Vigna sinensis* var. Chinese red × Iron) used in this experiment.

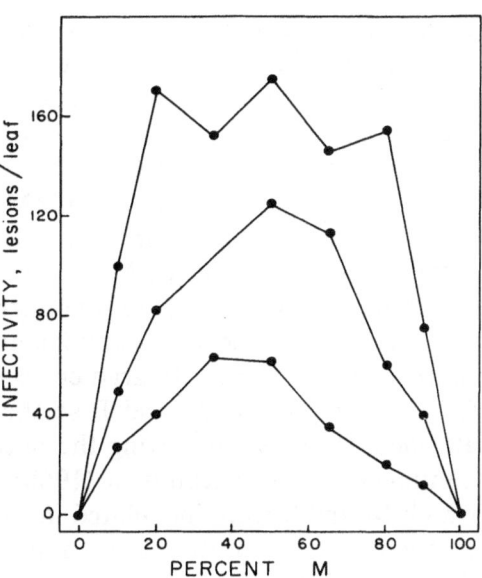

bility of some infections being initiated by single pairs of M and B particles or RNAs. Bruening and Agrawal (1967) increased, by transfer to a systemic host, virus from several of the lesions derived from their separated M and B preparations. The original SB isolate from which the M and B components had been separated did not form top component. However, three out of 19 lesions from "B" inoculum gave virus producing top component. None out of four lesions from "M" inoculum and none out of seven lesions from unfractionated virus gave virus producing top component. It is known (see Section 3.6) that the production of top component is under the control of M. Probably all preparations of CPMV-SB have some M particles capable of engendering T (i.e., SB is a mixture of strains). Only when a B preparation (i.e., a mixture of B and M with a very high B:M ratio) is the inoculum can "cloning" of M particles be accomplished, because some infections will be initiated by a single M particle plus several B particles. In other cases, several M particles presumably enter almost every cell which subsequently becomes infected, and cloning of M particles is less probable.

When two particles are partially resolved by sucrose density gradient centrifugation, the more rapidly sedimenting particle will be more heavily contaminated with the more slowly sedimenting particle than *vice versa*. This situation and the strong boost in infectivity obtained by adding even a trace of one component to a nearly pure preparation of the other tended to foster the view that the B component is more infective than the M component. Bancroft (1962) found that the highest specific infectivity for BPMV, partially resolved on a sucrose gradient, was associated with component B. Van Kammen (1967) obtained a similar result with CPMV. However, Wood and Bancroft (1965) found the highest specific activity to be associated with a region between the centers of the M and B zones for both BPMV and CPMV; Bruening and Agrawal (1967) confirmed these results for CPMV. Van Kammen (1968) and van Kammen and van Griensven (1970) combined sucrose and CsCl density gradient centrifugation steps to further purify CPMV components M and B so that an activation ratio of > 200 was attained, strongly supporting the notion that M and B are individually noninfectious. Van Kammen (1968) also confirmed, in experiments in which M and B were inoculated in various proportions, that particles in a roughly 1:1 proportion are maximally infectious and that variation in the concentration of the minority component in a mixture has the most powerful effect on the observed number of lesions. The conclusion of Agrawal (1964), that middle component is more infectious than bottom, is probably due to improper identification of the zones in the CsCl gradients used to resolve the components. What was interpreted by him to be M probably was a mixture of M and B_U and what was interpreted as B probably was B_L.

Infectivity activation ratios obtained with components of other comoviruses are 24 for RCMV after two cycles of sucrose density gradient centrifugation (Valenta and Marcinka, 1968); 4–9 for BPMV after two or three cycles (Moore and Scott, 1971); 17–55 for RaMV, type strain, and > 200 for RaMV-Kv, after two cycles (Kassanis et al., 1973); ~5 for BBSV after two cycles (Moghal and Francki, 1974); and 90–280 for BBSV and 19–29 for BBTMV using conservatively cut fractions after a single cycle of sucrose density gradient centrifugation (Govier, 1975).

Little information is available on the infectivity of these viruses as a function of concentration, with the M:B ratio constant. Kassanis et al. (1973) state that statistical analysis of the infectivity dilution curve of RaMV-KV on *Chenopodium quinoa* "fitted a theoretical two-hit curve very well, but could not be fitted to a one-hit curve." CPMV-SB lesion counts were found to vary as the first power of the virion concentration with either *Chenopodium amaranticolor* (Bruening and Agrawal, unpublished observations) or a *Vigna sinensis* variety (Beier and Bruening, unpublished observations) as local lesion host.

3.6. Hybrid Comoviruses

Since the RNAs of the M and B components are almost certainly the two chromosomes of the virus, it should be possible to derive hybrid viruses by inoculating mixtures of M from one virus and B from another. The isolation of tobravirus hybrids (Section 2) has been facilitated by the independent replication of the L-rod RNA in unstable infections. L-rod RNA from such an unstable infection assuredly will be free of S-rod RNA. For the comoviruses, difficulties have been encountered in sufficiently resolving the components, and no biological method for obtaining a pure component is available.

The usual purpose of a virus hybridization experiment is to discover whether a particular character of the virus is specified by M-RNA or by B-RNA. In order to interpret the results of a hybridization experiment, it is hlepful to know the infectivities of M and B preparations as compared to the infectivities of the homologous M + B mixtures (infectivity activation ratio) and whether one or the other of the two possible heterologous M + B mixtures is significantly more infectious. If several "crosses" are performed and the results are consistent, more reliable conclusions about the inheritance of specific characters can be drawn.

Two forms of CPMV-SB, one of which produces top component (SB-24), were used in the first demonstration of hybrid formation with a comovirus (Bruening, 1969). The M and B (i.e., M and B_U or B_L) components of SB-2 and SB-24 were purified by sucrose and CsCl density gradient centrifugation steps. The infectivity activation ratios were equal to or in excess of 200. When homologous component mixtures, i.e., SB-24 M + SB-24 B and SB-2 M + SB-2 B, were inoculated to a systemic host, the progeny virus produced top component in the former case but not the latter, as expected. Heterologous and homologous M plus B mixtures were equally infectious. The results after inoculation of the heterologous mixtures are shown in Table 2.

TABLE 2

Top Component Formation by Hybrid CPMVs

Inoculum	Trials in which T was formed	Trials in which T was not formed	Total number of trials
SB-2 M + SB-24 B	1	7	8
SB-24 M + SB-2 B	9	0	9

Except for the single example of T being formed after inoculation of SB-2 M + SB-24 B, the results are consistent with the middle component RNA specifying whether or not T is formed in the infected tissue, as indicated in Fig. 5. The single exception could have been due to insufficient purification of the SB-24 B component preparation. Virus from plants inoculated with SB-24 M plus SB-2 B was fractionated and the M component was mixed with SB-2 B. The progeny virus produced T, as expected for a "back cross" experiment of this type.

De Jager and van Kammen (1970) treated CPMV-SB with nitrous acid and obtained a mutant, SB-N3, which produced more T than M when propagated in cowpeas, and systemically infected Beka beans very poorly or not at all at 22–24°C. The wild-type SB produced less T than M, and in most cases it readily and systemically infected Beka beans, producing definite symptoms. Reactions of other hosts to SB and SB-N3 were very similar. The infectivity activation ratios of the components were about 12 for SB and >300 for SB-N3. Homologous and heterologous component mixtures were equally infectious. Since SB occasionally produced only a very mild instead of a severe systemic infection, the phenotype cannot be absolutely scored in every case. The total number of trials, given in Table 3, exceeds the number of trials scored because equivocal cases were ignored in the scoring.

The inability of the mutant SB-N3 to cause systemic infection of Beka beans (or the ability of SB to cause a systemic infection) appears to be controlled by the middle component. The amounts of top component which formed in the primary leaves of Beka beans inoculated with the heterologous component mixtures indicated that this

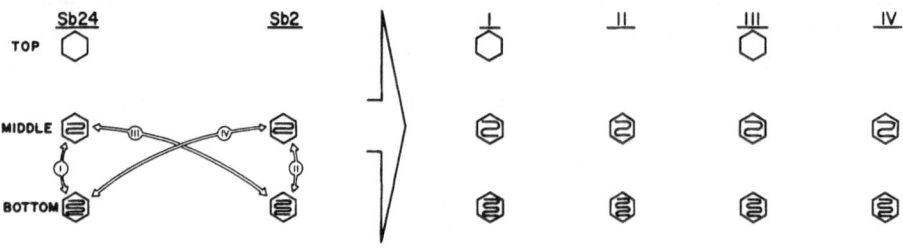

Fig. 5. Inheritance of top component forming ability. The middle component of cowpea mosaic virus specifies whether top component will be produced in the infected tissue. The M and B components of the top component-forming isolate SB24 and an isolate apparently free of top component, SB2, were inoculated in the four possible combinations. Only after inoculation of the two combinations with M derived from SB24 was (with the exception of a single experiment) T recovered from the infected tissue (Bruening, 1969).

TABLE 3

Systemic Infection by Hybrid CPMVs

Inoculum	Symptoms on Beka beans		Total number of trials
	Number of trials systemic	Number of trials not systemic	
SB M + SB-N3 B	14	0	15
SB-N3 M + SB B	0	13	15

character also is under the direction of the middle component, in agreement with the results of Bruening (1969). At 30°C, SB-N3 was able to systemically infect Beka beans, and produced the smaller amount of T characteristic of the wild-type SB. This is an important observation since the similar temperature sensitivity of these two characters implies a possible causal connection between high T production and inability to systemically infect this particular host.

Moore and Scott (1971) studied the type and J-10 strains of BPMV. The J-10 and type strains could be distinguished with antiserum to the type strain but not with antiserum to J-10. A weak spur formed in immunodiffusion tests against type strain antiserum, with type strain and J-10 virions in adjacent wells. This spur formation provided a test for J-10 antigenic character (i.e., for the lack of certain type strain antigen(s) in J-10). The M and B components of both viruses were purified by two or three cycles of sucrose density gradient centrifugation. The authors indicate that these components proved difficult to separate completely. The infectivity activation ratios were ~9 for J-10 components and ~4 for the type strain components. Homologous and heterologous component mixtures were equally infectious. Heterologous mixtures were inoculated on Pinto bean and local lesions were transferred to soybean. Soybean tissue was tested serologically for the presence of J-10 antigenic characters indicated above (Table 4).

The preponderance of results favors assignment of control over

TABLE 4

Serological Character of Hybrid BPMVs

Inoculum	Trials showing a spur	Trials not showing a spur	Total number of trials
Type M + J-10 B	9	46	55
J-10 M + type B	36	13	49

expression of the J-10 antigenic character to the middle component. Therefore, it is likely that at least one of the two kinds of capsid polypeptides is specified by the middle component RNA. However, as the authors acknowledge, the technical difficulties encountered in puri-fying the components have not allowed a clean result to be obtained.

Wood (1972) used nitrous acid to induce mutants of CPMV-VU which showed altered local lesion types when inoculated on Pinto beans. Two of these, VU-3d and VU-7b, were increased, and the components were separated by multiple cycles of sucrose density gradient centrifugation. Components of VU, VU-3d, and VU-7b showed infectivity activation ratios of only 3–4, based on local lesion counts on Pinto bean (a focal assay). When infectivity was measured by counts of the numbers of cowpea plants infected by serial dilutions of the components and component mixtures (a quantal assay), the infectivity activation ratio was about 40 for VU-3d and 100 for UV-7b. Homologous and heterologous component mixtures were equally infectious (by both assays) within experimental error. The lesions of VU, VU-3d, and VU-7b on Pinto bean were all of reproducible and of distinct types. None of these isolates produced detectable amounts of top component. The ratio of M to B was less than one for VU and VU-3d, but greater than one for VU-7b. In experiments in which one to four trial inoculations (serial dilutions on cowpeas, virus recovered from plants infected by the most dilute dose) were made of each of the nine possible M plus B mixtures, the results of trials corresponding to eight of the mixtures were consistent with the M-to-B component ratio being controlled by the source of B. Results from the ninth mixed inoculum (VU M plus VU-7b B) were not consistent. For seven out the the eight mixtures giving consistent results with regard to component ratio (including VU M plus VU-3b B and VU-3b M plus B), the lesion type was determined by the source of B. However, the inoculum VU-7b M plus VU-3d B induced VU-type local lesions (i.e., wild-type local lesions unlike those induced by either 3d or 7b). This appears to be due to an interaction between the M and B in the infected tissue rather than to a genetic reversion or to genetic recombination. Components were separated from virus recovered from tissue inoculated with VU-7b M plus VU-3d B. These were "backcrossed" with components of the mutants and wild-type VU. The results indicated that the component VU-3d B had retained its genetic character regardless of with which M component it had been associated or in what order it had been associated with the various M components. The characters of lesion type and component ratio never segregated in these experiments. Wood (1972) also reported that preliminary tryptic peptide maps of proteins (a mixture of S and L polypeptides) from the mixed component isolate VU-7b M plus VU-3d B (presumably compared with VU-3d and VU-7b proteins) indicated that the middle component "codes for one of the coat proteins" (peptide maps not presented). This is in agreement with the work of Moore and Scott (1971).

De Jager (1976) studied three nitrous acid-induced mutants of CPMV-SB. The mutants and wild-type virus all induced distinct symptoms on Pinto bean, and some of the viruses could be distinguished on other hosts as well. Infectivity activation ratios of about 80 and 170 were observed for CPMV-SB and the mutant N163, respectively. The heterologous mixtures showed comparable infectivity, and the local lesion type on Pinto bean (and symptoms on three other hosts as well) was controlled by the source of middle component. Mutants N123 and N140 increased in inoculated plants to a low level only, and sufficient amounts of purified components could not be obtained. Therefore, de Jager applied a "supplementation" test in which purified M or B component of the wild-type virus was coinoculated with unfractionated mutant virus. The restoration of wild-type symptoms for the mixture containing one of the wild-type components (but not the other) was taken as evidence for control of the symptoms by that component. From these experiments, the N123 mutation appears to lie in component M and the N140 mutation in component B. These results were supported by observing that mixtures of N140 with N123 or N163 gave rise to wild-type symptoms whereas an inoculum of N123 plus N163 did not. Virus behaving as wild type was subcultured from the plants receiving the mixed inoculum. The recovery of actively replicating wild-type virus from a mixture of two mutants which replicate poorly provides a simple test of whether the two mutations are likely to be in different components. However, the results of Wood (1972) described in the previous paragraph show that in at least one case it was possible to have wild-type symptoms from a mutant genotype virus. The simple test must be interpreted with caution.

Kassanis *et al.* (1973) found that the heterologous M and B component mixtures from RaMV-HZ and RaMV-KV were more infectious than the individual component preparations. The infectivity activation ratio for RaMV-KV was greater than 200. The corresponding data for RaMV-HZ were not given. However, the data for the heterologous mixtures were

20 μg/ml HZ M	0 lesions/half leaf
20 μg/ml KV B	1
20 μg/ml each of HZ M and KV B	345

25 μg/ml KV M	0
25 μg/ml HZ B	29
25 μg/ml each of KV M and HZ B	111

Thus the heterologous combination KV M plus HZ B appeared to be significantly less infectious than the reciprocal combination. The lesion counts indicate that the HZ B preparations were significantly contaminated with HZ M, due to technical difficulties in separating the components of this strain. Lesions from *Chenopodium quinoa* plants inoculated with the above mixtures were transferred to turnip seedlings, a good host for RaMV-HZ (Stefanac and Mamula, 1971) and one which has a more severe reaction to KV than to HZ infection (Kassanis *et al.*, 1973). Tissue samples from infected plants were analyzed by immunodiffusion against RaMV-KV antiserum (Table 5). Spur formation by RaMV-KV in an adjacent well was taken as a positive test for RaMV-HZ in the test well.

An obvious interpretation of the results is that the HZ serological character of the virions is determined by both the M and B components. A second character of HZ is that the virions tend not to form large aggregates, whereas KV virions do. All 31 isolates listed in the second column of Table 5 formed no or very few aggregates, as expected because of their HZ serological character. The one remaining isolate from KV M plus HZ B (third column) formed numerous aggregates. The authors concluded that the dual inheritance of the capsid characteristics, through both components M and B, can be explained if it is assumed that each one of the two capsid proteins is specified by each of the two component RNAs.

A possible alternative explanation of the data is that the 20 out of 21 isolates (derived from the KV M plus HZ B inocula) which had HZ capsid character were really derived from HZ M plus HZ B, the HZ M component of which was contaminating the HZ B preparation. If it is true that most comovirus infections are initiated by a mixture of M and B components (not just a pair), then most of the lesions which were

TABLE 5

Serological Character of Hybrid RaMVs

Inoculum	Trials showing a spur	Trials not showing a spur	Total number of trials
HZ M + KV B	11	0	11
KV M + HZ B	20	1	21

transferred to turnip seedlings would have contained KV M, HZ M, and HZ B. The HZ M could be expected to replicate more readily in the seedlings because of the poorer infectivity shown by KV M plus HZ B (i.e., presumably poorer than that shown by HZ M plus HZ B). Therefore, the hypothesis that the two capsid proteins of RaMV are coded for by two different viral RNA molecules is by no means proved.

Siler *et al.* (1976) treated RNA of CPMV-SB with the mutagen sodium bisulfite and then inoculated it on a variety of cowpea which is immune to CPMV-SB. Sap from the immune variety was used to inoculate a susceptible variety. The cycle of passage in the immune variety and in the susceptible variety was repeated. The virus recovered after the second cycle of passage was increased. When it was harvested 9 days after innoculation of susceptible plants, the virus consisted of fast electrophoretic form only, whereas the wild-type CPMV-SB produced about equal amounts of the slow and fast forms. The mutant, designated SB-Bi*l*, did have slow form when harvested 5 days after inoculation. At all times after inoculation, the ratio of fast to slow electrophoretic forms was greater for SB-Bi*l* than for SB. SB-Bi*l* produced no symptoms on the cowpeas, which are immune to SB, and could be detected in the inoculated plants only by transfer of infectivity to fully susceptible cowpeas. The mutant and wild-type viruses could not be distinguished by SB antiserum. The components of SB and SB-Bi*l* were separated by sucrose and CsCl density gradient centrifugation steps and gave infectivity activation ratios of >300. The two reciprocal heterologous M plus B inocula were not equally infectious:

1.25 μg/ml SB M	0 lesions/leaf
1.25 μg/ml SB-Bi*l* B	0
0.36 μg/ml each of SB M and SB-Bi*l* B	238
1.25 μg/ml SB-Bi*l* M	0
1.25 μg/ml SB B	0
0.36 μg/ml each of SB-Bi*l* M and SB B	122
0.36 μg/ml each of SB-Bi*l* M and SB-Bi*l* B	239
0.36 μg/ml each of SB M and SB-B	98

However, the lower infectivity of the combination SB-Bi*l* M plus SB B, as compared to SB M plus SB-Bi*l* B, cannot be explained on the basis of incompatibility of the components because the infectivities are in the same range as those found for the homologous component pairs. In three trials using a local lesion host and one trial using a serial dilution (quantal) assay, the infectivity for inoculum combinations which contained SB-Bi*l* B was two- to threefold greater than the infectivity for combinations which contained SB B, regardless of the source of M. Cowpea plants were inoculated with the two heterologous M plus B combinations and tissue was harvested after 5 days. Virus progeny from the inoculum SB M plus SB-Bi*l* B showed the high ratio of fast to slow electrophoretic forms which is characteristic of SB-Bi*l*; virus derived from the reciprocal inoculum did not (i.e., it was like SB). Therefore, the properties of higher infectivity and of more rapid conversion of slow to fast electrophoretic form both seem to be specified by component B RNA. The latter could be explained if the mutation were in the structural gene for the S capsid polypeptide and the mutant S polypeptide from the slow electrophoretic form of the virion is more susceptible to proteolytic cleavage (perhaps by the enzymatic activity studied by Lee *et al.*, 1975*a*). Alternatively, the mutation could alter the amount or specific activity of a virus-specified protease. The authors favored the latter explanation.

The hybrid comoviruses which have been recovered were all derived by inoculating components from closely related virus strains. The data of Wood and Bancroft (1965) show infectivity activation ratios of close to 1 (i.e., no activation) for heterologous M plus B mixtures from CPMV and BPMV and from CPMV and SqMV. Similar results were obtained with Nigerian and Trinidad CPMV (van Kammen, 1968), and for BBTMV and BBSV (Govier, 1975).

3.7. *In Vitro* Protein Synthesis

Davies and Kaesberg (1974) analyzed the polypeptides formed in a cell-free protein-synthesizing system from wheat germ to which a mixture of CPMV RNAs from M and B had been added. A spectrum of polypeptides, ranging from approximately 10,000 to 60,000 in apparent molecular weight, was found. Two out of five major zones migrated as would be expected for CPMV capsid polypeptides. No further identification was made of the material in these zones.

Recently Pelham and Jackson (1976) analyzed the products synthesized in a cell-free system from rabbit reticulocytes, which had been treated to reduce the endogenous incorporation. High molecular weight polypeptides were not apparent if no messenger RNA was added to the system. Partially resolved preparations of CPMV M RNA and B RNA both stimulated the synthesis of polypeptides in a spectrum of sizes. The largest polypeptides, as judged by electrophoretic mobility in gels, were of molecular weights 220,000 and 120,000. The former apparently is translated from B-RNA and the latter from M-RNA. The large polypeptides presumably are expressions of most of the coding capability of these RNAs. If so, then the capsid proteins and possibly other functional polypeptides may be derived *in vivo* by specific proteolysis, in analogy with poliovirus and similar small animal virus systems. (See Chapter 4 for further discussion.)

3.8. Nucleotide Sequence Relationships

The base ratios for total RNA of several comoviruses have a characteristically high uridylic acid content, typically 30% or greater (Mazzone *et al.*, 1962; Semancik and Bancroft, 1964; Bruening and Agrawal, 1967; Gibbs *et al.*, 1968). RNA from viruses of the BBWV group has about 27% uridylate (Doel, 1975). Van Kammen (1967) showed that the RNAs of M and B have similar but definitely distinct base ratios.

Van Kammen's group has reported extensively on the double-stranded RNAs isolated from CPMV-infected plants and on the use of those RNAs in hybridization experiments. Double-stranded RNAs corresponding in size to M-RNA and to B-RNA have been observed. Both direct hybridization and competition hybridization experiments indicate that few or no nucleotide sequences are common to the two virion RNAs. Melted double-stranded RNA from the larger of the two size classes seemed to hybridize only with B-RNA. The experiments have been well summarized by Jaspars (1974) and Jaspars and van Kammen (1972).

El Manna and Bruening (1973) carried out cycles of periodate oxidation and beta-elimination on CPMV RNAs, expecting to find the 3′-terminal nucleotide sequence . . . CCA-OH or . . . CC-OH, as had been found for other plant virus RNAs. Instead, they found . . . AAA-OH for the RNAs of CPMV-SB components M, B_U, and B_L. ^{32}P-labeled RNA was digested with a mixture of pancreatic ribonuclease A and ribonuclease T_1 to hydrolyze all but the polyadenylate sequences. The same size distribution, that of the surviving polyadenylate sequences, was found for M-RNA, B-RNA, and unfractionated CPMV RNA, and the weight average degree of polymerization was about 200 residues. The polyadenylate was demonstrated to be 3′-terminal and no internal oligoadenylate sequences were found. Semancik (1974) found polyadenylate sequences in both M-RNA and B-RNA of BPMV by molecular hybridization with [^{3}H]polyuridylate. He estimated the degree of polymerization to be 70–100 residues. Oxefelt (1976) recovered polyadenylate after digestion of B-RNA, but not of M-RNA, of RCMV.

3.9. Infection-Associated RNA Polymerase Activity

Zabel *et al.* (1974) have studied an RNA polymerase activity from CPMV-infected primary leaves of cowpeas. Tissue harvested 4 days after inoculation was homogenized in a low-ionic-strength pH 7.4 buffer and centrifuged at 1000*g* for 10 min to remove a strong, actinomycin D-sensitive RNA polymerase activity. Glycerol was added to the supernatant to a final concentration of 20% (v/v). The supernatant was centrifuged at 31,000*g* for 30 min and the sedimented material was washed with a buffer containing 10 mM magnesium ions and 5% glycerol. This insoluble fraction contained an apparently membrane-bound RNA polymerase activity which was nearly insensitive to actinomycin D at 20 μg/ml or deoxyribonuclease at 30 μg/ml. The corresponding fraction from uninoculated leaves did not have this activity. The infection-related activity had a broad and unusually high optimum magnesium ion concentration range of 8–20 mM. The reaction product (labeled by incorporation of [^{3}H]uridine triphosphate) was disrupted with sodium dodecylsulfate and analyzed by sucrose density gradient centrifugation. Four broad zones were found which correspond approximately in sedimentation coefficients to the values expected for the single-stranded and double-stranded RNAs of CPMV. The former two, but not the latter two, zones were almost completely sensitive to ribonuclease at high ionic strength. Thus the enzymatic activity catalyzed incorporation into both single-stranded RNA and RNA which, after detergent treatment, behaved as double-stranded RNA.

Zabel *et al.* (1976) were able to solubilize the RNA polymerase activity by extracting the material initially sedimenting at 31,000*g* with a pH 8.4 buffer free of magnesium ions and containing glycerol at a final concentration of 25% (v/v). The extraction procedure solubilized and stabilized the enzymatic activity, which was further purified by chromatography on a diethylaminoethyl-agarose column. Most of the activity eluted with the first ultraviolet-absorbing material to be displaced from the column by a gradient of KCl solution. It was almost completely dependent on added (viral) RNA. With added RNA, the reaction ([^{3}H]UMP incorporation) was linear for at least 9 h, indicating unusually high stability for a plant virus-related polymerase.

3.10. Events in Replication

Because mixtures of M-RNA and B-RNA are infectious, it can be assumed that at least one of them is a messenger RNA rather than the complement of a messenger RNA. However, this hypothesis has yet to be supported by a demonstration of the synthesis of an authentic comovirus protein in a cell-free protein-synthesizing system under the direction of viral RNA. The isolation of double-stranded RNAs from infected tissues indicates that the replication of both RNAs proceeds by means of complementary strands.

Owens and Bruening (1975) concluded that both capsid poly-peptides of CPMV-SB are synthesized principally or wholly on 80 S cytoplasmic ribosomes rather than on organelle ribosomes. Infected leaf slices were infiltrated with cycloheximide or chloramphenicol. Concentrations of cycloheximide which effectively inhibited the incor-poration of radioactive amino acids into both S and L capsid polypeptides also inhibited incorporation into the small polypeptide of ribulose diphosphate carboxylase, a polypeptide known to be synthesized on 80 S ribosomes. Concentrations of chloramphenicol which inhibited the incorporation of amino acids into the large subunit of ribulose diphosphate carboxylase (a polypeptide known to be synthesized on 70 S ribosomes) failed to reduce incorporation into the S or L polypeptides of CPMV. Hibi *et al.* (1975) found that CPMV increase in cowpea protoplasts was inhibited by cycloheximide but not by chloramphenicol.

Magyarosy *et al.* (1973) found that though the number of chloro-plasts in SqMV-infected leaves was decreased, the chloroplasts which remained could not be distinguished from the chloroplasts of uninocu-lated tissue on the basis of several structural and biochemical criteria. Langenberg and Schroeder (1975) and de Zoeten *et al.* (1974) were un-able to find viruslike particles inside chloroplasts of cowpea plants infected with CPMV. However, lipid globules were seen in the chloro-plasts of the infected plants.

Lockhart and Semancik (1968, 1969) found that actinomycin D inhibited the increase of CPMV in inoculated cowpea hypocotyls if it was applied (at a concentration of 10 μg/ml) at from 2 to about 16 h after inoculation but not later. The inhibitory effect at early post-inoculation times was also found if the inoculum was CPMV RNA, indicating that the inhibitory action of the actinomycin D was not at (or before) the step of virion uncoating. A similar inhibitory effect at early postinoculation times was found for cowpea chlorotic mottle virus and tobacco mosaic virus (a bean strain) in cowpea hypocotyls and CPMV in Cherokee Wax beans. However, BPMV increase was not inhibited in Cherokee Wax bean hypocotyls, although it was in Pencil Pod Wax bean hypocotyls. Certain other inhibitors of DNA replication and transcription had little or no effect on CPMV replication in cowpea hypocotyls. Actinomycin D at 10 μg/ml reduced [^{32}P]phosphate incorporation into cowpea hypocotyl RNA by 75–85%, and the actinomycin effect on CPMV replication was nearly the same regardless of whether the accumulation of infectivity in the tissue was measured as extracted virions or extracted RNA (i.e., after extraction with phenol). The authors concluded that for some virus–host combinations, the transcription of new host RNA early in infection is apparently needed in order for virus replication to proceed efficiently.

The only evidence for an increase in a specific host protein in response to infection by a comovirus comes from the work of Niblett *et al.* (1974). They found that aspartate transcarbamylase activity increased more than fivefold in CPMV-SB-infected cowpea hypocotyls as compared to mock-inoculated hypocotyls at 6 days after inoculation. Similar results were obtained with green leaves (Lee *et al.*, 1975b). Since the enzyme catalyzes the synthesis of ureidosuccinate, an intermediate in the pathway to pyrimidines, the increase could be related to the synthesis of virion RNA precursors. No qualitative difference was found in the enzyme from infected and uninoculated tissue. Magyarosy *et al.* (1973) found decreases in phosphopyruvate, glucose, and sucrose concentrations in SqMV-infected tissue, whereas glutamate, malate, and alanine concentrations were increased. Both Magyarosy *et al.* (1973) and Niblett *et al.* (1974) found an increase in the amounts of 80 S ribosomes in infected tissue.

Most of the RNA in infected cells which can be hybridized to ^{3}H-labeled CPMV virion RNA is associated with a "chloroplast" fraction recovered after centrifugation of extracts on discontinuous sucrose gradients (de Zoeten *et al.*, 1974; Assink *et al.* 1973). When the "chloroplast" fraction was centrifuged on a second (more shallow) discontinuous gradient, several fractions were obtained. The fractions were analyzed for hybridizable RNA and examined in the electron microscope. Chloroplasts were concentrated in the higher-density fractions. "Cytopathological structures" of variable shape and appearance (frequently traversed by vesicles) had been observed in thin sections of intact cells. Materials which appear to have been derived from the cytopathological structures were enriched in the lower-density fractions, as was the hybridizable RNA. On the basis of these results and autoradiographic studies, the authors concluded that the vesicles of the cytopathological structures may be sites of CPMV-RNA synthesis.

The subcellular sites of virus accumulation, the aggregated states of the accumulated virions, and the modifications of the cell structure have been studied by van der Scheer and Groenewegen (1971), Kim *et al.* (1974), and Langenberg and Schroeder (1975) for CPMV; by Kim and Fulton (1973) and Kim *et al.* (1974) for BPMV; by Honda and Matsui (1972) and Hooper *et al.* (1972) for RaMV; and by Sahambi *et al.* (1973), Hull and Plaskitt (1973/1974), and Milicić *et al.* (1974) for viruses of the BBWV group.

4. NEPOVIRUSES

In those cases where it has been tested, the minimum infectious entity for the nepoviruses seems to be two RNA molecules. The arrangement of the two RNA molecules in virions varies, however, from virus to virus. Virions containing one RNA molecule and others containing two have been observed for specific members of the group, whereas other members of the group have only virions with single RNA molecules. Genetic and some other properties of nepoviruses have been reviewed by Jaspars (1974) and by Gibbs and Harrison (1976).

Specific nematodes are capable of transmitting various nepoviruses (reviewed by Harrison *et al.*, 1974*a*), and the virus can persist for weeks in nematodes. Many are seed transmitted (e.g., Yang and Hamilton, 1974; Shepherd, 1972). Most members have wide host ranges.

4.1. Members of the Nepovirus Group

The type member is considered to be tobacco ringspot virus (Harrison *et al.*, 1971). Members of the group include the following:

Arabis mosaic virus	AraMV
Cherry leaf roll virus	CheLRV
Cocoa necrosis virus	CocNV
Grapevine chrome mosaic virus	
Grapevine fanleaf virus	GraFV
Mulberry ringspot virus	MulRSV
Myrobalan latent ringspot virus	MyrLRSV
Peach rosette mosaic virus	
Raspberry ringspot virus	RasRSV
Strawberry latent ringspot virus	StrLRSV
Tobacco ringspot virus	TobRSV
Tomato black ring virus	TomBRV
Tomato ringspot virus	TomRSV
Tomato top necrosis virus	TomTNV

Several serotypes have been observed for several of the viruses listed. However, there are only a few demonstrated serological relationships between the viruses listed (e.g., AraMV and GraFV, Cadman *et al.*, 1960, and Murant, 1970; CocNV and TomBRV, Kenten, 1972; MyrLRSV and TomBRV, Delbos *et al.*, 1976). Inclusion of several of the viruses in the group is tenuous, being based on the appearance of virions in the electron microscope, seed transmission (Hanada and Harrison, 1976), the virus being soil borne, and the induction of the ringspot or mottle symptoms and/or shock and recovery phases of infection which seem to be characteristic of some nepoviruses. Similarities in RNA and protein molecular weights for members of this group are discussed below.

4.2. Chemical Composition of Multiple Centrifugal Components

The multicomponent nature of nepoviruses was first revealed by the works of Steere (1956) and Stace-Smith *et al.* (1965) on TobRSV. Stace-Smith *et al.* (1965) observed three sedimenting boundaries. In order of decreasing relative amounts, these were the 128 S bottom component, 94 S middle component, and 53 S top component. The B and M components were found to be nucleoproteins; the top component had a spectrum expected for an RNA-free protein. Diener and Schneider (1966) observed that RNA from unfractionated TobRSV had two major components with sedimentation coefficients of 24 S and 32 S, the former being more abundant. That is, there were observed both two ribonucleoproteins and two RNAs for TobRSV. However, the more slowly and the more rapidly sedimenting forms of each of these did not occur in the same relative proportions. Diener and Schneider (1966) separated the M and B components and isolated RNA from them. Only the 24 S RNA was recovered from M; both 24 S and 32 S RNA were recovered from B, thus explaining the relatively large amount of 24 S RNA which was recovered from unfractionated TobRSV. The authors proposed that there are two kinds of TobRSV B components: those with one molecule of 32 S RNA and those with two molecules of 24 S RNA. Similar results and a similar model for the distribution of RNA molecules among ribonucleoprotein particles have been presented by Murant *et al.* (1972) for RasRSV. The two RNAs have been designated RNA 1 and RNA 2. However, there seems to be no consensus about which of the two is RNA 1 and which is RNA 2 (*cf.* Murant *et al.*, 1972; Rezaian and Francki, 1974). For the purposes of this chapter, the RNA of component M will be referred to as "M-

RNA." The smaller RNA of the bottom component will be "2B-RNA" and the larger "1B-RNA. The two major size classes of RNA from unfractionated virus will be referred to as "RNA 2" and "RNA 1" for the smaller and larger RNAs, respectively. This follows the convention widely accepted for the three-component covirus systems. RNAs of nepoviruses have been isolated by pronase digestion of the capsid in the presence of detergent and by various phenol extraction procedures (Murant *et al.*, 1972; Rezaian and Francki, 1973).

The reported sedimentation coefficients of various viruses considered to be in the nepovirus group are listed in Table 6. The ratios of sedimentation coefficients are also listed since the ratios ought to be less variable from analysis to analysis than the absolute values of the sedimentation coefficients. The sedimentation coefficient ratios for M/B have a larger range than those for B/T, relative to the mean values of the respective ratios. This implies that a corresponding large range of molecular weights should be observed for the M RNAs of the viruses. The larger RNAs (RNA 1) of TobRSV, RasRSV, TomBRV, and CheLRV have molecular weights (estimated by polyacrylamide gel electrophoresis) of 2.3×10^6, 2.4×10^6, 2.5×10^6, and 2.3–2.4×10^6, respectively. The molecular weights of the corresponding RNA 2's are

TABLE 6
Reported Sedimentation Coefficients of Nepoviruses[a]

Virus	T	M	B	M/B	B/T	Reference[b]
StrLRSV	58	—	126	—	2.2	a
RasRSV	52	92	130	0.71	2.5	b
TobRSV	53	91	126	0.72	2.4	c
AraMV	53	93	126	0.74	2.4	d
MulRSV	50	96	126	0.76	2.5	e
CocNV	54	101	129	0.78	—	f
GraCMV	—	92	117	0.79	—	g
TomBRV	55	97	121	0.80	2.2	h
TomTNV	52	102	126	0.81	2.4	i
MyrLRSV	—	115	135	0.85	—	j
CheLRV	52	115	130	0.89	2.5	k
TomRSV	53	119[c]	127[c]	0.94	2.4	l

[a] All sedimentation coefficients are in Svedbergs.
[b] a, Mayo *et al.* (1974a); b, Murant *et al.* (1972); c, Schneider and Diener (1966); d, Stace-Smith, as cited by Murant (1970b); e, Tsuchizaki (1975); f, Kenten (1972); g, Martelli and Quacquarelli (1972); h, Murant (1970a); i, Bancroft (1968); j, Dunez *et al.* (1971); k, average of values from Walkey *et al.* (1973) and Jones and Mayo (1972); l, Schneider *et al.* (1974a).
[c] The components listed as M and B in this table are designated B1 and B2, respectively, by Schneider *et al.* (1974a).

1.4 × 10⁶, 1.4 × 10⁶, 1.5 × 10⁶, and 2.1 × 10⁶ (Murant *et al.*, 1972, 1973; Jones and Mayo, 1972; Walkey *et al.*, 1973). The RNAs of TomRSV have sedimentation coefficients of 31 and 33 S and the apparent molecular weights of both RNAs are close to 2.3 × 10⁶ (Schneider *et al.*, 1974a). For both CheLRV and TomRSV, the smaller RNA is too large, apparently, for two copies to be housed in one capsid, and there is no 2B-RNA.

The estimated RNA contents of the bottom components, calculated (Reichmann, 1965) from the B/T sedimentation coefficient ratios in Table 6, are 38–43%. Chemical analysis of TobRSV yielded 42% RNA (Stace-Smith *et al.*, 1965). The tendency of the nucleoprotein particles to aggregate seems to be characteristic of several nepoviruses (StrLRSV, Mayo *et al.*, 1974a; TobRSV, Rezaian and Francki, 1973; RasRSV, Mayo *et al.*, 1973). Bancroft (1968) resolved two components of TomTNV by immunoelectrophoresis but did not attempt to relate these to the centrifugal components. Single electrophoretic forms have been found for RasRSV, StrLRSV, TobRSV, and TomRSV (Murant *et al.*, 1972; Mayo *et al.*, 1974a; Stace-Smith, 1970a,b; Schneider *et al.*, 1974a). The centrifugal components of RasRSV, TobRSV, and TomTNV could not be distinguished serologically (Murant *et al.*, 1972; Stace-Smith *et al.*, 1965; Bancroft, 1968).

Both TobRSV and RasRSV B components form two (partially resolved) zones during equilibrium centrifugation in CsCl density gradients (Mayo *et al.*, 1973; Schneider *et al.*, 1972a; Murant *et al.*, 1972). The M components formed a single zone in CsCl gradients. Under some circumstances, only one zone of RasRSV component B was found on CsCl gradients, and this was attributed to aggregation of the two density forms. Presumably the higher-density form of B will be the one with the larger RNA content. From the molecular weight values cited above, TobRSV and RasRSV particles with two 2B-RNAs would be expected to be more dense than particles with one 1B-RNA. However, I. R. Schneider (personal communication) has pointed out that the higher-density form of component B of TobRSV is generally present in lesser amount than the low density form (Schneider *et al.*, 1972a), whereas 2B-RNA generally exceeds 1B-RNA in amount (Diener and Schneider, 1966). It is possible that the RNA molecular weights are not correct or that the particle densities are not monotonically related to the RNA contents because of irregular binding of Cs ions (see Section 3.2). No firm conclusion about the nature of the two buoyant density forms of B can be drawn at this time. (See Section 4.6 for further discussion of the RNA contents of TobRSV particles.) The M and B components of CheLRV and TomRSV (which have no 2B-RNA) seemed to form just one zone each in CsCl gradients (Jones and Mayo, 1972; Schneider *et al,* 1974*a*).

Ultraviolet irradiation of RasRSV component B, but not component M, induced the apparent dimerization of the smaller RNA molecules to form species migrating slightly more slowly than 1B-RNA during electrophoresis in polyacrylamide gels (Mayo *et al.,* 1973), further supporting the notion that two 2B-RNAs are present in some B particles.

Mayo *et al.* (1974*a*) have summarized the apparent molecular weights of the capsid protein from six nepoviruses (all estimated by disruption of the virions with sodium dodecylsulfate, followed by gel electrophoresis in the presence of the detergent). They range from 54,000 to 59,000 with only a single zone for each virus (however, see Section 4.5). Mayo *et al.* (1971) have shown that a capsid composed of 60 copies of the capsid polypeptide is most consistent with the properties of AraMV, RasRSV, and TobRSV components. Assuming 60 polypeptides and one RNA 1 molecule per B component (low density form), particle weights of $5.5–5.9 \times 10^6$ for B can be calculated from the apparent polypeptide and RNA molecular weights cited above. This range is consistent with the sedimentation coefficients, estimated percentage of RNA, buoyant densities in CsCl gradients, and dimensions of the well-studied nepovirus B components. However, no exact information about nepovirus particle weights is available.

4.3. Component and RNA Infectivities; Hybrid Viruses

Bancroft (1968) was the first to demonstrate an enhancement of infectivity upon mixing two nucleoprotein components of a virus from the nepovirus group. TomTNV particles were separated by sucrose density gradient centrifugation (a single cycle, recovering B only from the lowest part of the zone). The observed infectivity activation ratios for the M and B component preparations (defined in Section 2.5), calculated from local lesion counts on *Chenopodium murales,* were about 10. Since the ratio of sedimentation coefficients of M/B is about $102/126 = 0.81$, it is possible that the smaller RNA has a molecular weight too high to have two of the smaller RNA molecules in one capsid (i.e., no 2B-RNA). The infectivity activation ratio, although not large, may be taken as tentative evidence for two kinds of RNA (1 and 2) being involved in initiating an infection. Similar results were obtained for CheLRV (infectivity activation ratio ~7; ratio of component sedimentation coefficients $115/130 = 0.89$, Jones and Mayo, 1972) and for

TomRSV (infectivity activation ratio ~ 4; ratio to sedimentation co-efficients 119/127 = 0.94, Schneider *et al.*, 1974*a*). For all three viruses, the bottom component preparations had higher levels of infectivity than the middle component preparations, probably because of the usual technical difficulties of sucrose density centrifugation. Whether pure M and/or B are noninfectious can only be surmised. The increasing similarity of M and B for the virus series TomTNV–CheLRV–TomRSV directs attention to the possibility that covirus systems exist which might go unrecognized because of the components being inseparable by the usual gradient centrifugation techniques.

For the nepoviruses which have two forms of bottom component (with one 1B-RNA or two 2B-RNAs), the bottom component preparations would, of course, be expected to be infectious. Diener and Schneider (1966), in the paper in which they reported the discovery of the two forms of bottom component of TobRSV, observed that in the analysis of TobRSV by sucrose density gradient centrifugation, infectivity was associated only with B (Infectivity of RasRSV is also definitely associated with component B only; Murant *et al.*, 1972.) In a similar analysis of the virion RNAs of TobRSV, the infectivity was associated with the 1B-RNA, although a shoulder on the slower-sedimenting side of the profile (Fig. 1B of Diener and Schneider, 1966) may be an indication that even in that experiment the infectivity-stimulating effect of the RNA 2 was being expressed.

Murant *et al.* (1972) found that heating RasRSV RNA in 8 M urea just before applying it to a polyacrylamide gel dissociated what apparently are RNA aggregates. After electrophoresis, the zones were more sharp for the heated RNA than for unheated RNA, and very little RNA migrated at other than the RNA 1 and RNA 2 positions. Harrison *et al.* (1972*a*) took advantage of this observation and were able to recover very highly purified RasRSV RNAs from gels. Infectivity activation ratios of about 80 were observed for the RNA 1 and RNA 2 so obtained, whereas values of only about 2–3 were found for RNA fractions obtained without the heating step prior to electrophoresis. Thus it is reasonable to assume that the pure RNAs are not infectious. An infectivity activation ratio of about 8 was obtained for TobRSV RNAs. Infectivity enhancement was not observed for heterologous mixtures of RasRSV RNA components with TobRSV RNA components. The addition of middle-component particles to bottom component (all RasRSV) caused a two- to fourfold stimulation of infectivity at M/B ratios of 7–90. Infectivity activation ratios of up to 8 were obtained with dilute inocula of the RNAs from TomBRV (Murant *et al.*, 1973).

Infectivity activation ratios of 2.2 and about 29 were obtained for RNAs from MyrLRSV and TomBRV, respectively, separated by sucrose density gradient centrifugation (Delbos *et al.*, 1976). MyrLRS virus seems to be an exception to the general trend in Table 6. It has a relatively high M/B ratio of sedimentation coefficients, and because of its position relative to TomTNV, CheLRV, and TomRSV in Table 6 it would be expected to have no 2B-RNA. However, MyrLRSV component B preparations contained RNA 2 in amounts too large to be explained by contamination with component M, whereas two strains of TomBRV had no detectable 2B-RNA (Delbos *et al.*, 1976).

The first hybrid nepoviruses were constructed from RasRSV strains. The English (E) and Scottish (S) isolates of RasRSV are serologically similar but not identical. Antiserum to strain S causes a spur to form next to a well with RasRSV-E when RasRSV-E and RasRSV-S are in adjacent wells; antiserum to S which has been absorbed with RasRSV-E is still capable of reacting with RasRSV-S. The two strains could also be distinguished because of the severe yellowing induced by RasRSV-E, but not S, on *Petunia hybrida*. Harrison *et al.* (1972*b*) separated the two RNAs of each RasRSV strain by gel electrophoresis. The infectivity activation ratios were about 50 for RasRSV-E but less than 10 for RasRSV-S because of the residual infectivity of the RasRSV-S RNA 1 preparation. The numbers of local lesions obtained from heterologous and homologous RNA mixtures from strains S and E were consistent with the homologous and heterologous combinations being about equally infectious. Some local lesions (on *Chenopodium amaranticolor*) were excised and transferred to *Chenopodium quinoa*. The resulting viruses were tested for serological specificity and for the kind of symptoms on *Petunia hybrida* (Table 7).

The results indicate that RNA 2 of RasRSV controls both the serological specificity of the virions and the yellowing systemic symptoms on *Petunia*. The single exception to this conclusion, a virus supposedly derived by inoculating the smaller RNA of strain E together with the larger RNA of strain S, can be explained if it is assumed that this virus is actually RasRSV-S which arose from the incompletely purified preparation of RasRSV-S RNA 1. Harrison *et al.* (1974*b*) showed that the yellowing symptoms on *Petunia* were associated with ultrastructural changes in the chloroplasts regardless of whether the inoculum was RasRSV-E or a hybrid of RasRSV strains E and S which gave yellowing symptoms. RasRSV-S and a hybrid with S properties did not cause the same ultrastructural changes. These

TABLE 7

Serological and Symptom Characters of Hybrid RasRSVs

RNA inoculum	Serological specificity		
	Trials showing a spur	Trials not showing a spur	Total number of trials
S (RNA 2) + E (RNA 1)	0	12	12
E (RNA 2) + S (RNA 1)	11	1	12
RNA inoculum	Symptoms on *Petunia hybrida*		
	Trials showing yellowing	Trials not showing yellowing	Total number of trials
S (RNA 2) + E (RNA 1)	0	8	8
E (RNA 2) + S (RNA 1)	11	1	12

authors also reported that the more efficient transmission by the nematode *Longidorus elongatus* which is exhibited by RasRSV-S, as compared to the less efficient RasRSV-E transmission, is also found for the hybrid derived by inoculating a mixture of RNA 2 of RasRSV-S plus RNA 1 of RasRSV-E. The inheritance of both the serological specificity and the efficiency of transmission by nematodes through the smaller of the two RasRSV RNAs (Harrison *et al.*, 1974a) implies that the RNA 2 carries the structural gene for the capsid protein.

Harrison *et al.* (1974b) extended the work of Harrison *et al.* (1972b) by performing crosses among four strains of RasRSV: the S and E strains used previously and the LG (named for its ability to infect Lloyd George raspberries) and D (from the Netherlands; induces yellowing in *Petunia,* as does E) strains. In all the crosses, the homologous and heterologous RNA mixtures were about equally infectious. Crosses of E with LG and S with LG generally confirmed the previous observation of serological specificity determined by the source of the smaller viral RNA. In back crosses from the LG and S hybrids, the original parental virus strains were regenerated. Ability to infect Lloyd George raspberries was determined by the source of RNA 1 in the hybrids of LG and S. That is, only virus with RNA 1 from RasRSV-LG was capable of infecting Lloyd George raspberries. For the mixed inoculations of RNA 2 from strain E or D with RNA 1 of strain LG, the resulting hybrid virus was expected to cause the systemic symptoms of yellowing on *Petunia hybrida*. However, the symptomless infection characteristic of RasRSV-LG was observed. In the case of the hybrid derived from E and LG, the serological reaction of the hybrid implies that the hybrid actually had formed. However, the composition of the hybrids was not established by backcrossing to regenerate the parental types. The authors interpret the lack of yellow symptoms on *Petunia* as being due to a suppression of the usual expression of a gene on the smaller RNA by a gene on the larger RNA of RasRSV-LG. They also present other examples of symptoms (on *Chenopodium*) being jointly controlled by the two viral RNAs or controlled by the larger RNA alone. The results are similar to those found by Wood (1972; see Section 3.6) for CPMV-VU. Experiments of Harrison and Hanada (1976) and by Hanada and Harrison (1976) showed that the rate at which RasRSV strains and hybrids of those strains invaded stem tips of inoculated plants and the ability of RasRSV and TomBRV strains to be seed transmitted were both controlled principally by RNA 1. However, the source of RNA 2 also influenced these properties, although in lesser degree. The genetic experiments described in this section support the notion that the genes of RasRSV, and probably also those of the other nepoviruses, are distributed on two different kinds of viral RNA.

4.4. Nucleotide Sequence Relationships

Rezaian and Francki (1973, 1974) isolated from tissue infected with TobRSV (by phenol extraction, salt precipitation, 2-methoxyethanol extraction, and digestion with deoxyribonuclease and ribonuclease) a fraction enriched in double-stranded RNA. As expected, the melted double-stranded RNA could be hybridized to radioactive TobRSV RNA. The amount of complementary RNA in this kind of preparation (as measured by hybridization to excess ^{14}C-labeled TobRSV RNA) was maximal at 3-4 days after the inoculation of cucumber cotyledons. RNA polymerase activity in a fraction from extracts of the same tissue was assayed in the presence of 2.5 μg/ml actinomycin D. This activity was maximal at 3 (2-4) days after inoculation. Neither complementary RNA nor the actinomycin D-resistant RNA polymerase activity was detected in uninoculated tissue. Accumulated virus infectivity was maximal at 5 days. These results implicate the complementary RNA as an intermediate in the replication of TobRSV. However, the double-stranded RNA was found by gel electrophoresis and sucrose density gradient centrifugation to be polydisperse in size and of molecular weights too small to correspond in length to either of the viral RNAs. Modifications of the isolation procedure (including omission of the nuclease digestion steps) did not result in the recovery of high-molecular-weight double-stranded RNA. TobRSV and a bean strain of tobacco mosaic virus were separately inoculated on French beans. The "double-stranded RNA fractions" were recovered and analyzed by sucrose density gradient centrifugation. Both preparations were polydisperse in the sedimentation rates of materials which, after melting, hybridized with the respective viral RNAs. However, the authors were able to isolate by their procedures ribonuclease-resistant RNA (containing sequences complementary to virion RNA) from the tobacco mosaic virus-infected tissue which did sediment as expected for high-molecular-weight double-stranded RNA. Nevertheless, it is likely that the molecular weight of the TobRSV double-stranded RNA does not represent the *in vivo* size of the strands of which it is composed because Schneider *et al.* (1974*b*) have reported briefly on the recovery of heterogeneous but high-molecular-weight double-stranded RNA from TobRSV-infected bean plants.

The low-molecular-weight double-stranded RNA has proved useful in establishing nucleotide sequence relationship between TobRSV virion RNAs (Rezaian and Francki, 1974). A fixed amount of radioactive total virion RNA was hybridized with increasing amounts of the double-stranded RNA preparation in different reaction mixtures. The amounts of ribonuclease-resistant radioactivity (after correction for the amount, 8%, of ribonuclease-resistant radioactivity found in the absence of added double-stranded RNA) fit an expected saturation curve. This result implies that all nucleotide sequences of the virion RNA are represented among the complementary sequences of the double-stranded RNA preparation. In competition hybridization experiments, unlabeled RNA 2 and RNA from purified component M were equally effective in competing with radioactive RNA 2 for sequences in the melted double-stranded RNA. However, RNA 2 and RNA 1 competed with each other much less effectively. Each heterologous competing RNA was considered to be "about 14% [as] efficient" as the homologous competing RNA. Therefore, the RNAs of TobRSV, like those of TRV CAM, seem to have significant amounts (several hundred nucleotides) of common sequences. The authors point out that it is possible that some of the RNA 2 sequences in the larger RNA are not really in RNA 1. That is, some RNA 2 molecules may be present as cross-linked dimers (even though no ultraviolet irradiation has been done) and therefore may be recovered in fractions containing the larger RNA molecules.

4.5. The Proteins and RNAs of Strawberry Latent Ringspot Virus

Among the viruses listed in Table 6 only StrLRSV lacked a recognizable component M. However, RNAs of apparent molecular weights 1.6×10^6 and 2.6×10^6 have been recovered from component B, and ultraviolet irradiation of the ribonucleoprotein caused a loss of material from the zone of the smaller RNA and a concomitant increase in material migrating as the larger RNA on polyacrylamide electrophoresis gels (Mayo *et al.*, 1974*a*). Thus the virus seems to be similar to, for example, RasRSV, except that all of the encapsidated smaller RNA is present as pairs of molecules, 2B-RNA. When intact StrLRSV and RasRSV virions were analyzed on polyacrylamide gels of three gel concentrations, the mobility of StrLRSV was retarded more by the higher gel concentrations than was the mobility of RasRSV. This result implies that the StrLRSV capsid is larger than that of RasRSV. The buoyant density on CsCl gradients implies a higher protein/RNA ratio in StrLRSV than in RasRSV. Analysis of virion protein was accomplished by disruption with sodium dodecylsulfate and electrophoresis in gels of 6%, 8%, and 10% polyacrylamide. Two major zones of polypeptides, with apparent molecular weights of about 29,000 and 44,000 (regardless of the gel concentration), were observed. Some preparations had an additional minor zone corresponding to a molecular weight of about 79,000. The pattern of the major polypeptides resembles to some extent the results obtained with the comoviruses. However, the molar amounts of the larger and smaller major polypeptides were in a ratio of about 1:1.3 (estimated from the intensity of staining of the zones in the gel) rather than the 1:1 ratio characteristic of the comoviruses. No serological relationship could be established to members of the comovirus group or to PV3 (a broad bean wilt virus). It is difficult to say whether StrLRSV should be considered a nepovirus. Mayo *et al.* (1974*a*) have put forth an interesting argument in favor of retaining StrLRSV in the group by stating that "One possibility is that nepovirus coat proteins are derived from a larger precursor molecule, and that both products of a 'maturation' cleavage occur in [StrLRSV] particles, whereas the precursor protein of other nepoviruses is cleaved in a different place and the smaller product is not found in the virus particles." The polypeptide ratio of $\sim$1:1.3 requires a differential loss of the two cleavage products, according to this theory, at some time before the electrophoretic analysis of the polypeptides of StrLRSV.

4.6.   Satellite Viruses (see also Chapter 3)

Schneider and co-workers have studied viruslike particles which were found to be associated with TobRSV. The particles form a broad zone sedimenting between and overlapping the M and B components of TobRSV (Schneider, 1971) when analyzed by sucrose density gradient centrifugation. On CsCl gradients the viruslike particles formed a series of discrete zones which ranged in density from less than that of TobRSV component M to greater than that for the more dense form of component B (Schneider et al., 1972a). In contrast to the heterogeneity of the particles, the RNA extracted from them proved to be a homogeneous material sedimenting at about 7.3 S.

The 7.3 S RNA is not infectious when inoculated alone but would give rise to the viruslike particles when inoculated together with a TobRSV which was free of the 7.3 S RNA or particles. Therefore, the particles seem to be the virions of a satellite virus of TobRSV (S-TobRSV) though they differ clearly from tobacco necrosis satellite in having the same protein coat as the helper. S-TobRSV particles from the low-density range or from the high-density range both gave rise, after inoculation, to the entire spectrum of S-TobRSV particle densities. S-TobRSV and the TobRSV with which it is associated could not be distinguished serologically. Schneider (1972) and Schneider and White (1976) showed that when the same strain of S-TobRSV was inoculated in combinations with two different strains of TobRSV, the serological character of the resulting S-TobRSV was determined by the strain of TobRSV with which it was mixed before inoculation and not by the host plant or by the strain of TobRSV with which the S-TobRSV had been associated in the previous infection. Thus the S-TobRSV capsid seems to be specified by the TobRSV genome. This result was expected because of the small theoretical coding capacity of (a 7.3 S) S-TobRSV RNA. At least two strains of S-TobRSV can be distinguished on the basis of symptoms induced upon coinoculation with the same strain of TobRSV (Schneider et al., 1972b).

Several estimates of the molecular weight of S-TobRSV RNA have been made. Schneider (1971) estimated a value of 86,000 from the sedimentation coefficient of 7.3 S (using an empirical formula); Diener and Smith (1973) found 77,000–84,000 by a comparison of the mobilities of formaldehyde-derivatized RNAs in formaldehyde-impregnated polyacrylamide gels; Sogo et al. (1974) calculated 115,000–125,000 by comparing the lengths of S-TobRSV RNA with the lengths of the RNAs of bacteriophage $Q\beta$ and carnation mottle virus on electron microscopic images. The heterogeneity of the S-TobRSV particles and their range of sedimentation coefficients and particle densities in CsCl solution can be explained most easily if it is assumed that each particle has several RNA molecules and that different particles have different numbers of RNA molecules. The more rapidly sedimenting S-TobRSV particles (on sucrose density gradients) produced the zones of higher densities on CsCl gradients, as expected according to this hypothesis. Because the multiple zones of S-TobRSV on CsCl gradients are uniformly spaced (density interval of about 0.0091 g/ml), and because the S-TobRSV capsids are probably the same as the TobRSV capsids, the S-TobRSV particles in the series probably differ only in that there is one additional RNA molecule in the particles of each succeeding zone. The particle series potentially can provide a scale linking the mass of RNA in the particle to the particle buoyant density. If the 14 S-TobRSV zones observed by Schneider *et al.* (1972*a*) in CsCl gradients are numbered from the lowest- to the highest-density zone, then TobRSV M has a density falling between S-TobRSV zones 2 and 3, and the two TobRSV B zones fall between zones 11 and 12 and just below the density of zone 13, respectively. Depending on whether one takes the low- or the high-density form of the B component to be the one with two copies of 2B-RNA (see Section 4.2), the density contribution of one molecule of RNA 2 would be equivalent to about nine or to just over ten molecules of the satellite RNA (assuming one RNA molecule per density increment). The molecular weight of RNA 2 is probably in the range of the 1.4×10^6 as an upper limit) estimated directly by gel electrophoresis to about half the value estimated for RNA 1, i.e., about 1.1×10^6 (as a lower limit). These numbers favor the molecular weight of S-TobRSV RNA estimated from electron microscopy, i.e., 115,000–125,000 (Sogo *et al.,* 1974). It must be recognized, however, that a direct relationship between RNA content and particle density has not been established.

Whether all of the 7.3 S RNA molecules of S-TobRSV are the same is not known. That is, it is possible that different 7.3 S RNAs have different nucleotide sequences and that the genome size is some multiple of the size of the 7.3 S RNA. Diener *et al.* (1974) irradiated TobRSV, S-TobRSV, and potato spindle tuber viroid (PSTV) with ultraviolet light. TobRSV was inactivated 70 times more readily than S-TobRSV and 90 times more readily than PSTV. (S-TobRSV RNA and PSTV have similar mobilities, after treatment with formaldehyde, during electrophoresis on polyacrylamide gels.) Under the usual considerations of "target size," these results imply that the biologically active unit of S-TobRSV is very small and that the genome of STobRSV could be a single 7.3 S RNA molecule. However, a quantitative interpretation is not possible because of technical difficulties (e.g., the multiple copies of S-TobRSV RNA per particle which might allow cross-linking of different molecules; there is a possibility of different degrees of photoreactivation for the TobRSV and S-TobRSV RNAs).

Oligonucleotides from T_1 ribonuclease digestion of S-TobRSV RNA form a simple pattern which is consistent with only a single nucleotide sequence for the 7.3 S RNA molecules (Schneider, 1976). The S-TobRSV genome probably is borne on single 7.3 S RNAs. Schneider and Thompson (1976) have isolated double-stranded RNA from tissue infected with TobRSV and S-TobRSV (but predominantly with the latter). This RNA was shown to contain RNA similar in size and biological activity to TobRSV virion RNA. Part of the double-stranded RNA appears to be larger than what would be expected for a double-stranded version of S-TobRSV RNA, implying the possibility of an unusual mode of replication.

Murant *et al.* (1973) observed in analyses of TomBRV RNAs a prominent zone of apparent molecular weight 500,000. The RNA was not infectious. TomBRV could be freed of the 500,000-molecular-weight RNA by inoculating the partially purified TomBRV (2.5×10^6) RNA 1 contaminated with a small amount of RNA 2. When the 500,000-molecular-weight RNA was coinoculated with the purified ("satellite-free") TomBRV, the former RNA again was found in the progeny virus. Thus the 500,000-molecular-weight RNA has the properties of a satellite. The corresponding particles were not isolated or characterized. Hanada and Harrison (1976) showed that the satellite can be seed transmitted. Delbos *et al.* (1976) found an RNA similar to the 500,000-molecular-weight RNA of TomBRV in both the middle and bottom components of MyrLRSV.

4.7. Events in Replication

As is the case with the comoviruses, the combination of two nepovirus RNAs is infectious, and it can be assumed that at least one of them is a messenger RNA rather than the complement of a messenger RNA. The purification of double-stranded RNA and actinomycin D-resistant RNA polymerase activity from TobRSV-infected tissue has been described in Section 4.4. The *in vitro* translation of a nepovirus virion RNA has not yet been reported.

Schneider and Diener (1966) observed the M and B components of

TobRSV to be synthesized at different rates at different times after inoculation. No significant change in the proteins of nepovirus-infected cells has been reported. Barker (1975) analyzed extracts of *Nicotiana* species infected with RasRSV by polyacrylamide gel electrophoresis in the absence of detergents. No zones were observed in the extracts of infected tissue which were not also present in the control tissue. Niblett *et al.* (1974) found only a 1.6-fold increase in aspartate trans-carbamylase activity in soybean hypocotyls infected with TobRSV (see Section 3.10). However, changes in nucleic acid synthesis have been reported. Atchison (1973) found that the rate of DNA synthesis in, and subsequently the mitotic index of, French bean root tip cells declined after invasion of those cells by TobRSV. In dual isotopic label experiments (^{3}H- and ^{14}C-labeled uridine incorporation into TobRSV-infected and control tissues), Rezaian and Francki (1973) found a decline in the synthesis of RNA migrating as 16 S and 23 S ribosomal RNAs in the infected tissues. The effects of virus infection on the ultrastructure of chloroplasts have been described by Harrison *et al.* (1974*b*). Other studies of changes in the ultrastructure of nepovirus-infected tissues include those of Yang and Hamilton (1974), Roberts and Harrison (1970), and Walkey and Webb (1970).

5. OTHER POSSIBLE TWO-COMPONENT SYSTEMS

This section deals briefly with the multicomponent aspects of the only animal coviruses (Nodamura and a virus from New Zealand black beetles), the isometric pea enation mosaic virus (PEMV), and two rod-shaped plant viruses of about 20 nm diameter and varying lengths, barley stripe mosaic virus (BSMV) [now classified as hordeiviruses (Fenner, 1976)], and soil-borne wheat mosaic virus (SBWMV).

Nodamura virus is an arthropod-borne virus which infects mosquitoes, ticks, moths, bees, and certain vertebrates and is the only virus infecting a vertebrate for which there is evidence of a genome composed of two single-stranded RNAs. Infectivity was found to be associated with, but not solely with, isometric particles sedimenting at about 135 S when partially purified virus was analyzed by sucrose gradient centrifugation. RNAs sedimenting at approximately 15 S and 22 S were recovered from purified virus. The two RNAs seem to reside in the same particle because they can be extracted in a linked form under mild conditions. Treatment of the linked RNAs with detergent or phenol yields RNA which sediments as distinct 22 S and 15 S components, implying that the linker may be proteinaceous. After sucrose density gradient centrifugation of the RNAs, infectivity was distributed in a broad zone extending across the zones corresponding to both RNAs. Infectivity activation ratios greater than 50 were observed for partially purified preparations of the two RNAs (Newman and Brown, 1973, 1976; Newman, personal communication). Longworth and Carey (1976) have characterized a virus from *Heteronychus arator* (New Zealand black beetle) which is very similar to Nodamura virus with respect to physical properties of the virions (137 S, 30 mm diameter, 20% RNA, one major and two minor polypeptides in the capsid). The virus infects a number of insects but not mice. Two RNAs, 15 S and 22 S, are present, probably in the same capsid.

The components of PEMV have been reported to have sedimentation coefficients ranging from 91 to 106 S (average, 97 S) for M and 107–122 S (average, 114 S) for B (summarized by Hull and Lane, 1973; Mahmood and Peters, 1973). The highest values (106 and 122 S: Izadpanah and Shepherd, 1966) may be the most reliable. The percentage of RNA (~28%) appears to be the same in both M and B since they have indistinguishable spectra (over the wavelength range 225–325 nm) and buoyant densities (in sucrose–D_2O gradients). These results imply that M and B should have different outside diameters. The electrophoretic mobilities of M and B in polyacrylamide gels were found to be different. The ratio of mobilities was more extreme in a gel of higher polyacrylamide concentration but was independent of the pH or voltage gradient (Hull and Lane, 1973), as would be expected for spherical particles of different outside diameters but similar surface charge density. German and de Zoeten (1975) have observed a bimodal distribution of particle diameters in the electron microscope. Thus PEMV seems to be a "spherical heterocapsidic virus" (van Vloten-Doting and Jaspars, this volume). There seems to be a general agreement on the existence of two different major virion RNAs (RNAs 1 and 2) with molecular weights greater than 1.3×10^6 and a minor RNA with a molecular weight less than 0.35×10^6 (summarized by German and de Zoeten, 1975); RNA 1 is associated with B but not with M. RNA 2 is associated with M; however, there is little agreement on whether or not RNAs 2 and 3 are present in B and on what the relationship is of RNAs 1 and 2 to infectivity.

Gonsalves and Shepherd (1972) separated M and B by multiple cycles of sucrose density gradient centrifugation; RNAs 1, 2, and 3 were recovered from B, but only RNA 2 was recovered from M. Infectivity seemed to be associated with RNA 2 but not with RNA 1 or 3. Both the M and B component preparations were found to be infectious, M having the higher specific infectivity (Izadpanah and Shepherd, 1966; Gonsalves and Shepherd, 1972; Mahmood and Peters, 1973). No enhancement of infectivity was observed upon mixing M and B. German and de Zoeten (1975) found principally RNAs with the mobilities of RNAs 1 and 2 when they analyzed PEMV RNA (from unfractionated virions) isolated at low temperature and under mild conditions. Only after heating or aging of the RNA preparation was RNA 3 (or, at least, an RNA with electrophoretic mobility in gel in the proper range for RNA 3) revealed. The authors observed a concomitant decrease in the size of the RNA 1 zone relative to the RNA 2 zone, with the appearance of the RNA 3 zone. The results are consistent with there being two forms of B, one with one RNA 1 per particle and the other with one RNA 2 and one RNA 3 per particle. This would explain the observation that both M and B were infectious. It is more difficult to explain how RNA 1 is formed if only RNA 2 is infectious since an RNA of an apparently higher molecular weight would have to be specified by one which is apparently smaller.

Hull and Lane (1973) came to different conclusions about PEMV. They observed infectivity activation ratios of up to 30 for M and B and up to 7 for RNA 1 and RNA 2. That is, they found strong evidence for two RNA molecules being required for infectivity. Very little RNA 3 was present in their preparations, and they concluded, from comparisons of the proportions of M and B and of RNA 2 and RNA 1, respectively, that M contains RNA 2 and B contains RNA 1. Heterologous mixtures of M and B from two PEMV variants were inoculated. The variants could be distinguished according to the electrophoretic mobilities of the virions and the relative amounts of M and B recovered from infected tissue. Both properties seemed to be specified by B. Hull and Lane (1973) found their strains of PEMV to be very closely serologically related to the strain utilized by Gonsalves and Shepherd (1972). It is very difficult to reconcile the results described in this and the preceding paragraphs without invoking experimental error of some kind or the possibility that serologically related viruses can have very different chromosome arrangements. Hull (personal communication) has recently repeated infectivity tests with M and B and concluded that both are required for infectivity.

De Zoeten *et al.* (1976) have studied the location of double-stranded RNA in pea cells infected with PEMV. *In situ* hybridization with ^{125}I-labeled PEMV virion RNA and solution hybridization to nucleic acids extracted from various subcellular fractions of infected and healthy tissue both showed the nucleus of infected cells to be the principal site for accumulation of RNA complementary to the virion RNA. Ferritin-labeled antibody to double-stranded RNA was observed to bind at a higher frequency to the nuclei of infected cells than to the nuclei of uninfected cells. Actinomycin D inhibited the incorporation of [^{3}H]uridine into nucleoli (detected by autoradiography) but not into the nucleoplasm of infected cells. All these results are consistent with the nucleoplasm as a site for PEMV RNA synthesis, in contrast to the RNA synthesis of most other plant viruses, which occurs in the cytoplasm.

The recent demonstration of the infection of aphid cells in culture with PEMV (Adam and Sander, 1976) may encourage some very interesting experiments with PEMV. (PEMV is transmitted in a persistent fashion by aphids.)

Concerning BSMV, Lane (1974) found that either two or three size classes could be displayed in polyacrylamide gels on which RNAs from various strains of BSMV and two related viruses had been electrophoretically analyzed. The RNAs are apparently in different virions, with capsids varying only in length. For the Rothamsted isolate of BSMV, for which three size classes were observed, all three RNAs were required for infection. It does not seem reasonable that both two-component and three-component systems would be found within a group of serologically related viruses, and, as Lane (1974) has stated, "The two-component strains could actually contain three components, two of which coelectrophorese, or one of which is present in very small amounts."

SBWMV forms rods of two distinct lengths. The amount of short (S) rods formed in infected tissue exceeds the amount of long (L) rods. Tsuchizaki *et al.* (1975) obtained, by multiple cycles of sucrose density gradient centrifugation, S-rod preparations which were not infective at the concentrations tested. L-rod preparations were infectious and were not free of S rods. No evidence of a defective (capsid protein-less) infection was obtained. Infectivity activation ratios of 2–4 were observed for the L- and S-rod preparations; that is, the noninfective S-rod preparations stimulated the infectivity of the L-rod preparations. (However, Powell, 1976, found evidence for infectivity-suppressing activity of S rods at high concentrations.) When the infectivity of a mixture of S and L rods was plotted vs. inoculum dilution, the slope of the curve was found to be close to that for a theoretical two-hit curve. Heterologous mixtures of S- and L-rod preparations from two SBWMV strains were inoculated to a local lesion host with the purpose of producing hybrid viruses. The S rods of SBWMV strain J-A are shorter (110 nm) than those of strain US-B (160 nm), and the two viruses can be distinguished serologically and on the basis of symptoms and host range (J-A infects tobacco but US-B does not). L rods of both J-A and US-B are 300 nm long. The lengths of S rods in individual local lesions from the plants receiving mixed inoculum were tested with the electron microscope, using a leaf dip technique. As expected (because of the S rods in the L-rod preparations), some lesions from both heterologous inocula had the longer S rods characteristic of US-B and others had shorter S rods characteristic of J-A. Virus was increased from lesions which had particles with S rods of the length expected if a hybrid virus had actually been obtained. In further tests on the two "hybrids" derived from J-A and US-B, as well as on the parental types and certain other hybrids, the serological character appears to be determined by the source of S rod, the ability to infect tobacco by the source of L rod, and the ability to produce certain symptoms by both S and L. Parental-type viruses were regenerated by heterologous mixed inoculation of S and L rods from the hybrids.

The results with SBWMV which are described in the previous paragraph are somewhat parallel to those obtained with TRV. However, the technical problems which have prevented the isolation of L rods free of detectable S rods make it impossible to firmly conclude that SBWMV is a two-component system. Most, perhaps all, of the results could be explained if, instead of hybrid viruses, mixtures of viruses had been formed in the mixed inoculation experiments. Histograms of the US-B rod lengths showed the predominant "peak" at 160 nm and no rods of less than 100 nm. The hybrid derived from plants inoculated with a mixture of preparations of US-B S rods and J-A L rods had the "peak" at 160 nm but also rods of lengths 100 nm and less (as is characteristic of J-A). That is, the "hybrid" might have been a mixture of US-B with a small amount of J-A.

SBWMV has not been shown to be serologically related to TRV; however, Powell (1976) has clearly demonstrated the similarity of SBWMV to tobacco mosaic virus by serological and other means. There is, of course, no evidence that tobacco mosaic virus is a two-component system. If further experiments support the notion that SBWMV is a two-component system, a comparison of the two related viruses might provide insight into the possible origin of the SBWMV two-component system. Alternatively, SBWMV may resemble more closely a cowpea strain of tobacco mosaic virus which produces noninfective short rods. In the latter system, highly purified L-rod RNA is infectious (in a nondefective mode), forming both long and shorter rods

(Bruening *et al.*, 1976; Whitfeld and Higgins, 1976). The properties of equally highly purified L rods or L-rod RNA of SBWMV must be determined before it can be concluded that SBWMV is or is not a two-component system. Another possibility is that SBWMV is a satellite virus system (Powell, 1976). (See Chapter 4 for details on the cowpea strain of TMV.)

ACKNOWLEDGMENTS

I am grateful to Brian D. Harrison, Richard M. Lister, John F. E. Newman, Irving R. Schneider, Lous Van Vloten-Doting, and Milton Zaitlin for comments and suggestions on various parts of the manuscript. Brian D. Harrison, John F. Longworth, John F. E. Newman, Charles A. Powell, and Irving R. Schneider very generously provided me with research results prior to their publication.

The writing of this chapter was initiated during the tenure of a fellowship from the John Simon Guggenheim Memorial Foundation. Research on two-component viruses in my laboratory has been benefited by long-term support from the National Science Foundation.

6. REFERENCES

Abou Haidar, M., Pfeiffer, P., Fritsch, C., and Hirth, L., 1973, Sequential reconstitution of tobacco rattle virus, *J. Gen. Virol.* **21**:83.

Adam, G., and Sander, E., 1976, Isolation and culture of aphid cells for the assay of insect-transmitted plant viruses, *Virology* **70**:459.

Agrawal, H., 1964, Identification of cowpea mosaic virus isolates, *Meded. Landbouwhogesch. Wageningen* **64–5**:1.

Agrawal, H., and Maat, D. Z., 1964, Serological relationships among polyhedral plant viruses and production of high-titred antisera, *Nature (London)* **202**:674.

Allen, T. C., 1967, Serological relationship between the Oregon strain of tobacco rattle virus and pea early browning virus. *Phytopathology* **57**:97.

Assink, A.-M., Swaans, H., and van Kammen, A., 1973, The localization of virus-specific double-stranded RNA of cowpea mosaic virus in subcellular fractions of infected *Vigna* leaves, *Virology* **53**:384.

Atchison, B. A., 1973, Division, expansion and DNA synthesis in meristematic cells of French bean (*Phaseolus vulgaris* L.) root-tips invaded by tobacco ringspot virus, *Physiol. Plant Pathol.* **3**:1.

Ball, E. M., 1973, Solid phase radioimmunoassay for plant viruses, *Virology* **55**:576.

Ball, L. A., Minson, A. C., and Shih, D. S., 1973, Synthesis of plant virus coat proteins in an animal cell-free system, *Nature (London) New Biol.* **246**:206.

Bancroft, J. B., 1962, Purification and properties of bean pod mottle virus and associated centrifugal and electrophoretic components, *Virology* **16**:419.

Bancroft, J. B., 1968, Tomato top necrosis virus, *Phytopathology* **58**:1360.

Barker, H., 1975, Effects of virus infection and polyacrylic acid on leaf proteins, *J. Gen. Virol.* **28**:155.

Beier, H., and Bruening, G., 1975, The use of an abrasive in the isolation of cowpea leaf protoplasts which support the multiplication of cowpea mosaic virus. *Virology* **64**:272.

Beier, H., and Bruening, G., 1976, Factors influencing the infection of cowpea protoplasts by cowpea mosaic virus RNA, *Virology* **72**:363.

Blevings, S., and Stace-Smith, R., 1976, *In vivo* and *in vitro* effects on the electrophoretic forms of particles of broad bean true mosaic virus, *J. Gen. Virol.* **31**:199.

Brown, F., and Hull, R., 1973, Comparative virology of small RNA viruses, *J. Gen. Virol.* **20S**:43.

Bruening, G., 1969, The inheritance of top component formation in cowpea mosaic virus, *Virology* **37**:577.

Bruening, G., and Agrawal, H. O., 1967, Infectivity of a mixture of cowpea mosaic virus ribonucleoprotein components, *Virology* **32**:306.

Bruening, G., Beachy, R. N., Scalla, R., and Zaitlin, M., 1976, *In vitro* and *in vivo* translation of the ribonucleic acids of a cowpea strain of tobacco mosaic virus, *Virology* **71**:498.

Cadman, C. H., 1962, Evidence for association of tobacco rattle virus nucleic acid with a cell component, *Nature (London)* **193**:49.

Cadman, C. H., 1963, Biology of soil-borne viruses, *Annu. Rev. Phytopathol.* **1**:143.

Cadman, C. H., and Harrison, B. D., 1959, Studies on the properties of soil-borne viruses of the tobacco-rattle type occurring in Scotland, *Ann. Appl. Biol.* **47**:542.

Cadman, C. H., Dias, H. F., and Harrison, B. D., 1960, Sap-transmissible viruses associated with diseases of grape vines in Europe and North America, *Nature (London)* **187**:577.

Campbell, R. N., 1964, Radish mosaic virus, a crucifer virus serologically related to strains of bean pod mottle virus, *Phytopathology* **54**:1418.

Casjens, S., and King, J., 1975, Virus assembly, *Annu. Rev. Biochem.* **44**:555.

Clark, M. F., and Lister, R. M., 1971, The application of polyethylene glycol solubility-concentration gradients in plant virus research, *Virology* **43**:338.

Cockbain, A. J., Cook, S. M., and Bowen, R., 1975, Transmission of broad bean stain virus and Echtes Ackerbohnenmosaik-Virus to field beans (*Vicia faba*) by weevils, *Ann. Appl. Biol.* **81**:331.

Cooper, J. I., and Harrison, B. D., 1973, The role of weed hosts and the distribution and activity of vector nematodes in the ecology of tobacco rattle virus, *Ann. Appl. Biol.* **73**:53.

Cooper, J. I., and Mayo, M. A., 1972, Some properties of the particles of three tobravirus isolates, *J. Gen. Virol.* **16**:285.

Crick, F. H. C., and Watson, J. D., 1956, Structure of small viruses, *Nature (London)* **177**:473.

Crowther, R. A., Geelen, J. L. M. C., and Mellema, J. E., 1974, A three-dimensional image reconstruction of cowpea mosaic virus, *Virology* **57**:20.

Darby, G., and Minson, A. C., 1972, The structure of tobacco rattle virus ribonucleic acids: Nature of the 3′-terminal nucleosides, *J. Gen. Virol.* **14**:199.

Darby, G., and Minson, A. C., 1973, The structure of tobacco rattle virus ribonucleic acids: Common nucleotide sequences in the RNA species. *J. Gen. Virol.* **21**:285.

Davies, J. W., and Kaesberg, P., 1974, Translation of virus m-RNA: Protein synthesis directed by several virus RNAs in a cell-free extract from wheat germ, *J. Gen. Virol.* **25**:11.

de Jager, C. P., 1976, Genetic analysis of cowpea mosaic virus mutants by supplementation and reassortment tests, *Virology* **70**:151.

de Jager, C. P., and van Kammen, A., 1970, The relationship between the components of cowpea mosaic virus. III. Location of genetic information for two biological functions in the middle component of CPMW, *Virology* **41**:281.

Delbos, R., Dunez, J., Barrau, J., and Fisac, R., 1976, The RNAs of three strains of tomato black ring virus, *Ann. Microbiol. (Inst. Pasteur)* **127A**:101.

de Zoeten, G. A., 1966, California tobacco rattle virus, its intracellular appearance, and the cytology of the infected cell, *Phytopathology* **56**:744.

de Zoeten, G. A., Assink, A. M., and van Kammen, A., 1974, Association of cowpea mosaic virus-induced double-stranded RNA with a cytopathological structure in infected cells, *Virology* **59**:341.

de Zoeten, G. A., Powell, C. A., Gaard, G., and German, T. L., 1976, *In situ* localization of pea enation mosaic virus double-stranded ribonucleic acid, *Virology* **70**:459.

Diener, T. O., and Schneider, I. R., 1966, The two components of tobacco ringspot virus nucleic acid: Origin and properties, *Virology* **29**:100.

Diener, T. O., and Smith, D. R., 1973, Potato spindle tuber viroid. IX. Molecular-weight determination by gel electrophoresis of formylated RNA, *Virology* **53**:359.

Diener, T. O., Schneider, I. R., and Smith, D. R., 1974, Potato spindle tuber viroid. XI. A comparison of the ultraviolet light sensitivities of PSTV, tobacco ringspot virus, and its satellite, *Virology* **57**:577.

Doel, T. R., 1975, Comparative properties of type, nasturtium ringspot and petunia ringspot strains of broad bean wilt virus, *J. Gen. Virol.* **26**:95.

Dunez, J., Delbos, R., Desvignes, J.-C., Marenaud, C., Kuszala, J., and Vuitteneg, A., 1971, Mise en evidence d'un virus de type ringspot sur *Prunus cerasifera, Ann. Phytopathol. Suppl.* **1971**:117.

Durham, A. C. H., and Klug, A., 1971, Polymerization of tobacco mosaic virus protein and its control, *Nature (London) New Biol.* **229**:42.

El Manna, M. M., 1968, Low molecular weight cations in cowpea mosaic virus, M.A. thesis, University of California at Davis, 83 pp.

El Manna, M. M., and Bruening, G., 1973, Polyadehylate sequences in the ribonucleic acids of cowpea mosaic virus, *Virology* **56**:198.

Fenner, F., 1976, The classification and nomenclature of viruses. Summary of results of meetings of the International Committee of Taxonomy of Viruses in Madrid, September 1975, *Virology* **71**:371.

Finch, J. T., 1965, Preliminary X-ray diffraction studies of tobacco rattle and barley stripe mosaic virus, *J. Mol. Biol.* **12**:612.

Fritsch, C., Witz, J., Abou Haidar, M., and Hirth, L., 1973, Polymerization of tobacco rattle virus proteins, *FEBS Lett.* **29**:211.

Fritsch, C., Mayo, M. A., and Hirth, L., 1976, *In vitro* translation of tobacco rattle virus RNA, *Ann. Microbiol. (Inst. Pasteur)* **127A**:93.

Frost, R. R., Harrison, B. D., and Woods, R. D., 1967, Apparent symbiotic interaction between particles of tobacco rattle virus, *J. Gen. Virol.* **1**:57.

Frowd, J. A., and Tombinson, J. A., 1972, Relationship between a parsley virus, nasturtium ringspot virus and broad bean wilt virus, *Ann. Appl. Biol.* **72**:189.

Fulton, J. P., Scott, H. A., and Gaméz, R., 1975, Beetle transmission of legume viruses, in: *Tropical Diseases of Legumes* (J. Bird and K. Maramorosch, eds.), Academic Press, New York.

Fulton, R. W., 1962, The effect of dilution on necrotic ringspot virus infectivity and the enhancement of infectivity by non-infective virus, *Virology* **18**:477.

Gaméz, R., 1972, Los virus del frijol en Centroamerica. II. Algunas propiedades y transmision por crisomelidos del virus del mosaico rugoso del frijol, *Turrialba* **22**:249.

Geelen, J. L. M. C., van Kammen, A., and Verduin, B. J. M., 1972, Structure of the capsid of cowpea mosaic virus. The chemical subunit: Molecular weight and number of subunits per particle, *Virology* **49**:205.

Geelen, J. L. M. C., Rezelman, G., and van Kammen, A., 1973, The infectivity of the two electrophoretic forms of cowpea mosaic virus, *Virology* **51**:279.

Gerhardson, B., and Petersson, J., 1974, Transmission of red clover mottle virus by clover shoot weevils, *Apion* spp., *Swed. J. Agr. Res.* **4**:161.

German, T. L., and de Zoeten, G. A., 1975, Purification and properties of the replicative forms and replicative intermediates of pea enation mosaic virus, *Virology* **66**:172.

Ghabrial, S. A., and Lister, R. M., 1973a, Anomalies in molecular weight determinations of tobacco rattle virus protein by SDS-polyacrylamide gel electrophoresis, *Virology* **51**:485.

Ghabrial, S. A., and Lister, R. M., 1973b, Coat protein and symptom specifications in tobacco rattle virus, *Virology* **52**:1.

Gibbs, A. J., and Harrison, B. D., 1964, A form of pea early-browning virus found in Britain, *Ann. Appl. Biol.* **54**:1.

Gibbs, A. J., and Harrison, B. D., 1976, *Plant Virology: The Principles*, Edward Arnold, London.

Gibbs, A. J., and McIntyre, G. A., 1970, A method for assessing the size of a protein from its composition: its use in evaluating data on the size of the protein subunits of plant virus particles, *J. Gen. Virol.* **9**:51.

Gibbs, A. J., Giussani-Belli, G., and Smith, H. G., 1968, Broad-bean strain and true broad-bean mosaic viruses, *Ann. Appl. Biol.* **61**:99.

Gillaspie, A. G., and Bancroft, J. B., 1965, The rate of accumulation, specific infectivity, and electrophoretic characteristics of bean pod mottle virus in bean and soybean, *Phytopathology* **55**:906.

Gonsalves, D., and Shepherd, R. J., 1972, Biological and biophysical properties of the two nucleoprotein components of pea enation mosaic virus and their associated nucleic acids, *Virology* **48**:709.

Govier, D. A., 1975, Complementation between middle and bottom components of broad bean stain virus and Echtes Ackerbonemosaik-virus, *J. Gen. Virol.* **28**:373.

Hanada, K., and Harrison, B. D., 1977, Effects of virus genotype and temperature on seed transmission of nepoviruses, *Ann. Appl. Biol.* **85**:79.

Haque, S. Q., and Persad, G. C., 1975, Some observations on the seed-transmission of beetle-transmitted cowpea mosaic virus, in: *Tropical Diseases of Legumes*, (J. Bird and K. Maramorosch, eds.), Academic Press, New York.

Harrison, B. D., 1966, Further studies on a British form of pea early-browning virus, *Ann. Appl. Biol.* **57**:121.

Harrison, B. D., and Crockatt, A. A., 1971, Effects of cycloheximide on the accumulation of tobacco rattle virus in leaf disks of *Nicotiana clevelandii, J. Gen. Virol.* **12**:183.

Harrison, B. D., and Hanada, K., 1976, Competitiveness between genotypes of raspberry ringspot virus is mainly determined by RNA-1, *J. Gen. Virol.* **31**:455.

Harrison, B. D., and Klug, A., 1966, Relation between length and sedimentation coefficient for particles of tobacco rattle virus, *Virology* **30**:738.

Harrison, B. D., and Nixon, H. L., 1959, Separation and properties of particles of tobacco rattle virus with different lengths, *J. Gen. Microbiol.* **21**:569.

Harrison, B. D., and Roberts, I. M., 1968, Association of tobacco rattle virus with mitochondria, *J. Gen. Virol.* **3**:121.

Harrison, B. D., and Woods, R. D., 1966, Serotypes and particle dimensions of tobacco rattle viruses from Europe and America, *Virology* **28**:610.

Harrison, B. D., Finch, J. T., Gibbs, A. J., Hollings, M., Shepherd, R. J., Valenta, V., and Wetter, C., 1971, Sixteen groups of plant viruses, *Virology* **45**:356.

Harrison, B. D., Murant, A. F., and Mayo, M. A., 1972a, Evidence for two functional RNA species in raspberry ringspot virus, *J. Gen. Virol.* **16**:339.

Harrison, B. D., Murant, A. F., and Mayo, M. A., 1972b, Two properties of raspberry ringspot virus determined by its smaller RNA, *J. Gen. Virol.* **17**:137.

Harrison, B. D., Robertson, W. M., and Taylor, C. E., 1974a, Specificity of retention and transmission of viruses by nematodes, *J. Nematol.* **6**:155.

Harrison, B. D., Murant, A. F., Mayo, M. A. and Roberts, I. M., 1974b, Distribution of determinants for symptom production, host range and nematode transmissibility between the two RNA components of raspberry ringspot virus, *J. Gen. Virol.* **22**:233.

Harrison, B. D., Kubo, S., Robinson, D. J., and Hutcheson, A. M., 1976, The multiplication cycle of tobacco rattle virus in tobacco mesophyll cells, *J. Gen. Virol.* **33**:237.

Hibi, T., Rezelman, G., and van Kammen, A., 1975, Infection of cowpea mesophyll protoplasts with cowpea mosaic virus, *Virology* **64**:308.

Higgins, T. J. V., Goodwin, P. B., and Whitfeld, P. R., 1976, Occurrence of short particles in beans infected with the cowpea strain of TMV. II. Evidence that short particles contain the cistron for coat-protein, *Virology* **71**:486.

Honda, Y., and Matsui, C., 1972, Electron microscopy of intracellular radish mosaic virus, *Phytopathology* **62**:448.

Hooper, G. R., Spink, G. C., and Myers, R. L., 1972, Electron microscopy of leaf enations on Chinese white winter radish infected with radish mosaic virus, *Virology* **47**:833.

Hull, R., and Lane, L. C., 1973, The unusual nature of the components of a strain of pea enation mosaic virus, *Virology* **55**:1.

Hull, R., and Plaskitt, A., 1973/74, The *in vivo* behavior of broad bean wilt virus and three of its strains, *Interviology* **2**:352.

Huttinga, H., 1973, Separation of long and short particles of tobacco rattle virus with polyethylene glycol, *Neth. J. Plant Pathol.* **79**:9.

Izadpanah, K., and Shepherd, R. J., 1966, Purification and properties of the pea enation mosaic virus, *Virology* **28**:463.

Jaspars, E. M. J., 1974, Plant viruses with a multipartite genome, *Adv. Virus Res.* **19**:37.

Jaspars, E. M. J., and van Kammen, A., 1972, Analysis of the genome constitution of cowpea mosaic and alfalfa mosaic viruses. *Proc. Eighth FEBS Meeting* **27**:121.

Johnston, J. P., and Ogston, A. G., 1946, A boundary anomaly found in the ultracentrifugal sedimentation of mixtures, *Trans. Faraday Soc.* **42**:789.

Jones, A. T., and Barker, H., 1976, Properties and relationships of broad bean stain virus and Echtes Ackerbohnenmosaik-Virus, *Ann. Appl. Biol.* **83**:231.

Jones, A. T., and Mayo, M. A., 1972, The two nucleoprotein particles of cherry leaf roll virus, *J. Gen. Virol.* **16**:349.

Juretić, N., and Fulton, R. W., 1974, Some characteristics of the particle types of radish mosaic virus, *Intervirology* **4**:57.

Kassanis, B., White, R. F., and Woods, R. D., 1973, Genetic complementation between middle and bottom components of two strains of radish mosaic virus, *J. Gen. Virol.* **20**:277.

Kenten, R. H., 1972, The purification and some properties of cocoa necrosis virus, a serotype of tomato black ring virus, *Ann. Appl. Biol.* **71**:119.

Kim, K. S., and Fulton, J. P., 1973, Plant virus-induced cell-wall overgrowth and associated membrane elaboration, *J. Ultrastruct. Res.* **45**:328.

Kim, K. S., Fulton, J. P., and Scott, H. A., 1974, Osmiophilic globules and myelinic bodies in cells infected with two comoviruses, *J. Gen. Virol.* **25**:445.

Kitajima, E. W., and Costa, A. S., 1969, Association of pepper ringspot virus (Brazilian tobacco rattle) and host cell mitochondria, *J. Gen. Virol.* **4**:177.

Köhler, E., 1956, Uber eine reversible, durch die Jahreszeit induzierte Virulenzanderung beim Tabak-Rattle-Virus, *Nachr. Itsch. Pflanzenschutzdienst. Brschw.* **8**:93.

Kubo, S., Harrison, B. D., Robinson, D. J., and Mayo, M. A., 1975, Tobacco rattle virus in tobacco mesophyll protoplasts: Infection and virus multiplication, *J. Gen. Virol.* **27**:293.

Lane, L. C., 1974, The components of barley stripe mosaic and related viruses, *Virology* **58**:323.

Langenberg, W. G., and Schroeder, H. F., 1975, The ultrastructural appearance of cowpea mosaic virus in cowpea, *J. Ultrastruct. Res.* **51**:166.

Lastra, J. R., Acosta, J. M., and de Uzcátegui, R., 1975, *Cucumis metuliferus* as a local lesion host for squash mosaic virus, *Plant Dis. Rep.* **59**:693.

Lawrence, C., and Thach, R. E., 1975, Identification of a viral protein involved in posttranslational maturation of the encephalomyocarditis virus capsid precursor, *J. Virol.* **15**:918.

Lee, F. N., and Walters, J. H., 1970, A virus isolate from *Desmodium* related to bean pod mottle virus, *Phytopathology* **60**:585.

Lee, R. F., Johnson, L. B., and Niblett, C. L., 1975a, Effect of host enzyme extracts on the electrophoretic forms and specific infectivity of cowpea mosaic virus, *Physiol. Plant Pathol.* **7**:59.

Lee, R. F., Johnson, L. B., and Niblett, C. L., 1975b, Aspartate transcarbamylase activity in healthy and virus-infected cowpea and soybean leaves, *Phytopathology* **65**:1079.

Lesnaw, J. A., and Reichmann, M. E., 1970, Determination of molecular weights of plant viral protein subunits by polyacrylamide gel electrophoresis, *Virology* **42**:724.

Lister, R. M., 1966, Possible relationships of virus-specific products of tobacco rattle virus, *Virology* **28**:350.

Lister, R. M., 1967, A symptomatological difference between some unstable and stable variants of pea early browning virus, *Virology* **31**:739.

Lister, R. M., 1968, Functional relationships between virus-specific products of infection by viruses of the tobacco rattle type, *J. Gen. Virol.* **2**:43.

Lister, R. M., 1969, Tobacco rattle, NETU, viruses in relation to functional heterogeneity of plant viruses, *Fed. Proc.* **28**:1875.

Lister, R. M., and Bracker, C. E., 1969, Defectiveness and dependence in three related strains of tobacco rattle virus, *Virology* **37**:262.

Lister, R. M., and Murant, A. F., 1967, Seed transmission of nematode-borne viruses, *Ann. Appl. Biol.* **59**:49.

Lockhart, B. E. L., and Semancik, J. S., 1968, Inhibition of the multiplication of a plant virus by actinomycin D, *Virology* **36**:504.

Lockhart, B. E. L., and Semancik, J. S., 1969, Differential effect of actinomycin D on plant-virus multiplication, *Virology* **39**:362.

Longworth, J. F., and Carey, G. P., 1976, A small RNA virus with a divided genome from *Heteronychus arator* (F.) [Coleoptera: Scarabaeidae], *J. Gen. Virol.* **33**:31.

Maat, D. Z., 1963, Pea early browning virus and tobacco rattle virus—two different but serologically related viruses, *Neth. J. Plant Pathol.* **69**:287.

Magyarosy, A. C., Buchanan, B. B., and Schurmann, P., 1973, Effect of a systemic infection on chloroplast function and structure, *Virology* **55**:426.

Mahmood, K., and Peters, D., 1973, Purification of pea enation mosaic virus and the infectivity of its components, *Neth. J. Plant Pathol.* **79**:138.

Makino, S., Woolford, J. L., Tanford, C., and Webster, R. E., 1975, Interaction of deoxycholate and of detergents with the coat protein of bacteriophage fl, *J. Biol. Chem.* **250**:4327.

Martelli, G. P., and Quacquarelli, A., 1972, Grapevine chrome mosaic virus, in: *CMI/ABB Descriptions of plant Viruses* (A. J. Gibbs, B. D. Harrison, and A. F. Murant, eds.), No. 103, Commonwealth Mycological Institute, Kew.

Mayo, M. A., and Cooper, J. I., 1973, Partial degradation of the protein in tobacco rattle virus during storage, *J. Gen. Virol.* **18**:281.

Mayo, M. A., and Robinson, D. J., 1975, Revision of estimates of the molecular weights Tobravirus coat proteins, *Intervirology* **5**:313.

Mayo, M. A., Murant, A. F., and Harrison, B. D., 1971, New evidence on the structure of nepoviruses, *J. Gen. Virol.* **12**:175.

Mayo, M. A., Harrison, B. D., Murant, A. F., and Barker, A., 1973, Cross-linking of RNA induced by ultraviolet irradiation of particles of raspberry ringspot virus, *J. Gen. Virol.* **19**:155.

Mayo, M. A., Murant, A. F., Harrison, B. D., and Goold, R. A., 1974a, Two protein and two RNA species in particles of strawberry latent ringspot virus, *J. Gen. Virol.* **24**:29.

Mayo, M. A., Robinson, D. J., and Perombelon, M. C. M., 1974b, Some properties of a bacterial protease with a specific effect on the protein in tobacco rattle virus particles, *J. Gen. Microbiol.* **85**:121.

Mayo, M. A., Fritsch, C., and Hirth, L., 1976, Translation *in vitro* of tobacco rattle virus RNA using wheat germ extracts, *Virology* **69**:408.

Mazzone, H. M., Incardona, N. L., and Kaesberg, P., 1962, Biochemical and biophysical properties of squash mosaic virus and related macromolecules, *Biochim. Biophys. Acta* **55**:164.

Miki, T., and Okada, Y., 1970, Comparative studies on some strains of tobacco rattle virus, *Virology* **42**:993.

Milicić, D., Wrischer, M., and Juretić, N., 1974, Intracellular inclusion bodies of broad bean wilt virus, *Phytopathol. Z.* **80**:127.

Minson, A. C., and Darby, G., 1973a, A study of sequence homology between tobacco rattle virus ribonucleic acids, *J. Gen. Virol.* **19**:253.

Minson, T., and Darby, G., 1973b, 3′-Terminal oligonucleotide fragments of tobacco rattle virus ribonucleic acids, *J. Mol. Biol.* **77**:337.

Moghal, S. M., and Francki, R. I. B., 1974, Occurrence and properties of broad bean stain virus in South Australia, *Aust. J. Biol. Sci.* **27**:341.

Moore, B. J., 1973, Quail pea mosaic virus: A new member of the Comovirus group, *Plant Dis. Rep.* **57**:311.

Moore, B. J., and Scott, H. A., 1971, Properties of a strain of bean pod mottle virus, *Phytopathology* **61**:831.

Morris, T. J., 1974, Two nucleoprotein components associated with the cowpea strain of TMV, *Proc. Am. Phytopathol. Soc.* **1**:83.

Morris, T. J., and Semancik, J. S., 1973a, Homologous interference between components of tobacco rattle virus, *Virology* **52**:314.

Morris, T. J., and Semancik, J. S., 1973b, In vitro protein polymerization and nucleoprotein reconstitution of tobacco rattle virus, *Virology* **53**:215.

Murant, A. F., 1970a, Tomato black ring virus, in: *CMI/AAB Descriptions of Plant Viruses* (A. J. Gibbs, B. D. Harrison, and A. F. Murant, eds.), No. 38, Commonwealth Mycological Institute, Kew.

Murant, A. F., 1970b, Arabis mosaic virus, in: *CMI/AAB Descriptions of Plant Viruses* (A. J. Gibbs, B. D. Harrison, and A. F. Murant, eds.), No. 16, Commonwealth Mycological Institute, Kew.

Murant, A. F., Mayo, M. A., Harrison, B. D., and Goold, R. A., 1972, Properties of virus and RNA components of raspberry ringspot virus, *J. Gen. Virol.* **16**:327.

Murant, A. F., Mayo, M. A., Harrison, B. D., and Goold, R. A., 1973, Evidence for two functional RNA species and a "satellite" RNA in tomato black ring virus, *J. Gen. Virol.* **19**:275.

Nelson, M. R., and Knuhtsen, H. K., 1973a, Squash mosaic virus variability: Epidemiological consequences of differences in seed transmission frequency between strains, *Phytopathology* **63**:918.

Nelson, M. R., and Knuhtsen, H. K., 1973b, Squash mosaic virus variability: Review and serological comparison of six biotypes, *Phytopathology* **63**:920.

Newman, J. F. E., and Brown, F., 1973, Evidence for a divided genome in Nodamura virus, an arthropod-borne Picornavirus, *J. Gen. Virol.* **21**:371.

Newman, J. F. E., and Brown, F., 1976, Absence of poly(A) from the infective RNA of Nodamura virus, *J. Gen. Virol.* **30**:137.

Niblett, C. L., and Semancik, J. S., 1969, Conversion of the electrophoretic forms of cowpea mosaic virus *in vivo* and *in vitro*, *Virology* **38**:685.

Niblett, C. L., and Semancik, J. S., 1970, The significance of the coat protein in infection by the electrophoretic forms of cowpea mosaic virus, *Virology* **41**:201.

Niblett, C. L., Johnson, L. B., and Lee R. F., 1974, Aspartate transcarbamylase activity in etiolated cowpea and soybean hypocotyls infected with cowpea mosaic virus or tobacco ringspot virus, *Physiol. Plant Pathol.* **4**:63.

Nixon, H. L., and Harrison, B. D., 1959, Electron microscope evidence on the structure of the particles of tobacco rattle virus, *J. Gen. Microbiol.* **21**:582.

Offord, R. E., 1966, Electron microscopic observations on the substructure of tobacco rattle virus, *J. Mol. Biol.* **17**:370.

Owens, R. A., and Bruening, G., 1975, The pattern of amino acid incorporation into two cowpea mosaic virus proteins in the presence of ribosome-specific protein synthesis inhibitors, *Virology* **64:**520.

Oxefelt, P., 1976, Biological and physiochemical characteristics of three strains of red clover mottle virus, *Virology* **74:**73.

Partridge, J. E., Shannon, L. M., Gumpf, D. J., and Colbaugh, P., 1974, Glycoprotein in the capsid of plant viruses as a possible determinant of seed transmissibility, *Nature (London)* **247:**391.

Paul, H. L., 1963, Untersuchungen über das Echte Ackerbohnenmosaik-Virus, *Phytopathol. Z.* **49:**161.

Pelham, H. R. B., and Jackson, R. J., 1976, An efficient mRNA-dependent translation system from reticulocyte lysates, *Eur. J. Biochem.* **67:**247.

Powell, C. A., 1976, The relationship between soil-borne wheat mosaic virus and tobacco mosaic virus, *Virology* **71:**453.

Reichmann, M. E., 1965, Determination of the ribonuleic acid content of spherical viruses from sedimentation coefficients of full and empty particles, *Virology* **25:**166.

Reijnders, L., Aalbers, A. M. J., van Kammen, A., and Thuring, R. W. J., 1974, Molecular weights of plant virus RNAs determined by gel electrophoresis under denaturing conditions, *Virology* **60:**515.

Rezaian, M. A., and Francki, R. I. B., 1973, Replication of tobacco ringspot virus. I. Detection of a low molecular weight double-stranded RNA from infected plants, *Virology* **56:**238.

Rezaian, M. A., and Francki, R. I. B., 1974, Replication of tobacco ringspot virus. II. Differences in nucleotide sequences between the viral RNA components, *Virology* **59:**275.

Rice, R. V., Lindberg, G. D., Kaesberg, P., Walker, J. C., and Stahmann, M. A., 1955, The three components of squash mosaic virus, *Phytopathology* **45:**145.

Roberts, I. M., and Harrison, B. D., 1970, Inclusion bodies and tubular structures in *Chenopodium amaranticolor* plants infected with strawberry latent ringspot virus, *J. Gen. Virol.* **7:**47.

Robinson, D. J., 1973*a*, Inactivation and mutagenesis of tobacco rattle virus by nitrous acid, *J. Gen. Virol.* **18:**215.

Robinson, D. J., 1973*b*, Properties of two temperature-sensitive mutants of tobacco rattle virus, *J. Gen. Virol.* **21:**499.

Robinson, D. J., 1974, Early events in local infection of *Chenopodium amaranticolor* leaves by mutant and wild-type strains of tobacco rattle virus, *J. Gen. Virol.* **24:**391.

Robinson, N. C., and Tanford, C., 1975, The binding of deoxycholate, Triton X-100, sodium dodecyl sulfate, and phosphatidylcholine vesicles to cytochrome b_5, *Biochemistry* **14:**369.

Sahambi, H. S., Milne, R. G., Cook, S. M., Gibbs, A. J., and Woods, R. D., 1973, Broad bean wilt and nasturtium ringspot viruses are related, *Phytopathol. Z.* **76:**158.

Sänger, H. L., 1968, Characteristics of tobacco rattle virus; evidence that its two particles are functionally defective and mutually complementing, *Mol. Gen. Genet.* **101:**346.

Sänger, H. L., 1969, Functions of the two particles of tobacco rattle virus, *J. Virol.* **3:**304.

Sänger, H. L., and Brandenburg, E., 1961, Uber die Gewinnung von Infektiosem aus "Wintertyp"-Pflanzen des Tabak-Rattle-Virus durch Phenolextraktion, *Naturwissenschaften* **48:**391.

Schneider, I. R., 1971, Characteristics of a satellite-like virus of tobacco ringspot virus, *Virology* **45**:108.

Schneider, I. R., 1972, Tobacco ringspot virus codes for the coat protein of its satellite, *Phytopathology* **62**:788 (abstract).

Schneider, I. R., 1976, Defective plant viruses, in: *Program and Abstracts, Beltsville Symposium on Virology in Agriculture*, p. 15, U.S. Department of Agriculture, Beltsville, Md.

Schneider, I. R., and Diener, T. O., 1966, The correlation between the proportions of the virus-related products and the infectious component during the synthesis of tobacco ringspot virus, *Virology* **29**:92.

Schneider, I. R., and Thompson, S. M., 1976, Double-stranded nucleic acids found in tissue infected with the satellite of tobacco ringspot virus, *Proc. Am. Phytopathol. Soc.* **3**:209.

Schneider, I. R., and White, R. M., 1976, Tobacco ringspot virus codes for the coat protein of its satellite, *Virology* **70**:244.

Schneider, I. R., Hull, R., and Markham, R., 1972a, Multidense satellite of tobacco ringspot virus: A regular series of components of different densities, *Virology* **47**:320.

Schneider, I. R., White, R. M., and Gooding, G. V., 1972b, Two new isolates of the satellite of tobacco ringspot virus, *Virology* **50**:902.

Schneider, I. R., White, R. M., and Civerolo, E. L., 1974a, Two nucleic acid-containing components of tomato ringspot virus, *Virology* **57**:139.

Schneider, I. R., White, R. M., and Thompson, S. M., 1974b, High molecular weight double-stranded nucleic acids from tobacco ringspot virus-infected plants, *Proc. Am. Phytopathol. Soc.* **1**:82.

Semancik, J. S., 1966a, Studies on electrophoretic heterogeneity in isometric plant viruses, *Virology* **30**:698.

Semancik, J. S., 1966b, Purification and properties of two isolates of tobacco rattle virus from pepper in California, *Phytopathology* **56**:1190.

Semancik, J. S., 1970, Identity of structural protein from two isolates of TRV with different length of associated short particles, *Virology* **40**:618.

Semancik, J. S., 1974, Detection of polyadenylic acid sequences in plant pathogenic RNAs, *Virology* **62**:288.

Semancik, J. S., and Bancroft, J. B., 1964, Further characterization of the nucleoprotein components of bean pod mottle virus, *Virology* **22**:33.

Semancik, J. B., and Bancroft, J. B., 1965, Stability differences between the nucleoprotein components of bean pod mottle virus, *Virology* **27**:476.

Semancik, J. S., and Kajiyama, M. R., 1967, Comparative studies on two strains of tobacco rattle virus, *J. Gen. Virol.* **1**:153.

Semancik, J. S., and Kajiyama, M. R., 1968, Enhancement of tobacco rattle virus stable form infection by heterologous short particles, *Virology* **34**:170.

Semancik, J. S., and Reynolds, D. A., 1969, Assembly of protein and nucleoprotein particles from extracted tobacco rattle virus protein and RNA, *Science* **164**:559.

Shepherd, R. J., 1963, Serological relationship between bean pod mottle virus and cowpea mosaic viruses from Arkansas and Trinidad, *Phytopathology* **53**:865.

Shepherd, R. J., 1972, Transmission of viruses through seed and pollen, in: *Principles and Techniques in Plant Virology* (C. I. Kado and H. O. Agrawal, eds.), pp. 267–292, Van Nostrand Reinhold, New York.

Shoulder, A., Darby, G., and Minson, T., 1974, RNA-RNA hybridization using ^{125}I-labelled RNA from tobacco necrosis virus and its satellite, *Nature (London)* **251**:733.

Siler, D. J., Babcock, J., and Bruening, G., 1976, The electrophoretic mobility and enhanced infectivity of a mutant of cowpea mosaic virus, *Virology* **71**:560.

Sogo, J. M., Schneider, I. R., and Koller, T., 1974, Size determination by electron microscopy of the RNA of tobacco ringspot satellite virus, *Virology* **57**:459.

Stace-Smith, R., 1970*a*, Tobacco ringspot virus, in: *CMI/AAB Descriptions of Plant Viruses* (A. J. Gibbs, B. D. Harrison, and A. F. Murant, eds.), No. 17, Commonwealth Mycological Institute, Kew.

Stace-Smith, R., 1970*b*, Tomato ringspot virus, in: *CMI/AAB Descriptions of Plant Viruses* (A. J. Gibbs, B. D. Harrison, and A. F. Murant, eds.), No. 18, Commonwealth Mycological Institute, Kew.

Stace-Smith, R., Reichmann, M. E., and Wright, N. S., 1965, Purification and properties of tobacco ringspot virus and two RNA-deficient components, *Virology* **25**:487.

Steere, R. L., 1956, Purification and properties of tobacco ringspot virus, *Phytopathology* **46**:60.

Stefanac, Z., and Mamula, D., 1971, A strain of radish mosaic virus occurring in turnip in Yugoslavia, *Ann. Appl. Biol.* **69**:229.

Swaans, H., and van Kammen, A., 1973, Reconsideration of the distinction between the severe and yellow strains of cowpea mosaic virus, *Neth. J. Plant Pathol.* **79**:257.

Tanford, C., 1961, *Physical Chemistry of Macromolecules*, p. 417, Wiley, New York.

Taylor, C. E., 1972, Transmission of viruses by nematodes, in: *Principles and Techniques in Plant Virology* (C. I. Kado and H. O. Agrawal, eds.), pp. 226–247, Van Nostrand Reinhold, New York.

Taylor, R. H., Smith, P. R., Reinganum, C., and Gibbs, A. J., 1968, Purification and properties of broad bean wilt virus, *Aust. J. Biol. Sci.* **21**:929.

Tollin, P., and Wilson, H. R., 1971, Some observations on the structure of the Campinas strain of tobacco rattle virus, *J. Gen. Virol.* **3**:433.

Tsuchizaki, T., 1975, Mulberry ringspot virus, in: *CMI/AAB Descriptions of Plant Viruses* (A. J. Gibbs, B. D. Harrison, and A. F. Murant, eds.), No. 142, Commonwealth Mycological Institute, Kew.

Tsuchizaki, T., Hibino, H., and Saito, Y., 1975, The biological functions of short and long particles of soil-borne wheat mosaic virus, *Phytopathology* **65**:523.

Valenta, V., and Gressnerova, M., 1966, Serological relationships among members of the cowpea mosaic virus group, *Acta Virol.* **10**:182.

Valenta, V., and Marcinka, K., 1968, Enhanced infectivity of combined bottom and middle components of red clover mottle virus, *Acta Virol. (Prague)* **12**:288.

van der Scheer, C., and Groenewegen, J., 1971, Structure in cells of *Vigna unguiculata* infected with cowpea mosaic virus, *Virology* **46**:493.

van Hoof, H. A., 1970, Some observations on retention of tobacco rattle virus in nematodes, *Neth. J. Plant Pathol.* **76**:329.

van Kammen, A., 1967, Purification and properties of the components of cowpea mosaic virus, *Virology* **31**:633.

van Kammen, A., 1968, The relationship between the components of cowpea mosaic virus. I. Two ribonucleoprotein particles necessary for the infectivity of CPMV, *Virology* **34**:312.

van Kammen, A., 1972, Plant viruses with a divided genome, *Annu. Rev. Phytopathol.* **10**:125.

van Kammen, A., and van Griensven, L. J. L. D., 1970, The relationship between the components of cowpea mosaic virus. II. Further characterization of the nucleoprotein components of CPMV, *Virology* **41**:274.

Walkey, D. G. A., and Webb, M. J. W., 1970, Tubular inclusion bodies in plants infected with viruses of the NEPO type, *J. Gen. Virol.* **7**:159.

Walkey, D. G. A., Stace-Smith, R., and Tremaine, J. A., 1973, Serological, physical and chemical properties of strains of cherry leaf roll virus, *Phytopathology* **63**:566.

Walters, H. J., 1969, Bettle transmission of plant viruses, *Adv. Virus Res.* **15**:339.

White, R. F., Kassanis, B., and Woods, R. D., 1973, Isopycnic banding of strains of radish mosaic virus in rubidium bromide solutions, *J. Gen. Virol.* **20**:387.

Whitfeld, P. R., and Higgins, T. J. V., 1976, Occurrence of short particles in beans infected with the cowpea strain of TMV. I. Purification and characterization of the short particles, *Virology* **71**:471.

Whitney, W. K., and Gilmer, R. M., 1974, Insect vectors of cowpea mosaic virus in Nigeria, *Ann. Appl. Biol.* **77**:17.

Wilson, H. R., Tollin, P., and Rahman, A., 1975, RNA conformation in rod-shaped viruses: A possible molecular model for RNA in Narcissus mosaic virus, *J. Theor. Biol.* **53**:327.

Wood, H. A., 1971, Buoyant density changes of cowpea mosaic virus components at different pH values, *Virology* **43**:511.

Wood, H. A., 1972, Genetic complementation between the two nucleoprotein components of cowpea mosaic virus, *Virology* **49**:592.

Wood, H. A., and Bancroft, J. B., 1965, Activation of a plant virus by related incomplete nucleoprotein particles, *Virology* **27**:94.

Wu, G.-J., and Bruening, G., 1971, Two proteins from cowpea mosaic virus, *Virology* **46**:596.

Yang, A. F., and Hamilton, R. I., 1974, The mechanism of seed transmission of tobacco ringspot virus in soybean, *Virology* **62**:26.

Zabel, P., Weenen-Swaans, H., and van Kammen, A., 1974, *In vitro* replication of cowpea mosaic virus RNA. I. Isolation and properties of the membrane-bound replicase, *J. Virol.* **14**:1049.

Zabel, P., Jongen-Neven, I., and van Kammen, A., 1976, *In vitro* replication of cowpea mosaic virus RNA. II. Solubilization of membrane-bound replicase and the partial purification of the solubilized enzyme, *J. Virol.* **17**:679.

Zinder, N. D., 1975, (ed.), *RNA Phages*, Cold Spring Harbor Laboratory, Cold Spring Harbor, N.Y.

CHAPTER 3

Defective and Satellite Plant Viruses

Joseph G. Atabekov

Department of Virology
and
Laboratory of Bioorganic Chemistry
Moscow State University and Academy of Agricultural Sciences
Moscow, U.S.S.R.

1. INTRODUCTION

By the term "complete virus" or "normal virus," we imply a virus capable of infecting susceptible cells and of replicating to yield progeny of infective particles. It is assumed that a normal virus is capable of performing certain functions thereby inducing production of new proteins in the infected cell which are essential for virus replication.

Two types of products arising due to virus infection and expression of viral genetic information can be considered: (1) virus-specific (or virus-coded) proteins, i.e., the proteins coded by the viral genome, and (2) virus-induced proteins, i.e., the proteins coded by the cell genome but appearing after virus infection. It can be assumed that the synthesis of virus-induced proteins is either stimulated or derepressed by infection. This may be exemplified with interferon formation in virus-infected animal cells.

The genome of certain RNA-containing viruses, e.g., RNA bacteriophage codes for three virus-specific proteins, each of which is essential for the production of normal progeny. Assuming that each of the virus-specific proteins is indispensable for viral RNA replication and/or formation of complete mature virus particles, it may be expected that a change in any gene resulting in a lack of virus-specific and functional protein production will lead to abortive infection, i.e., transformation of a normal virus to a defective one. One can assume that the defective virus possesses a complete set of genes required for replication, but that one (or more) of them is mutationally changed. On the other hand, the term "deficient virus" usually connotes a virus with incomplete genome, i.e., a virus in which part of the genetic information required for replication is missing. It is quite clear that deficient viruses cannot multiply alone, but must depend on another virus which codes for the products which the deficient virus cannot induce by itself.

One more possibility should be anticipated, namely, when a defective virus contains a complete set of genes similar to that of the wild-type virus but the mutation(s) affects the expression of some part of the viral genome [e.g., the translation of some gene(s) becomes impossible]. Formally, such a virus should be grouped with the defectives, although this results in the absence of a relevant virus-coded product, which is equivalent to the absence of a gene in the genome of the deficient virus. This hypothetical example illustrates how tentative is the classification of "defective" and "deficient" viruses. Furthermore, a deficient virus is defective in a sense, as infection may be abortive. Thus I do not regard the subdivision of nonfunctional viruses into "defective" and "deficient" as terminologically advantageous, and will hereafter use only the term "defective virus."

To describe those functions of a virus which, if lacking, may render it defective, the possibility of existence of so-called nontranslatable nucleotide sequences in viral RNA must be considered. Examination of the primary structure of bacteriophage RNAs has shown that an appreciable part of the polynucleotide chain is not translated directly into protein. It is more or less clear now that at least part of the nontranslated sequences serve as the sites recognized by appropriate virus-specific proteins or by ribosomes in the course of translation and replication of viral RNA. Presumably, part of the nontranslated regions of bacteriophage RNA will create a specific secondary structure at certain regions of the molecule essential for the performance of a definite function. The role of the nontranslated regions of mRNA, however, is speculative. Nevertheless, it may be assumed that RNAs of different viruses, including plant viruses, have nontranslated regions, and that a mutational alteration in such regions may make it impossible to perform the function of that sequence, thus leading to formation of a virus defective in this function. In other words, it may be possible that defective viruses exist in nature whose defectiveness results from an alteration not in a structural gene but in nontranslated regions of the viral RNA.

Defectiveness of a virus can appear at different stages of infection depending on which of the virus-coded products is defective. A majority of defective plant viruses described so far carry the defect in their coat protein gene leading to inability of the coat protein to be assembled with viral RNA to yield normal virions (see below).

It should be emphasized that not only grouping of one or another virus with *defective* or *deficient* ones but also its classification as *normal* is quite tentative. For example, tobacco mosaic virus (TMV) infective for tobacco can be regarded as defective in nonhost plants, e.g., cereals. It was reported (Dodds and Hamilton, 1972; Hamilton and Dodds, 1970) that TMV replication can be activated in barley plants by a certain strain of barley stripe mosaic virus (BSMV). Therefore, it can be suggested that BSMV complements TMV in mixedly infected barley cells, compensating for its defectiveness under these conditions.

On the other hand, it cannot be excluded that even such a classically defective virus as the satellite of tobacco necrosis virus (STNV, see below) may turn out to be infective and act as a normal virus in some plant.

Until recently, virologists were inclined to regard as defective those viruses with a "divided" or "segmented" genome, i.e., with the genome consisting of two or more fragments, each containing only part of the genetic information of the virus and enclosed in a physically independent and usually noninfectious particle. The replication of the entire virus genome (the total of all RNA fragments) is subject to mutual complementation of genome fragments, each of which is noninfective by itself (see Chapters 1 and 2 of this volume).

Obviously, the specific infectivity of viruses with fragmented genomes will be less than that of a virus containing a single full complement of genome (TMV RNA), since the probability of simultaneous entrance of all fragments in an infected cell decreases with an increasing number of genome fragments. Will it be correct on this basis to regard viruses having a fragmented genome as defective? Probably not, for nature probably had sound reasons to let such viruses survive in time even though they possessed certain characteristics which may seem to be disadvantageous.

Likewise, a comparative description of many other properties of plant viruses may be considered. For example, it is well known that some plant viruses are capable of multiplication in the generative cells of host plants, whereas others are not. This may be regarded as sufficient ground in itself to consider the latter viruses as defectives. Thus the problem under discussion is frequently the result of subjective estimation of certain properties of a virus.

2. DEFECTIVE VIRUSES

Defective viruses are important tools in studies on the genome structure of many viruses and of the mechanisms responsible for the expression of their genetic information. A comparative study of a defective virus and the wild type gives an idea of the function performed by the protein product of the respective gene.

Except for the conditionally lethal viruses, identification of defective viruses and their isolation and subculturing inevitably are fraught with technical difficulties. The possibility of selection of conditionally lethal mutants among plant viruses, however, has so far been confined only to temperature-sensitive strains.

Defectiveness of a virus may be manifested as interruption of its reproduction at some phase of the infection cycle, as decreased productivity of virus multiplication as compared to the normal virus, or as low specific infectivity of the progeny virus.

2.1. Productivity of Virus Infection

Different strains of a virus vary in the amount of virus progeny they yield (Veldee and Fraenkel-Conrat, 1962). TMV strains differ greatly in this respect, but it is important that common TMV turns out to be much more productive than many of its chemically induced mutants. When nitrous acid-treated TMV was assayed on a local lesion host, it was found that some of the local lesions contained no transmittable virus (the "miss" phenomenon discussed by Siegel, 1965). As was noted by Matthews (1970), almost all chemically induced mutant viruses can be regarded as defective in the sense that they are incapable of multiplying as efficiently as the parent strain. Apparently, different mutational alterations can cause a decrease in virus productivity, with ensuing unfavorable changes at different stages of virus multiplication.

Productivity of the virus is an inherited characteristic, yet the degree of productivity of unrelated viruses can hardly be held as a criterion for the assessment of a virus as normal or defective. For example, the productivity of turnip yellow mosaic virus (0.5–2.0 mg/g fresh weight) markedly exceeds that of barley yellow dwarf virus (BYDV) (usually less than 100 μg/liter juice) (Rochow, 1970), yet this is hardly indicative of BYDV being defective.

2.2. Specific Infectivity of the Virus

Specific infectivity (infectivity per unit weight) may vary widely in different viruses depending on the sensitivity of the host plant and the properties of the virus. Different strains of the same virus may vary in their specific infectivity for a given host. For example, on *Nicotiana glutinosa,* the cowpea strain of TMV produced about 10 times more local lesions than the bean strain (Bawden and Pirie, 1956). Similarly, TMV-HR appears to be much less infectious than common TMV (Fraenkel-Conrat and Singer, 1957).

The reasons for the lower infectivity of some virus strains are obscure, but it seems possible that some peculiarities of the coat protein may be responsible. This is in agreement with the observations of Fraenkel-Conrat and Singer (1957), who showed the differences in the infectivity of common TMV and TMV-HR strain to reflect differences in the properties of their coat proteins. The specific infectivity of hybrid virus particles mixedly reassembled from HR RNA and common TMV protein was several times higher than the infectivity of HR itself. Therefore, the low infectivity of HR (which seems to be indicative of the relative defectiveness of this virus) must be due to an aberrant functional behavior of HR coat protein during initial stages of infection (adsorption, uncoating).

Some further indications of the indefinite and tentative meaning of the concept of virus defectiveness come from the studies of BSMV. The specific infectivity of BSMV for *Chenopodium amaranticolor* (Coste) Reyn is much lower than that of TMV. Purified preparations of BSMV frequently possess little or no infectivity (Atabekov and Novikov, 1966, 1971), inasmuch as some variants of BSMV become difficult or even impossible to transfer by sap inoculations (McKinney and Greeley, 1965). Therefore, at least some isolates of BSMV could be regarded as being defective in comparison to such highly infective viruses as TMV.

However, when the RNAs were isolated from the low-infectivity or completely noninfective BSMV, they were invariably infectious (Atabekov and Novikov, 1966, 1971). These data suggest that inability of some BSMV preparations to infect *Ch. amaranticolor* is due to changes in its coat protein structure which render it unable to perform certain functions at initial infection stages. This initial barrier can be overcome by the use of free BSMV RNA as an inoculum (for review, see Atabekov, 1975).

The foregoing discussion has dealt with cases where the infectivity of virus particles was low or lacking, although the virus was potentially infective, possessing a complete genome. Certain cases of the production of viruslike particles containing incomplete viral RNA will be discussed below.

2.3. Defective Particles in Preparations of Normal Viruses

Defective virus particles probably occur in the preparation of any virus. Many or even all animal viruses produce defective particles when repeatedly passed at high multiplicity. Huang and Baltimore (1970) list the following properties of biologically active, defective animal virus particles: (1) they contain normal structural protein(s); (2) they contain only part of the normal viral genome (i.e., are deficient); (3) they are not infective by themselves but can replicate in the presence of a helper virus; and (4) they interfere with homologous normal virus. Therefore, the defective particles of this kind were named "defective interfering" (DI) particles (see their chapters in Volume 10 of this series).

It was suggested by Huang and Baltimore (1970) that DI particles play a significant role in viral diseases. Poliovirus DI particles have been isolated and described (Cole *et al.*, 1971; Cole and Baltimore, 1973*a*). These particles lack about 15% of the poliovirus genome, carrying a deletion in the part of the RNA molecule coding for the structural proteins. The DI particles need the functional help of normal particles in the infected cell to yield progeny DI particles. In cells infected by DI, only capsid proteins are missing, other poliovirus-specific polypeptides being found (Cole and Baltimore, 1973*a,b*).

It seems logical to suggest that, upon plant virus infection, defective particles generally similar to DI particles of animal viruses may be produced. Thus purified preparations of any plant virus may contain a certain amount of noninfective incomplete particles, the origin of which remains unclear.

2.3.1. Incomplete Particles of Turnip Yellow Mosaic Virus (TYMV)

During the fractionation of TYMV preparations in density gradients, a set of noninfective nucleoprotein particles and empty shells (top component) were found in addition to the normal virus. The properties of these particles were described in detail by Matthews in his reviews (Matthews and Ralph, 1966; Matthews, 1970). The noninfective nucleoprotein particles and top component appeared to be identical in structure and antigenic specificity to intact infectious virus.

It was suggested by Matthews and Ralph (1966) that all minor fractions of noninfective TYMV nucleoprotein "represent abortive virus synthesis." Despite the fact that these noninfectious virus-like nucleoprotein particles were described many years ago, it is still not evident whether or not they can replicate in an infected cell with the help of complete TYMV. Consequently, their similarity to the DI particles described by Huang and Baltimore (1970) cannot be ascertained. Their presence, however, is not necessary for the replication of normal TYMV.

2.3.2. Satellite Virus of Tobacco Ringspot Virus

Tobacco ringspot virus (TRSV) preparations yield three individual zones upon centrifugation in sucrose density gradients, designated as top, middle, and bottom components. Top component lacks RNA and has a sedimentation coefficient of 53 S. Middle nucleoprotein component contains 28% RNA with reported s values of 91–94 S. Bottom component contains 42% RNA and its sedimentation coefficient is about 126–128 S (Stace-Smith *et al.*, 1965; Schneider and Diener, 1966).

Middle component contains 24 S RNA with a molecular weight of 1.4×10^6. Bottom component consists of two types of particles, one containing 32 S infectious RNA (molecular weight 2.3×10^6) and the second containing two molecules of 24 S RNA per particle (Diener and Schneider, 1966). These two particles differ from each other in buoyant density (Schneider *et al.*, 1972a).

The 32 S RNA is infectious and constitutes a complete TRSV genome. Partial homology was revealed in the nucleotide sequence between the 24 S RNA from the middle and bottom components (Rezaian and Francki, 1974). However, the main part of the nucleotide sequences differed in the 32 S and 24 S RNA molecules. Therefore, the 24 S RNA molecules are not the precursors of 32 S full-length RNA (Rezaian and Francki, 1974).

The actual principles of the TRSV genome arrangement and function are not clear. In accordance with the observations of Harrison *et al.* (1973), this virus may have a divided genome. The authors showed that the infectivity of the large RNA was increased by the addition of the small RNA, which was not infective by itself. They suggested that these two types of TRSV RNA "carry different pieces of genetic information." All three TRSV components have seemingly identical isometric protein capsids composed of the same protein (Schneider *et al.*, 1972a) (see Chapter 2 for further discussion of this virus).

An additional component was found in the virus preparations isolated from TRSV-infected bean plants (Schneider, 1969, 1971). In shape, size, and antigenicity, the new particles were indistinguishable from TRSV. In contrast to TRSV, however, these particles were not infectious by themselves, but were capable of replicating in the presence of normal TRSV and were thus originally called "satellite-like" (Schneider, 1969) and later called "satellite" of TRSV (S-TRSV) (Schneider *et al.*, 1972a). S-TRSV represents a heterologous population of particles distinguishable by their buoyant density value and sedimentation properties (Schneider, 1971; Schneider *et al.*, 1972a). These S-TRSV particles contain within their capsid numerous short, single-stranded RNA molecules sedimenting at 7.3 S (Schneider, 1969, 1971; Schneider *et al.*, 1972a). The heterogeneity of S-TRSV is due to the unequal numbers of RNA molecules encapsidated in different particles in a S-TRSV population. The molecular weight estimates for S-TRSV RNA fell within the range of $0.77-1.25 \times 10^5$ in different analyses (Schneider, 1969, 1971; Schneider *et al.*, 1972a; Diener and Smith, 1973; Sogo *et al.*, 1974).

The 7 S RNA fragments contained by a S-TRSV particle have approximately the same size but not necessarily identical genetic information, and possibly there may be different sets of 7 S fragments. At present, it is evident that at least part of these small strands are biologically active, i.e., capable of replicating in the presence of TRSV genome. Under conditions of mixed infection, S-TRSV interferes with the replication of normal TRSV, and the progeny of mixed infection can predominantly be S-TRSV particles (Schneider, 1969, 1971).

The presence of S-TRSV was not apparent in the original STRV preparations used in the experiments (Schneider and Diener, 1966; Diener and Schneider, 1966). The actual origin of S-TRSV remains obscure. Schneider (1969, 1971) and Schneider *et al.* (1972a) suggested that S-TRSV possibly originated from TRSV during the period of experimentation; i.e., its formation in the stocks of the virus is a "recent event" (Schneider, 1969, 1971). If this suggestion is correct, the appearance of S-TRSV can be tentatively regarded as an example of the production of defective interfering particles in the culture of a plant virus. The key question remaining to be answered is whether or not there is homology between the nucleic acid(s) of S-TRSV and a portion of the genome of the TRSV from which it may be derived.

The RNA of S-TRSV does not code for its own coat protein, since the S-TRSV capsid is identical with that of the helper TRSV strain (Schneider, 1972; Schneider *et al.,* 1972*b*; Schneider and White, 1976). In this respect, this system differs from the classical case of the interaction of the satellite of tobacco necrosis virus (STNV) with its helper, tobacco necrosis virus (TNV) (see below).

2.3.3. Fragments of Helical Viruses

The process of isolation of rod-shaped virus particles from an infected cell is inevitably accompanied by their fragmentation. These fragments contain only part of the RNA genome, and are probably defective. Elucidation of the origin of such particles in virus stocks faces serious difficulties. No definite answers can be given to the questions of whether the particles shorter than normal length play any part in the replication and whether they are formed in appreciable amounts during the infection or appear only after cell destruction and virus isolation.

The results of Hulett and Loring (1965) and Francki (1966) suggest that short, noninfective TMV fragments can contribute to the process of infection, i.e., that their genetic information can be expressed in the infected cell in the presence of normal TMV rods. Random fragments found in the preparations of rod-shaped viruses (such as TMV, potato virus X) probably contain different pieces from different parts of the RNA molecule and carry different sets of genes (or portions of genes). It can hardly be expected that the majority of random fragments of viral RNA are efficiently translated or replicated in the infected cell, considering the well-known high specificity of the interaction of ribosomes with the regions of initiation of RNA translation and the template specificity of RNA replicase. In other words, it seems unlikely that the products of random fragmentation of viral RNA will be able to replicate in the infected cell. Yet, it cannot be excluded that some fragments present in purified preparations of such virus as TMV may replicate in the presence of intact virus, and be considered as DI particles. Reports indicate that the cowpea strain of

TMV carries short rods containing the coat protein gene besides the full-length particles (Morris, 1974; Bruening *et al.*, 1976) (see Chapter 4).

2.4. Peculiarities of Winter Wheat Mosaic Virus Infection

Almost 40 years ago, a cereal disease caused by winter wheat mosaic virus (WWMV) was described (Zashurilo and Sitnikova, 1939). WWMV is not mechanically transmissible, although it is transmissible by leafhoppers. Suckov (1943) reported that needlelike crystals (believed to be composed of virus particles) may be isolated from plant extracts of WWMV-infected wheat, oat, and millet. It appeared later that the paracrystals isolated from the infected plants contained only the WWMV-protein antigen but not any nucleic acid (Atabekov *et al.*, 1968).

The needlelike crystals of WWMV antigen are made up of individual fibrillar structures. WWMV protein can exist in a number of molecular forms, depending on solvent conditions: (1) globular form—a protein subunit $s_{20,w}^0 = 2$ S; (2) aggregate 5 S; (3) fibrillar form—a linear aggregate of protein monomers; or (4) helical form—an aggregate form of helically packed subunits (rodlike particles with helical structure and internal hole). The polymerization of WWMV protein is reversible, and all the aggregates can be dissociated into 2 S monomers (Atabekov *et al.*, 1968).

The functional significance of different forms of WWMV protein is not yet clear. We cannot ascertain that *in vitro* aggregation of WWMV protein is correlated with the assembly of virus particles, as the structure of the WWMV particles is not known. Nevertheless, the similarity of the helical form of WWMV protein aggregates to the structure of several known viruses and the high concentration of this protein in infected plants suggest that a viruslike structure is reassembled when WWMV protein repolymerizes.

Numerous attempts to find viruslike particles in the extracts or in the ultrathin sections of WWMV-infected millet leaves have failed so far.* Thus it may be concluded that systemically infected millet plants that contain large amounts of WWMV antigen do not contain any

---

* Razvjazkina *et al.* (1968) found viruslike bacilliform particles in WWMV-infected wheat plants. However, this is not sufficient grounds for identification of these particles as WWMV virions. Contamination of WWMV infection by some other virus(es) was not excluded since the virus stock was taken from field infected plants. Besides, the bacilliform particles were absent from WWMV-infected millet plants.

virions. This leads us to suggest that WWMV is a defective virus, yet additional work is needed to obtain insight into WWMV infection.

2.5. Missense Mutations and Nonfunctionality of the Virus-Coded Products (Defective and Temperature-Sensitive Phenotypes)

The functionality of a protein molecule depends on its unique conformation, and relatively fine variations of the secondary and tertiary structure of a polypeptide chain are reflected in its functional activity (e.g., enzymatic activity, capability of assembly into a correct quaternary structure). The slightest changes in the primary structure of a protein may also affect its activity and conformational stability.

It is widely accepted that the functionally active conformation of a protein can be altered into a nonfunctional state *in vivo* (as well as *in vitro*) by changes in the environmental conditions, and that different proteins vary in the degree of their stability in respect to particular factors (e.g., temperature).

The natural strains of a virus are usually superior in that they are more stable than its mutants induced by artificial mutagenesis. Natural selection seems to ensure stability of the major strain(s) in a population of virus particles, generally discriminating these from the mutants defective in some virus-specific function.

Mutational changes in the viral genome leading to the formation of a defective virus-specific protein may be expressed differently: (1) conformational changes in the virus protein (the defective product of the mutated gene) are so pronounced that the protein loses its solubility and forms an insoluble precipitate *in vivo*; (2) conformational changes brought about by a mutation render the virus-coded protein nonfunctional, although it remains soluble; (3) the defective protein remains soluble and is apparently functional under certain conditions only. However, it is made nonfunctional under slightly changed conditions, nonpermissive for this mutant but not for the wild-type virus.

The aforementioned mutations are assigned to missense mutations. Nonsense mutations common in bacteria have not been found in eukaryotic organisms so far. A mutation rendering the virus defective may, seemingly, arise in any of the genes essential for the replication of the virus. However, most easily identified are the mutations of the coat protein gene, which can be detected by several tests including serological analysis and/or the direct analysis of the amino acid content (or sequence) of the coat protein.

2.5.1. Coat Protein Mutants of TMV

The bulk of the information on defective plant viruses is available from studies of different TMV strains. Assuming that the entire TMV RNA molecule (molecular weight about 2×10^6) contains translatable genetic information, then the TMV genome could code for about nine to twelve small-size proteins. Yet until now, only three functional genes in the TMV genome have been identified.

1. It is more or less clear that the TMV genome must contain a separate gene (or perhaps a group of genes) responsible for the local lesion production in *Nicotiana sylvestris* Speg and Comes. Common TMV produces a systemic reaction in *N. sylvestris,* but many nitrous acid-induced TMV mutants have acquired the ability of inducing local lesions in this host. Several years ago, localization of this local lesion gene in TMV RNA was studied by Kado and Knight (1966), who reported evidence that this gene was located in the 5'-terminal part comprising about 30% of the TMV RNA molecule.* This local lesion-inducing gene(s) is not indispensable for virus multiplication, and defective mutants can hardly arise from the mutation in this gene.

2. A RNA replicase gene is probably needed in the replication of viral RNA in a host cell. Clearly, mutations in this gene can be the reason for the defectivity of a plant virus.

3. Obviously, a relatively small part of the TMV genome is engaged in the coding for coat protein; 474 nucleotides out of the total of 6300 residues in TMV RNA should be involved in the coding for the 158 amino acid residues of the coat protein of common TMV strain. If the coat protein has no other functions besides the structural one, then a mutation in this gene does not seem to have much influence on the expression of other viral genes. In the absence of the active structural protein, the RNA of many viruses can replicate, yielding infective daughter RNA molecules, yet it remains unprotected from the action of ribonucleases (RNases) in the cell sap. Hence the infective principle is unstable in the absence of the coat protein. Various forms of "defective" mutations in the coat protein gene are described below.

---

* It now appears probable that this gene is located in the 3'-terminal third (see Chapter 4).

Siegel *et al.* (1962) isolated two unusual mutants of TMV which were defective in the capacity to produce mature TMV particles. No viruslike nucleoprotein particles could be isolated from the infected plants. The cells infected by these mutants contained infective viral RNA unprotected (or incorrectly protected) by the coat protein. These coat protein mutants were designated as "PM2" and "PM1."

The symptoms produced by different defective TMV mutants are essentially similar. The primary symptoms appear as chlorotic spots at initial infection sites approximately a week after inoculation. The defective mutants move slowly from cell to cell and usually are confined to the inoculated leaves. Yellow spots increase in size and develop preferentially in the regions along the veins. Systemic spread of infection from the lower to upper leaves occurs very slowly (Siegel *et al.*, 1962; Sarkar, 1967; Kapitsa *et al.*, 1969c; Bhalla and Sehgal, 1973). In Samsun tobacco, systemic movement of defective mutants causes vein clearing, yellow mottle, and typical oakleaf patterns.

2.5.1a. Soluble Coat Protein Mutants

In soluble coat protein mutants, the coat protein is unable to copolymerize with the infectious virus RNA, but remains soluble. Several defective TMV strains belonging to this group have been described: PM2 (Siegel *et al.*, 1962; Zaitlin and McCaughey, 1965), Ni 2204 (Jockusch, 1966b,c), PM5 (Hariharasubramanian and Siegel, 1967, 1969), PM6 (Hubert and Zaitlin, 1972), and the so-called Turin strain (Kassanis and Conti, 1971). The defective TMV mutant reported by Bhalla and Sehgal (1973) also falls in this category. In all these cases, the virus coat protein can be isolated from the infected cells by an ingenious procedure (Siegel *et al.*, 1962; Zaitlin and McCaughey, 1965; Hariharasubramanian and Siegel, 1969) based on its partially retained ability of reversible pH-dependent polymerization–depolymerization. The protein soluble in the pH 7.0 phosphate buffer remains in the supernatant after centrifugation at 100,000g for 30–60 min and can be polymerized at about pH 5.0, forming aggregates readily sedimented upon centrifugation. Several repeating cycles of polymerization at pH 5.0 and clarification at pH 7.0 by centrifugation enable one to obtain a purified preparation of defective coat protein (Zaitlin and McCaughey, 1965).

The changes in polypeptide chain conformation of the coat protein caused by amino acid replacements can manifest themselves by unusual polymerization and anomalous macromolecular aggregate formation *in vitro* and *in vivo*. It was originally reported by Zaitlin and Ferris (1964) that instead of normal TMV-like aggregates with a helical structure the PM2 protein polymerizes *in vitro* into open single- and double-helical aggregates, as visualized by electron microscopy. Examination of the fine structure of these aggregates (Siegel *et al.*, 1966) revealed that they exist in several different forms. The forms of the PM2 protein aggregates produced *in vitro* upon polymerization at pH 5.2 are as follows: (1) *Single helices*. It can be seen from Fig. 1a that aggregation of the protein leads to the formation of groups of closely packed helices and separate single helices of the same pitch (20–29 nm). The diameter of the helices in the closely packed groups was 12 nm. (2) *Double helices* consisting of two tightly packed single strands (Fig. 1b). It was suggested by Siegel *et al.* (1966) that such structures would not be produced by the combination of two preformed single helices and that different types of aggregates would be initiated upon polymerization of defective protein either as single or as double helices. (3) *Double-double helices* seemingly consisting of two double helices plectonemically coiled (Fig. 1c,d).

The preparations obtained by dipping epidermal strips of the infected plant into negative stain contained long crystal-like structures consisting of tightly packed single helices (Siegel *et al.*, 1966). The authors claimed these structures to correspond to PM2 protein aggregates formed *in vivo* in PM2-infected cells. Using optical phase microscopy, Bald (1964) observed in PM2-infected cells some unusual inclusions resembling striate loops and needles. These inclusions appear similar to the crystal-like aggregates of single helices reported by Siegel *et al.* (1966). Thus two amino acid replacements in the PM2 polypeptide chain give rise to a protein subunit which polymerizes into an open rather than into a compact TMV helix. Besides the anomalous aggregation properties, PM2 protein can be differentiated antigenically from the common strain; at least this was the case with PM2 protein in the depolymerized form (Rappaport and Zaitlin, 1967).

As mentioned above, the coat protein defectiveness could be due to widely different amino acid substitutions, and the proteins of different mutants might differ markedly in their degree of defectiveness. The coat protein of the PM2 series mutants is soluble but is nonfunctional in the sense that it is not capable of forming stable nucleoprotein rods.

Despite the defectiveness of PM2 protein, a small but significant part of the infectious material remains viable in the homogenates of PM2-infected leaves after incubation at 30–37°C for about 1 h (Siegel

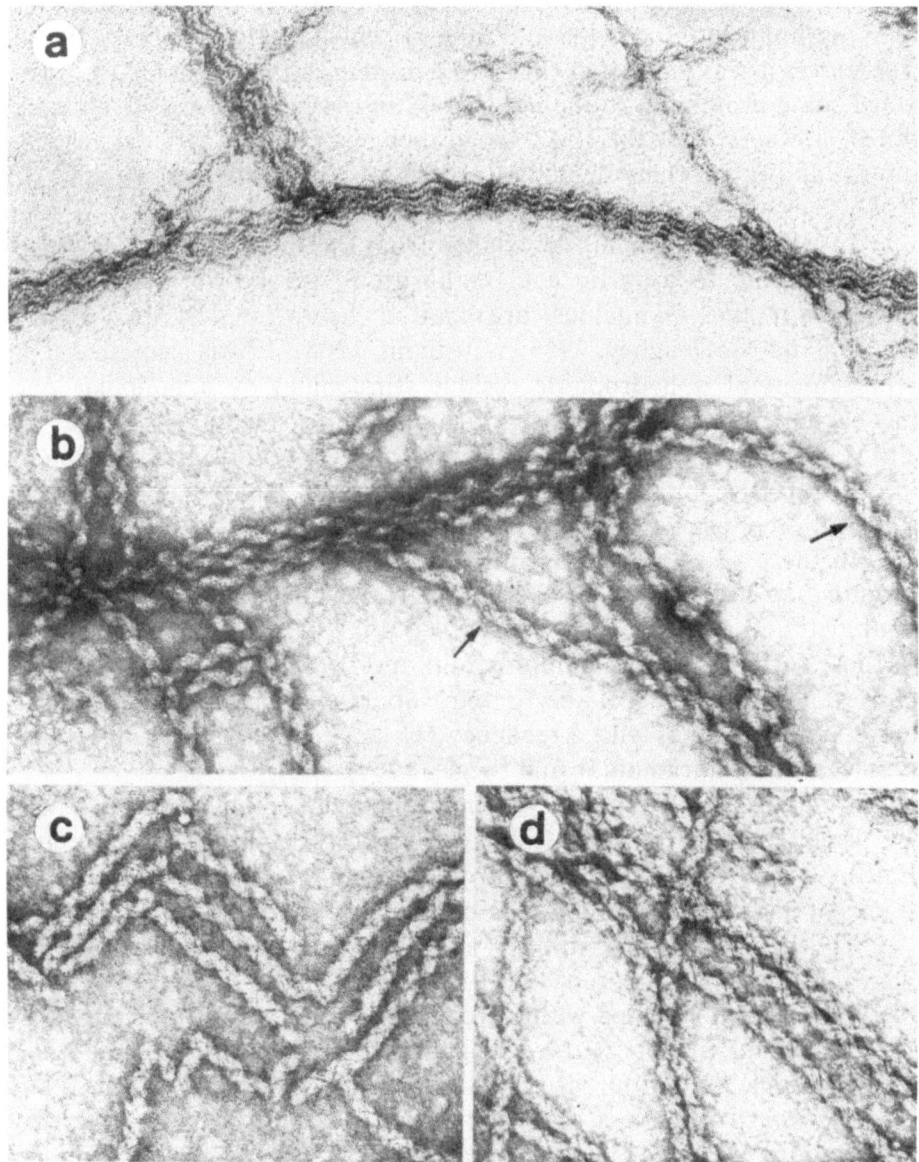

Fig. 1. Aggregates of PM2 protein formed *in vitro*. a: Closely packed groups of single helices. Double helices are also seen. b: Double helices. Arrows point to regions of distinct doubleness. c,d: Double-double helices shown under two different staining conditions. Regions of double helix are also visible. ×200,000. Courtesy of R. Markham from Siegel *et al.* (1966).

et al., 1962; Sarkar and Jockusch, 1968). The infective material was associated with some "coarse particles" of the cell homogenate sedimenting upon low-speed (8000–12,000*g*) centrifugation (Sarkar, 1967). Therefore, it was suggested that PM2 protein, although defective, provided some protection to the viral RNA in the infected cell. It must be noted, however, that the PM2 group includes mutants differing widely in the ability of their defective protein to copolymerize with TMV RNA.

In PM2 coat protein, the change from threonine to isoleucine and from glutamic to aspartic acid at positions 28 and 95, respectively, resulted in the anomalous aggregation behavior described above (Zaitlin and McCaughey, 1965; Wittmann, 1965). It was suggested that replacement of a hydrophilic residue (threonine) by a nonpolar one (isoleucine) would be more significant for the structural changes of TMV protein subunits and transformation of the normal coat protein into a defective one (Zaitlin and McCaughey, 1965) than would the substitution of aspartic for glutamic acid.

In the case of the PM5 mutant, a single amino acid replacement (arginine to cysteine at position 112) in the coat protein rendered it nonfunctional. PM5 protein produced rodlike particles roughly similar to those formed by the common strain upon polymerization at pH 5.1. However, the packing of the protein subunits in these aggregates was loose and imperfect, with a tendency for stacked-disk structure formation (Hariharasubramanian and Siegel, 1969).

Another defective strain with nonfunctional soluble protein, PM6, was isolated after nitrous acid treatment of U1-TMV (Hubert and Zaitlin, 1972). The PM6 coat protein could aggregate *in vitro* into stacks of disks without production of helical rodlike particles.

The defectiveness is still less marked in the mutant described by Sehgal (1973). This mutant was isolated from the progeny of TMV RNA (strain U1) treated with nitrous acid. Unlike the PM1 and PM2 strains, the mutant reported by Sehgal (1973) was capable of producing a considerable amount of virus particles. The productivity of this strain was, however, much less than that of the parent strain. The purified preparations of this mutant contained 3.5% RNA on the average instead of 5% as in normal TMV. The bulk of the preparation consisted of particles shorter than TMV carrying fragmented RNA, but the infectivity was associated only with the particles of the same buoyant density as the parental strain. The polypeptide chain of this mutant possessed three replacements as compared to the parental strain. The mutant contained two extra arginines and one glycine but lacked one residue of glutamic acid (or glutamine), serine, and threonine. Sehgal

(1973) concluded that the heterogeneity of the mutant preparations resulted from *in vitro* fragmentation of the mutant during purification. The mutant particles were considerably more sensitive to thermal and urea denaturation than the parental strain. These observations indicate that the mutant does not form a sufficiently stable nucleoprotein complex upon assembly, which may be due to the partially denatured state of the mutant protein. Thus a considerable amount of "free" coat protein accumulates in the mutant-infected cells. This protein is either inactive in virus assembly, or if it is active there must be some other reason(s) for the low productivity of this TMV mutant. All these observations permit us to formally assign Sehgal's mutant to the group of defective TMV strains capable of producing soluble coat protein. In this case, however, the mutant protein retains at least partial ability to assemble, with viral RNA yielding fragile particles with a distinct tendency to break.

Several TMV strains have been described which possess low infectivity compared to the wild-type strain and which are only slightly more infective than PM2 (Kassanis and Woods, 1969). These viruses were defective because they occurred in negligible amounts in the infected cells and produced broken and abnormally short particles.

2.5.1b. Insoluble Coat Protein Mutants

When the first insoluble coat protein mutant (PM1) was described by Siegel *et al.* (1962), it was held that it did not produce structural protein since no virus antigen could be detected with the common serological tests. Using phase contrast microscopy, Bald (1964) found that the cytoplasm of PM1-infected cells contained gel-like masses not detected in healthy cells or in cells infected with nondefective TMV strains. It was thus suggested that the gel-like masses corresponded to PM1-coded defective coat protein.

Rappaport *et al.* (1964) succeeded in detecting virus-related antigen in PM1-infected plants, using antisera prepared against disaggregated TMV (U1) protein, and PM2 protein. Absorbing the antisera with extracts from PM1-infected plants produced considerable inhibition of the ability of these antisera to neutralize the infectivity of TMV (Table 1). It can be seen from Table 1 that antigenically active material was present in PM1- as well as in PM2-infected plants. The PM1 antigen could be detected using antisera to the proteins of TMV and PM2, but not by anti-TMV sera.

TABLE 1

Detection of a Virus-Related Antigen in Plants Infected with
Defective TMV Mutants[a]

Rabbit antiserum 1/1000	Absorbed with plant extract	Survival (%) of TMV upon reaction with absorbed serum
Anti-TMV protein	Healthy	8.6
	PM1 infected	24
	PM2 infected	100
Anti-PM2 protein	Healthy	21
	PM1 infected	100
	PM2 infected	100
Anti-TMV	Healthy	3.4
	PM1 infected	2.7
	PM2 infected	100

[a] Antisera to TMV protein, PM2 protein, and intact TMV were mixed with the indicated plant extracts. The mixtures were incubated at 37°C for 90 min and then at 2°C for 24 h followed by centrifugation at 105,000g for 30 min. The supernatant solutions of absorbed antisera were mixed with equal volumes of TMV (1 μg/ml) and the mixtures assayed for infectivity (Rappaport *et al.*, 1964).

With fluorescent antibody technique, Nagaraj (1965) arrived at essentially similar conclusions, although he reported existence of a weak reaction between PM1 antigen and anti-TMV serum. It follows from both reports that there is an antigenic relationship between TMV (or PM2) depolymerized protein and PM1 coat protein present in the infected plant cells in a denatured state. There is a very weak, if any, antigenic relationship between intact TMV and PM1 protein. Thus PM1 protein has no (or almost no) antigenic determinants in common with TMV protein subunits packed within intact TMV.

Insoluble and serologically active PM1 coat protein was shown to be associated with the leaf homogenate fraction sedimenting at 12,000g. The highly aggregated PM1 antigen was insoluble in sodium deoxycholate and Triton X-100, but could be at least partially solubilized when the infected leaves were homogenized in concentrated formic acid or in 67% acetic acid. The defective protein became insoluble again upon removal of the acetic acid (Parish and Zaitlin, 1966).

Several other defective TMV strains with properties generally similar to those of PM1 were reported, i.e., PM4 (Zaitlin and Keswani, 1964; Zaitlin and Hariharasubramanian, 1968), PM2I (Hariharasubramanian *et al.*, 1973), DM (Kapitsa *et al.*, 1969a,b), and the so-called English PM2 variant isolated by Kassanis and Bastow (1971a) from the original PM2. Recently, Sarkar isolated two spontaneous mutants,

TABLE 2

Amino Acid Analysis of the Insoluble, Defective Coat Proteins of TMV Mutants[a]

Amino acid	PM1 Subisolate D		PM4 Subisolate A		PM4 Subisolate C		PM21 Subisolate B	
	Integral Value	Change from TMV	Integral Value	Change from TMV	Integral Value	Change from TMV	Integral Value	Change from TMV
Cysteine[b]	—		1		1		—	
Aspartic acid	17	−1	17	−1	17	−1	17	−1
Threonine	15	−1	14	−2	14	−2	16	
Serine	16		14	−2	15	−1	16	
Glutamic	16		16		16		16	
Proline	8		8		8		8	
Glycine	7	+1	8	+2	8	+2	6	
Alanine	14		14		14		14	
Valine	14		13	−1	13	−1	14	
Isoleucine	9		9		9		8	−1
Leucine	13	+1	14	+2	13	+1	12	
Tyrosine	4		4		4		4	
Phenylalanine	8		8		8		8	
Lysine	3	+1	3	+1	3	+1	3	+1
Arginine	11		12	+1	12	+1	12	+1

[a] Values given relative to glutamic acid (16 residues/molecule). In all cases, the values for histidine and methionine were too small to measure accurately and were less than 0.1 residue/molecule. From Hariharasubramanian et al. (1973).
[b] Cysteine not determined in some mutants. Tryptophan not determined in all samples.

DT1 and DT2 (defective mutants of Tübingen), both producing insoluble coat protein (Sarkar, personal communication). The defective protein could in this case be solubilized in the presence of 0.1% SDS. The solution of the defective protein in 0.1% SDS was stable and could be centrifuged at 140,000g at room temperature for clarification.

A relatively simple procedure of extraction of purified preparations of the defective PM1 coat protein was proposed by Hariharasubramanian *et al.* (1973) on the basis of the above-described properties. Final purification was achieved by gel filtration of the protein solubilized in the presence of 0.1% SDS, with subsequent fractionation by electrophoresis in polyacrylamide gel. The major protein band was isolated from the gel and analyzed.

The results of amino acid analysis of several such protein preparations are presented in Table 2. These data show that subisolates A and C of PM4 strain have six and five amino acid replacements, respectively. On the other hand, it is well known that TMV mutants obtained by nitrous acid treatment have typically only one or two (and never more than three) amino acid replacements in the coat protein (Tsugita and Fraenkel-Conrat, 1962; Funatsu and Fraenkel-Conrat, 1974; Wittmann and Wittmann-Liebold, 1966). Zaitlin and Hariharasubramanian (1968) suggested that it is unlikely that the PM1 and PM4 mutants had been induced by nitrous acid, since the nature and the number of amino acid replacements in their coat proteins are inconsistent with the classical view of nitrous acid-induced mutagenesis. Nitrous acid treatment causes deamination of adenine to hypoxanthine, which may pair like G, and cytosine is converted into uracil ($C \rightarrow U$) (Schuster and Schramm, 1958; Siegel, 1965). Singer and Fraenkel-Conrat (1974) reported that about 90% of their observed amino acid substitutions resulting from nitrous acid-induced mutagenesis could be accounted for by $A \rightarrow G$ and $C \rightarrow U$ exchanges.

The nature of the amino acid replacements revealed in the coat protein of the insoluble defective strains (Table 2), however, is frequently inconsistent with this specificity of base conversion and resulting amino acid replacement as derived from the triplet genetic code. For example, the replacement of threonine by glycine, leucine, and arginine, as observed in the coat protein of subisolates A and C of PM4 and subisolate D of PM1, cannot be interpreted in terms of changes due to nitrous acid.

This concerns not only defective strains with insoluble coat protein but also strains of PM2 type. As mentioned in the foregoing, the coat protein of the mutant described by Sehgal (1973) possessed three amino acid replacements: it lacked glutamic acid (or glutamine), serine, and threonine, but contained two additional residues of arginine and one of glycine. The conversion of the Gln → Arg (CAA → CGA) and Ser → Gly (AGU → GGU) can be attributed to nitrous acid (A → G), but the Thr → Arg conversion (ACU, ACC, ACA, ACG codons for threonine and AGA, AGG, CGU, CGC, CGA, CGG codons for arginine) cannot. These observations led Sehgal (1973) to suggest that his mutant was not a nitrous acid-induced variant but occurred as a spontaneous contaminant in the original TMV-U1 population.

The replacement in PM2 of glutamic acid (coded by GAA or GAG) by aspartic acid (coded by GAU or GAC) also cannot result from nitrous acid treatment. Thus it seems probable that the origin of the mutants of the PM series may not be connected directly to nitrous acid treatment. Two alternatives of their origin were discussed by Hariharasubramanian *et al* (1973): (1) PM strains contaminate U1 isolates and survive through the nitrous acid treatment. This implies that contaminations of the U1 stock cannot be removed by passage of the virus through a local lesion at high dilution, which seems to be unlikely. (2) The genesis of PM strains could start from the original nitrous acid-induced mutation(s), with subsequent selection based on spontaneous mutations during subculturing.

More recently, a similar phenomenon was described by Bald *et al.* (1974) for two natural TMV strains. TMV strain U5 (*Nicotiana glauca* form of TMV) differs from U1 strain in several respects (namely, host range, symptoms produced in different hosts, amino acid content of the coat protein). Under certain conditions of culturing and several transfers of U1 in *N. glauca,* a strain indistinguishable from U5 was isolated. The newly isolated strain (M5) differed by 15 amino acid substitutions from U1-TMV and corresponded with natural U5 strain in its host range (Bald *et al.,* 1974). The authors considered a possible mechanism of U1 → U5 transition consisting of original mutations and the subsequent "process that allows exchange of information or alteration of the message, segregation of different variants and rigid selection among them by the host cells." In this process, some intermediate strains, unstable and similar to defective TMV strains of the PM series, might be produced. Clearly, the U1 → U5 transition not only includes the fundamental change in the coat protein gene but also involves the gene(s) responsible for host-range specificity (U5 is unable to infect tomato) and host reaction control.

Therefore, in both cases (PM mutants and M5) we have to deal with the unusual phenomenon of genetic transition which cannot represent a single mutation but rests on considerable changes in the viral genome. As suggested by Bald (1964), defective mutants produce "submutant" forms of TMV and "seem to be more subject of variation than TMV-U1, the parent strain."* In line with this concept, back mutations to normal TMV appear not to occur with PM1 and PM2 (Bald, 1964). This is also in agreement with the observations of Sehgal (1973), who noticed no reversions of his mutant to the wild-type parent strain during 6 years of culturing in plants (discussed above). Contrastingly, Hubert and Zaitlin (1972) reported conversions of defective PM6 mutant to the normal virus with functional coat protein. Thus the questions of the origin of defective mutants and their amino acid replacements remain obscure.

Quite clearly, different amino acid substitutions responsible for the coat protein defectiveness may or may not change its solubility properties. Insofar as the fine structural changes of the polypeptide chain of TMV protein rendering it nonfunctional as a result of different amino acid substitutions are concerned, these are purely speculative. The two so-called immutable regions in the coat protein gene (e.g., see Fraenkel-Conrat, 1969) code for the amino acid residues 87–95 and 113–122. It is noteworthy that the proteins of two defective strains of the PM2 series (PM2 and PM5) have substitutions just within the edge of one of the "immutable" regions (PM2 in position 95 and PM5 in position 112). Presumably, the coat protein molecule has certain sites in which amino acid substitutions render the protein defective.

Hariharasubramanian *et al.* (1973) suggested that the coat protein of the defective mutants of the PM1 series had extra positive charges as a result of substitution of neutral amino acids by lysine and arginine and a decrease in the aspartic acid content. Caspar (1963) postulated that two abnormally titrating groups in TMV protein would correspond with carboxyl–carboxylate pairs located in radii of 2.5 and 8.4 nm from the particle axis. The latter pair was supposed to function as a negative switch to control the virus protein aggregation into a helix (in the absence of RNA), thus playing a significant role in TMV assembly. This feature is common to different TMV strains (Butler and Durham, 1972), so it was reasonably suggested that defectiveness of the PM1 mutant protein was due to the lack of a carboxylic group at this critical position in the polypeptide chain (Hariharasubramanian *et al.*, 1973). In accordance with this suggestion, it was shown that the protein of

* *Editor's comment:* The occasional occurrence of gross changes in chemically mutagenized TMV U1 leading to other known strains was similarly explained by Tsugita and Fraenkel-Conrat (1962).

several defective strains had less aspartic acid (asparagine) residues than wild-type TMV (Table 2).

2.5.2. Temperature Dependence of Viruses

Quite clearly, the functional activity of any protein will depend on the temperature, and different temperatures are optimal for their activity.

Temperature-sensitive (*ts*) mutations are assigned to the class of missense mutations. This is the case when base substitution results in the change of the codon message and substitution of one amino acid for another in the polypeptide chain. As a result, the synthesized polypeptide chain may differ from normal protein of the wild type by its conformational properties, and, consequently, by its functional activity at elevated temperature.

As was mentioned, replication of virus in the infected cell depends on certain functions coded by the viral genome and performed by the virus-specific proteins. Virus-specific proteins of different viruses and viral strains may differ markedly in the degree of temperature sensitivity and in the temperature optimal for their activity. The implication is that the proteins have two levels of temperature sensitivity, i.e., sensitivity to heating and to cooling. The terms "temperature sensitivity" and "cold sensitivity" usually imply sensitivity to heating and cooling, respectively. A nonpermissive temperature for a virus can render certain virus-specific protein(s) nonfunctional which are essential for virus multiplication.

Strictly speaking, failure of the virus to multiply at elevated (for temperature-sensitive viruses) and at lower (for cold-sensitive viruses) temperatures may not necessarily be proof that a virus- and not a host cell-coded function is temperature sensitive. One can imagine a hypothetical situation in which virus replication is blocked not because of direct inactivation of a virus-specific protein but because of the temperature sensitivity of a certain cell-coded system(s) essential for virus replication but nonessential for host-plant survival at this temperature. Yet is should be noted that if such situations are real, they have not been described so far. Therefore, failure of virus replication at nonpermissive temperatures may be treated as evidence of the temperature sensitivity of the virus-coded function(s).

The notion of defective or normal viruses based on their different temperature sensitivities is quite tentative. This is strengthened by the fact that, on the one hand, at lower temperatures *ts* virus is capable of replication yielding progeny, and, on the other, many of those viruses which we regard as "normal," i.e., temperature-resistant (*tr*), may also prove to be "defective" at unusually high temperatures at which the plant still survives.

An optimal temperature for common TMV is about 20–25°C. At 35°C, the virus concentration in the infected tissues dropped and the coat protein accumulated in the form of disks and rodlike aggregates of varying length (Lebeurier and Hirth, 1966). At 38°C, a considerable amount of denatured TMV (U1 strain) coat protein was found in the infected plant (Hariharasubramanian and Zaitlin, 1968).

The tentative character of the subdivision of viruses into "normal" and "defective" with respect to their temperature sensitivity is further strengthened by the existence of so-called thermophilic viruses. For example, the LB strain of TMV isolated by Lebeurier and Hirth (1966) replicated more actively at 36°C than at 24°C; dolichos enation mosaic virus (DEMV) produced many defective short particles at 20°C but not at 32°C (Kassanis and McCarthy, 1967); the TC strain of TMV (Lebeurier and Wurtz, 1968) isolated from LB also produced more infective virus at 35°C than at 20°C (see also Kassanis and Bastow, 1971*c*).

Despite some limitations in the assignment of temperature-sensitive and thermophilic strains to the category of defective viruses, some other observations lend support to the assertion that they are virtually defective as compared to the common TMV. It was reported by Kassanis and Bastow (1971*c*) that many broken particles of varying length were present in the preparation of *ts* strain Ni 118 isolated from plants infected even at the permissive temperature (20°C).

Similar observations are indicative of a certain defectiveness of thermophilic TMV strains. For example, the thermophilic strain TC produced a certain amount of structurally defective particles at the temperature optimal for its replication (35°C) (Lebeurier and Wurtz, 1968; Kassanis and Bastow, 1971*c*). Purified preparations of the TC strain had an unusually low E_{260}/E_{280} value, reflecting the presence of a considerable amount of protein not bound to RNA. The authors suggested that TC protein "coated its RNA in a rather inefficient way, especially when multiplying at 20°." Thus it can be concluded that, at least in the cases discussed above, both *ts* mutants and thermophilic strains can be regarded as defective compared to common TMV.

2.5.2a. Temperature-Sensitive (*ts*) Coat Protein Mutants of TMV

Jockusch (1964, 1966*a,b,c*) was the first to systematically describe various TMV mutants and strains with respect to their temperature sensitivity. He compared the *tr* or *ts* behavior of these viruses *in vivo* in the infected plant with the properties of their coat protein preparations isolated from the virus and tested *in vitro*.

For the assessment of the degree of the *in vivo* temperature stability of the virus, Jockusch (1966*b*) proposed the use of the infectivity ratio value of the extracts from plants inoculated at 32°C and 23°C (coefficient Q in Table 3). He assigned those strains with $Q \leq 0.5$ to the *ts* group and those with $Q > 0.5$ to the *tr* group. Of the 21 TMV mutants tested, 14 were *ts* according to this criterion. Only seven mutants and four natural wild strains were *tr*. As shown by Jockusch (1966*b*), the *ts* group falls into two classes considered at length below.

TABLE 3

Temperature Dependence of Different TMV Strains[a]

Strain	Temperature dependence of virus multiplication in *N. tabacum* (Q)[b]	Type of strain
vulgare	1–2	*tr*
Ni 103	0.2	*ts*
Ni 105	1.0	*tr*
Ni 106	1.4	*tr*
Ni 109	1.0	*tr*
Ni 118	0.01	*ts*
Ni 1688	0.5	*ts*
Ni 1927	1.5	*tr*
CP 415	0.3	*ts*
flavum	0.01	*ts*
necans	0.2	*ts*
reflavescens	0.01	*ts*
A 14	1.2	*tr*
Ni 458	0.2	*ts*
Ni 511	0.02	*ts*
Ni 606	0.01	*ts*
Ni 696	0.01	*ts*
Ni 1193	1.5	*tr*
Ni 1196	0.5	*ts*
Ni 2516	0.2 (a)	*ts*
Ni 2519	0.15 (a)	*ts*
dahlemense	1.0 (a)	*tr*
U2	1.0 (a)	*tr*
HR	0.73 (a)	*tr*

[a] From Jockusch (1966*b*).
[b] Q is the ratio of the infectivity (number of lesions per *N. tabacum* var. Xanthinc) of the extracts from *N. tabacum* var. Samsun at 32°C to that of 23°C. Inoculated plants were exposed for 4 days, except (a) cases exposed for 6 days. The virus was regarded as *ts* if $Q \leq 0.5$, and as *tr* if $Q > 0.5$.

The *ts* mutants of class I are represented typically by Ni 118 and *flavum* and possess the following characteristics: (1) At nonpermissive temperatures viral particles are formed in negligible amounts; the infectivity of extracts at 30–35°C is low (Kassanis and Bastow, 1971*b*) or entirely lacking (Atabekov *et al.*, 1970). Under nonpermissive conditions, cells infected with *ts* I mutants accumulate infectious viral RNA unprotected by the protein (Jockusch, 1966*b*); i.e., the situation is in principle similar to that reported for plants infected by defective mutants of the PM series (see above). (2) Infection is unable to spread in the infected plant at high temperature. (3) Shift of the infected plants from high to permissive temperature results in a rapid accumulation of appreciable amounts of infective mature virus particles.

Presumably, on infection by *ts* mutants at 32°C, the infective material accumulates in the form of free or partially protein-bound RNA. Shift from nonpermissive (30–35°C) to permissive (20°C) temperature leads to rapid incorporation of this RNA into mature viral particles. It may be suggested that in the cell infected by *ts* I-type mutants there may be a preformed pool of coat protein molecules nonfunctional at 32°C but renatured (at least partly) at 20°C.

It is apparent that at 30–35°C the host cells infected by *ts* I strains do not contain any appreciable amounts of soluble coat protein. Extracts of such plants do not react with antiserum to Ni 118. Yet, the *ts* mutations of this type do not seem to reduce the amount of coat protein produced at restrictive temperatures. Moreover, the typical I-class mutant (Ni 118) produced more coat protein at 35°C than at 23°C (Jockusch, 1968*b*).

It was shown by Jockusch (1966*a,c*) that the coat protein preparation isolated from the *ts* I virus displayed the *ts* properties *in vitro*. The protein was stable at 23°C but denatured rapidly at 30–35°C, whereas the protein preparations of *vulgare* remained native. Thermal denaturation of the coat protein of *ts* I-class mutants is followed by the formation of insoluble material both *in vitro* and *in vivo*.

A convenient experimental test of the *ts* behavior of coat protein was offered by Jockusch (1966*a,c*). It is well known that low molecular weight TMV protein can be polymerized *in vitro* at pH 5.0 into rodlike particles with helical structure and that these aggregates can be dissociated at a pH of about 8. Thermal denaturation of the coat protein was shown to be attended by the loss of the protein's capacity to produce these rodlike aggregates. Instead of the regular rodlike aggregates soluble at pH 5.0 ($s_{20,w}$ = 100 S and more) which are produced by coat protein preparations of *tr*-TMV, the Ni 118 protein treated at 30°C formed an insoluble precipitate (Jockusch, 1966c) at pH 5.0 which could be removed by low-speed centrifugation. It could be solubilized with 67% acetic acid or 9–10 M urea (Joskusch, 1966c). On the other hand, at 20°C, the Ni 118 coat protein was polymerized into normal soluble aggregates upon acidification of the solution to pH 5.0.

A clear-cut distinction of the behavior of the coat protein of *ts* I and *tr*-TMV strains was demonstrated with denaturation kinetics (Fig. 2A,B). Denaturation of the *ts* protein becomes evident within minutes, while the *tr* protein remains soluble within hours of heating. Almost all mutants tested (see Fig. 2A) were obtained from *vulgare* and contained a single substitution in the coat protein. The only exception was *reflavescens*, which originated from *flavum* through the *necans* strain. It can be seen from Fig. 2A that the *reflavescens* coat protein occupies an intermediate position between *tr* and *ts* strains with respect to the degree of temperature sensitivity. The most clear-cut correlation of *ts* properties *in vitro* and *in vivo* was observed with the Ni 118 protein.

Similar results were obtained with the *in vitro* denaturation kinetics of the structural protein of the mutants derived from strain A14 (Fig. 2B). The bottom line in Fig. 2B corresponds to the data for the protein of the defective Ni 2204 strain which produced insoluble coat protein at both temperatures (24°C and 30°C). The properties of *ts* mutant Ni 2519 will be considered below.

The mutant *ts*38 described by Hariharasubramanian *et al.* (1970) should also be grouped with *ts* I mutants. The coat protein of *ts*38 mutant was unstable at high temperatures *in vitro* and *in vivo* at high ionic strength.

It must be noted that polymerization of *ts*38 protein into rodlike aggregates is difficult. Different conditions favoring TMV protein polymerization that were tested by the authors caused flocculation of the *ts*38 protein from solution. Therefore, the *ts*38 mutant can be regarded as a defective virus with altered aggregation characteristics and reduced thermal stability of the coat protein.

It was only natural to try to compare the *tr* and *ts* behavior of the coat protein of different TMV strains with the position and character of amino acid substitutions in the polypeptide chain. Relevant information was presented by Jockusch (1966c) (see Fig. 3).

The *ts* properties of two typical *ts* I mutants are determined by a single amino acid replacement which leads to the *tr* → *ts* transition of the coat protein (see also Table 3). From the comparison of amino acid substitutions in the coat protein of different *ts* I strains with the amino

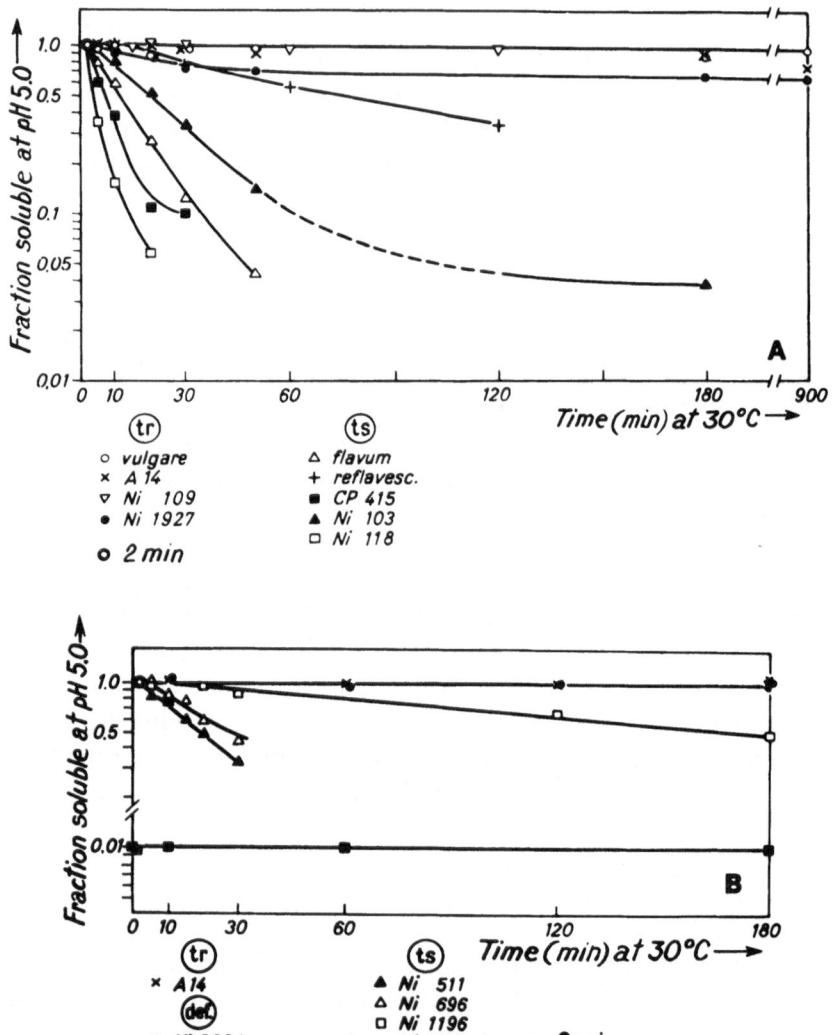

Fig. 2A,B. Loss of solubility at pH 5.0 after incubation of the coat protein of different TMV strains at 30°C, pH 7.0, ionic strength 0.1. Courtesy of H. Jockusch from Jockusch (1966b).

acid sequence of wild-type *tr* strain, it followed that the proline residues at positions 20 and 63 were essential for the normal (*tr*) conformation of TMV coat protein. It was suggested by Jockusch (1966c) that the Asp-Pro sequence at positions 19–20 is essential for the stabilization of the site of folding of the polypeptide chain in the TMV subunit.

The coat protein of *ts*38 mutant (not shown in Fig. 3) contains two amino acid substitutions, namely, threonine to alanine at position 81 and serine to phenylalanine at position 143. Of the two substitutions, the first (Thr → Ala at position 81) has been reported several times with functional TMV strains 344, 383, 344 (Funatsu and Fraenkel-Conrat, 1964), suggesting that this change alone is insufficient for appearance of the *ts* I phenotype. The second substitution (Ser → Phe at position 143), alone or in combination with the first one, appears to be responsible for the *ts* behavior of *ts*38 protein (Hariharasubramanian *et al.*, 1970).

Unfortunately, no simple rules have been deduced so far to explain the *tr* → *ts* conversion of the TMV coat protein. Quite obviously, the effect of amino acid replacements on the thermal stability of TMV coat protein cannot be understood before the exact conformation of the protein subunit within the TMV rod is known. It must be noted that within the helical rodlike aggregate, the thermal stability of the subunit increased sharply (Jockusch, 1966*a,c*). The coat protein of any TMV strain (including *ts* I mutants) is more temperature resistant than the identical protein in a disaggregated form (Jockusch, 1966*a,c*).

2.5.2b. Temperature-Sensitive Non-Coat Protein Mutants

We do not know how many other genes TMV RNA contains besides the coat protein gene. Obviously, any of the nonstructural pro-

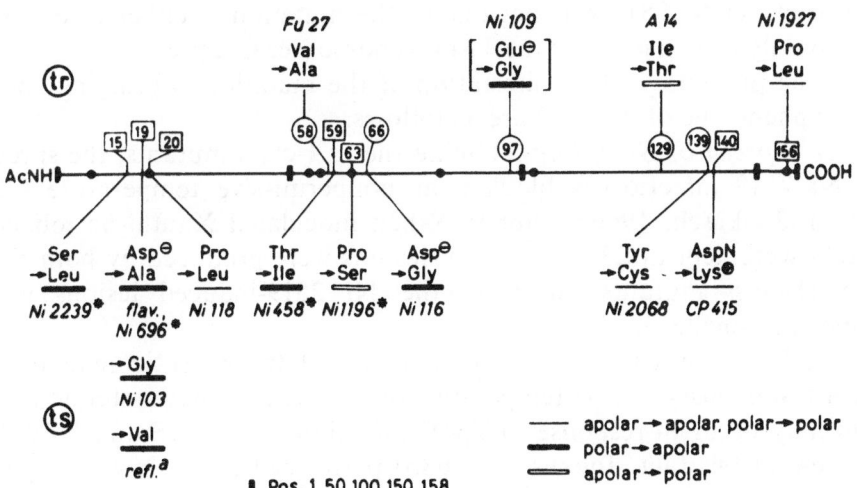

Fig. 3. Amino acid replacements in coat protein and *ts*, *tr* behavior of several TMV mutants. The line represents the polypeptide chain of *vulgare*, consisting of 158 amino acid residues. Figures above the line refer to the positions of the replacements. *Amino acid substitutions which lead to the observed behavior in the presence of the A14 substitution. Courtesy of H. Jockusch from Jockusch (1966*c*).

tein genes may give, as a result of a mutational change, a *ts* virus-coded product. Therefore, it may be expected that during mutagenesis of TMV, *ts* mutants for non-coat protein genes will be formed at a frequency comparable to that ·of appearance of *ts* I mutants. This is probably the case, although most *ts* mutants of TMV have been shown to produce thermally labile structural protein (i.e., they belong to *ts* I class). Unfortunately, in those rare cases when the mutant may be assigned to the *ts* II class in Jockusch's terminology we cannot identify, with any assurance, the affected gene(s). Only one noncoat protein *ts* mutant of TMV (Ni 2519) has been examined thoroughly (Wittmann-Liebold *et al.*, 1965; Jockusch, 1966*a,b,c*; Bosch and Jockusch, 1972). Quite clearly, the *ts* behavior of Ni 2519 is not due to a mutation in its coat protein gene. It was shown by direct analysis that the primary structure of Ni 2519 coat protein and that of the virus (A14) from which it was derived were the same (Wittmann-Liebold *et al.*, 1965). In complete agreement, the coat protein of Ni 2519 proved to be temperature resistant in the *in vitro* experiments (Fig. 2B). Further, coat protein synthesis proceeded at a normal rate in Ni 2519-infected tobacco cells at restrictive temperature (35°C) (Bosch and Jockusch, 1972). The second important TMV-coded function, the replication of viral RNA, was also not blocked at temperatures restrictive for this mutant (Jockusch, 1966*b*; Bosch and Jockusch, 1972). Thus temperature sensitivity of Ni 2519 was not due to the mutation in either of the two supposedly known genes of the TMV genome (see Chapter 4).

The physiological manifestation of the mutation(s) bringing about the *ts* phenotype of Ni 2519 are as follows:

1. Spread of Symptoms. Unlike the *ts* I-class mutants, the spread of Ni 2519 infection is blocked at nonpermissive temperature (32–35°C) (Jockusch, 1966*b*, 1968*b*). When inoculated Xanthi-nc tobacco plants were kept at 23°C for 36 h, lesions were produced by both *ts* I- and II-class mutants, although the Ni 2519-induced lesions were somewhat smaller in size.

It has been known for a long time that the necrotic reaction of local lesion hosts can be temperature-sensitive, i.e., that systemic reaction may occur in response to TMV infection at 35°C (Samuel, 1931). In view of this fact, Jockusch (1968*b*) performed the following experiment to test the inhibition of spreading of Ni 2519 in Xanthi-nc tobacco plants at 35°C. The plants were inoculated with Ni 2519, using Ni 118 as control. They were kept for 36 h at 23°C, then transferred to 35°C for 24 h, and finally returned to 23°C for 24 h. Under these conditions, local lesions arose initially (at 23°C) with both the *ts* II- and I-class mutants; the infection then spread at 35°C in Ni 118-infected plants, and finally it was localized again (at 23°C). As a result, Ni 118-produced lesions appeared to increase considerably in diameter at 35°C (like the common type *tr* strain), whereas the Ni 2519 lesions did not spread at 35°C.

2. Maturation of the Virions. The formation of intact nucleoprotein Ni 2519 particles was inhibited in infected cells at high temperature, although coat protein and RNA syntheses took place. The coat protein of Ni 2519 is identical in the primary structure to the A14 *tr* strain, hence it must be functionally active in reassembly with the viral RNA. However, it was shown by Bosch and Jockusch (1972) that the stages of Ni 2519 maturation and encapsidation of the RNA in the protein were temperature-sensitive.

Recently it has been shown that the specificity of the protein-RNA interaction can be very high *in vivo* upon maturation of TMV particles (Atabekova *et al.*, 1975). We have found no genomic masking or phenotypic mixing effects in tobacco plants doubly infected with two TMV strains (*vulgare* and U2). The implication is that under the conditions of mixed infection when viral RNAs and coat proteins of both strains are present, the homologous RNA and protein of each strain can specifically recognize one another, and discriminate against the heterologous components.

The specificity of the protein-RNA interaction has been repeatedly studied in the *in vitro* experiments on TMV reconstitution. It has been established that the process of TMV reassembly is initiated by the interaction of TMV protein with a specific nucleotide sequence, at a now known location on TMV RNA. Thus a TMV RNA molecule possesses at least one reconstitution initiating site displaying a high affinity for TMV protein. If that is the only region of the TMV RNA molecule available for coat protein recognition, then TMV assembly would depend on two main factors: (1) specificity of the nucleotide sequence in the site which controls the degree of TMV RNA affinity for the coat protein and (2) specificity of the secondary and tertiary structure of the polynucleotide chain controlling accessibility of that site of the molecule for the protein.

It may be assumed that in some extreme cases mutations in the initiation segment or in certain other critical sites of the RNA molecule will cause complete loss of its affinity or availability for the viral protein. As a result, a strain may arise which is defective not because of the thermal lability of a certain virus-coded protein but because of the *ts* behavior of the TMV RNA molecule itself, or, to be more precise, of a certain site(s) of the RNA which affects its affinity or accessibility to the protein. As suggested by Bosch and Jockusch (1972), such a "critical segment" of the RNA molecule may be affected by the Ni 2519 *ts* mutation.

One more peculiar feature of the Ni 2519 mutant should be noted. The inoculum of Ni 2519 contained about 0.5–0.8% wild-type virus contaminants even when the virus was isolated by two single-lesion passages in *N. tabacum* var. Xanthi-nc (Jockusch, 1968*b*; Bosch and Jockusch, 1972). The reasons for the continuous presence of *tr* contamination in Ni 2519 isolates are not yet clear.

Several other groups of workers presented indirect experimental evidence suggesting that other TMV strains may be *ts* in non-coat protein genes. For example, it was demonstrated by Lebeurier and Hirth (1966) that the common TMV strain multiplies more actively at 28°C than at 35°C. At high temperature, the accumulation of free viral coat protein took place without parallel accumulation of free viral RNA. These observations led them to suggest that the TMV-specific RNA replicase was less active at 35°C than at 24°C; i.e., it was *ts*. Similar observations were made by Kassanis and Bastow (1971*c*) on four TMV strains. Infectivity of both the intact virus and the free RNA extracts was markedly higher at 20°C than at 35°C. The authors claimed that high temperature inhibited the viral RNA replication, hence all four TMV strains tested could be regarded as *ts* for the RNA replication (three of them had defective coat proteins). Kapitsa *et al.* (1970) also suggested that their DM strain of TMV was *ts* in the RNA replicase gene, since it produced less infective RNA at 36.5°C than at 28°C. This interpretation is, however, not unambiguous, for it is based only on infectivity data.

2.6. Defective Viruses and Genome Masking

It can be assumed that any virus culture does not consist of only virions of a single strain, but represents a mixed population of the major virus and a certain number of spontaneous mutant particles. Thus, among the mutants contaminating the major strain, different defective mutants may well be present. The form of interaction between the genomes of the major virus and the contaminating mutants is difficult to predict. It is not excluded that under certain conditions the defective mutant is complemented by the wild-type virus and hence can survive in nature.

It was reported by several groups of authors (Schaskolskaya *et al.*, 1968; Sarkar, 1969; Atabekov *et al.*, 1970; Kassanis and Bastow, 1971*a,b*; Kassanis and Conti, 1971; Atabekova *et al.*, 1975) that under the conditions of mixed infection the *ts* coat protein mutants of TMV as well as mutants producing defective coat protein could be complemented by different *tr* helper strains. It was proved (Atabekov *et al.*, 1970; Kassanis and Bastow, 1971*a,b*; Atabekova *et al.*, 1975) that the complementation between the defective and normal strain was due to the formation of "hybrid" particles, i.e., to the masking of the genome of the defective virus within the coat protein of the helper TMV strain. In all aforementioned cases, the phenomenon of genome masking was observed under the conditions when the infected cell contained RNAs from two strains but functional protein from only one, the protein of the second strain being either defective or nonfunctional at the high temperature employed. In other words, the RNA of the defective or *ts* coat protein mutant did not encounter the homologous protein and was enclosed in a heterologous envelope upon maturation of viral particles. Supposedly, this type of interaction between *ts* and *tr* viruses may lead to the formation of an artificial, high-temperature-stable satellite-helper system ensuring survival of the *ts* virus at high temperature. These aspects of genomic masking have been discussed in greater detail by Okada and Ohno in Volume 6 of *Comprehensive Virology*.

2.7. Unstable Variants of Tobacco Necrosis Virus

Different questions concerning the properties of tobacco necrosis virus (TNV) and its association with satellite virus will be discussed later. In the present section, we shall deal only with defective forms of infection, when the virus is incapable of producing a functional coat protein even though infective RNA is synthesized.

It was found by Babos and Kassanis (1962) that there were great differences in the infectivity of extracts from individual TNV-induced lesions. While generally the extracts from individual lesions were highly infective, i.e., contained "stable" variants of the virus, some cultures of TNV also produced "unstable" variants. One out of the 20 lesions induced by TNV preparations contained the virus in apparently low-infective (unstable) form. However, extraction with phenol or other agents which inactivate or remove RNase from the preparation was capable of stabilizing the infectivity of unstable TNV variants (Babos and Kassanis, 1962; Kassanis and Welkie, 1963).

A characteristic feature of unstable TNV is thus the increase in infectivity (ten- to a hundredfold) upon phenol extraction of infected leaves, as compared to sap expressed from such leaves, whether it was subsequently extracted with phenol or not. In contrast, the infectivity of phenol-extracted leaves infected with normal TNV was only one-fifth that of expressed sap (Babos and Kassanis, 1962).

When the sap from leaves infected with unstable TNV was tested with antiserum to normal TNV, no serological reaction was produced. All these observations indicate that unstable variants exist in the infected cell in the form of free RNA unprotected (or protected incompletely) by the coat protein, and thus susceptible to degradation by RNase released upon leaf homogenization. The authors concluded that most of the RNA of unstable TNV is free and "not bound to any large host component," as was suggested for RNAs of unstable tobacco rattle virus by Cadman (1962) and for RNA of defective TMV strains by Siegel et al. (1962).

The reasons for the transition of normal TNV into the unstable variant are unclear. It should be noted that the frequency of unstable variant production is quite high (5%). It is not ruled out that during the infection unstable variants can produce insignificant amounts of stable particles as a result of reversion. However, it was reported by Babos and Kassanis (1962) and Kassanis and Welkie (1963) that unstable variants do not seem to revert to stable ones in the course of subculturing.

Small amounts of complete particles found in the extracts from plants infected with unstable TNV do not necessarily mean that they were produced by the unstable variant itself rather than by normal residual TNV contaminating the unstable variant (see below).

It can be suggested that in the case of unstable TNV variants the coat protein gene is either deeply repressed or deleted. It must be noted, however, that some defective strains of tobacco mosaic virus producing insoluble coat protein were also repeatedly regarded as not producing any coat protein, and only by closer examination was their structural protein found in infected cells.

Thus in cells infected with unstable TNV variants the product of the coat protein gene is either lacking or nonfunctional. The other TNV genes seem to be active, as suggested by the following two facts: (1) infective viral RNA replicates and accumulates in cells infected with unstable variants, and (2) unstable TNV is capable of activating the satellite of tobacco necrosis virus (STNV) (see below for details) in mixed infections (Babos and Kassanis, 1962); i.e., the products of genes essential for the complementation of STNV can be produced by unstable TNV.

2.8. Unstable Variants of Tobacco Rattle Virus and Pea Early-Browning Virus

The essential distinction of unstable forms of tobacco rattle virus (TRV) and pea early-browning virus (PEBV) from the above mentioned TMV strains defective in their coat protein is that "instability" (i.e., sensitivity to RNase action in the expressed sap) of the TRV and PEBV variants is due to the lack and not the nonfunctionality of the coat protein upon infection.

The peculiarities of TRV reproduction have been exhaustively discussed (Lister, 1969; Matthews, 1970; van Kammen, 1972; see also Chapter 2 of this volume); therefore, we shall confine ourselves to a brief account of this system. Purified TRV preparations contain two major rodlike virus particles: long particles (180–210 nm, $s_{20,w}$ = 300 S) and short particles (45–115 nm, $s_{20,w}$ = 143–155 S, depending on the isolate). In the purified viral suspensions, shorter particles are also present, but they appear to be degradation products of longer particles and probably play no functional role in TRV multiplication. The RNA extracted from TRV preparations has sedimentation coefficients 12–20 S (molecular weight 0.7–1.0 $\times$ 10^6) and 26 S (molecular weight about 2.3 $\times$ 10^6) (Harrison, 1970). Only long particles (and, respectively, the 26 S RNA) were found to be infective, but the infectivity was unstable: infected tissues contained no detectable virus particles or viral antigens. It must be noted that, unlike the unstable variants of tobacco necrosis virus described above which are inactivated in the expressed sap immediately after leaf homogenization, the unstable TRV remains infective for several hours (Cadman, 1962). A similar phenomenon was reported for defective TMV mutants (Siegel *et al.*, 1962).

Investigations conducted for several years by many researchers have shown that, during typical TRV replication, complementary interaction between the short and the long particles occurs. The RNA of the long particles lacks the genetic information for the coat protein, which accounts for the labile infection in plants inoculated with the long particles alone. The coat protein gene is carried by the RNA of the short particles, as shown by complementation experiments. This was confirmed also with *in vitro* translation studies which showed that the short RNA directed the synthesis of TRV coat protein in a cell-free protein-synthesizing system (Ball *et al.*, 1973, etc., see Chapter 4).

As with most of the questions concerning the evolution and relationships of viruses under natural conditions, we lack information on the origin of the short particles and the pathways in which the symbiosis of the components of tobacco rattle virus has become possible. Unstable forms of TRV can be cultivated continuously without giving rise to the stable form of infection (Lister, 1969). Apparently, the genome of the long particles completely lacks the structural protein gene.

Pea early-browning virus preparations also contain particles of the two lengths (Bos and van der Want, 1962; Harrison, 1966). The functional relationships between the short and long PEBV particles are similar to those described for TRV (Huttinga, 1969; Gibbs and Harrison, 1964; Lister, 1966, 1967; see Chapter 2 for more details on TRV and PEBV).

3. SATELLITISM IN PLANT VIRUSES

Viral satellitism is an example of a more general phenomenon, that of complementational interaction between seemingly unrelaxed viruses.

In the infected cell, satellite viruses are unable to perform certain function(s) essential for their independent replication. However, a satellite virus can multiply under conditions of mixed infection in the presence of a certain normal virus (helper), utilizing for its replication the virus-specific product(s) coded for by the helper virus.

To discuss the problem in more concrete and specific terms, it is necessary to define the phenomenon of satellitism in viruses. We group with satellite viruses those which lack some genetic information essential for their replication but are capable of multiplication in certain types of cells in the presence of the normal helper virus. Formally, the fact that infective virus acts as helper (i.e., complementation has one-sided but not reciprocal character) represents one important characteristic of satellitism and satellite-virus definition. The fact that both satellite and helper viruses code independently for their structural proteins, i.e., contain heterologous coat protein gene(s), represents the second characteristic. The fact that the satellite–helper system is stable and both viruses can readily multiply in the course of joint infection and numerous successive passages may be regarded as a third characteristic of satellitism.

We are aware of the fact that all these criteria are very formal, but they are convenient, since they permit distinction of viral satellitism from such related phenomena as interaction between the components of viruses with a divided genome, synergism between normal viruses, and genomic masking described above. The above definition suggests that satellite virus is *deficient* in the parts of its genetic information. However, it can be assumed that satellitelike interactions may occur between two viruses, one of which is normal (helper) and the second of which *defective* in a certain function(s) (i.e., produces a nonfunctional virus-specific product).

It follows that under natural conditions various satellite viruses may occur, their different functions depending on the helper virus. In a consideration of different possible types of satellitism, it seems reasonable to assume that a certain satellite virus may exist which is incapable of multiplying in certain cells not because of its inability to code for some virus-specific protein(s) but because of its inability to give rise to the virus-induced (cell-specific) products required for its multiplication, but this product is induced by the helper virus. The examples of such type of satellitism are not available so far.

Typical examples of satellitism in viruses are set by the interactions between (1) tobacco necrosis viruses (TNV) with the virus satellite of tobacco necrosis virus (STNV) and (2) adenoviruses with adeno-associated viruses. Below we will consider only the first example.

3.1. Association between Tobacco Necrosis Virus and Its Satellite: General Description

Smith and Bald (1935) were the first to recognize tobacco necrosis as a virus disease. The experimental host range of TNV is very wide, including 88 plant species from 37 families (Kassanis, 1964). Different TNV strains produce varying symptoms in host plants, the most common symptom being veinal necrosis.

TNV was isolated not only from plants showing necrosis but also from the roots of apparently healthy plants. Thus, the so-called potato culture of TNV was originally isolated from the roots of an apparently healthy potato plant (Bawden and Pirie, 1942). Kassanis (1964) suggested that the name "tobacco necrosis virus" should be restricted to the viruses serologically related to the original "potato culture."

One TNV culture known as "Rothamsted culture" (Bawden, 1941; Bawden and Pirie, 1942, 1945) was the object of many studies. About 40 years ago, Pirie *et al.* (1938) found that purified preparations of that

TNV culture (later named the "Rothamsted culture") consisted of two fractions, one amorphous and the other crystallizing as thin plates. The so-called crystallizable nucleoprotein (Bawden and Pirie, 1945) was the major component of the virus preparation. However, it was noninfectious.

A unique feature of purified preparations of the TNV "Rothamsted culture" was the presence of two kinds of virus particles of different sizes: 30 nm and 17 nm in diameter (Bawden and Pirie, 1950). Initially, the origin of the two kinds of particles was not clear and they were believed to be antigenically identical. Therefore, it was supposed that the small particles represented either a stage in synthesis or a degradation product of the larger virions. However, Kassanis and Nixon (1960) studied critically the properties of this TNV culture and, practically speaking, established the notion of virus satellitism.

With sucrose density gradient centrifugation of Rothamsted TNV, two and sometimes three components were isolated. The top component ($s_{20,w}$ = 45 S) corresponded to small particles (17 nm in diameter); the middle component ($s_{20,w}$ = 116 S) contained large particles (30 nm in diameter); and the third, bottom component ($s_{20,w}$ = 216 S) if present, consisted of aggregates of small particles (Kassanis and Nixon, 1960). An important further finding was that large and small particles were antigenically unrelated (Kassanis and Nixon, 1960). The large particles were infective and multiplied in the inoculated plants in the absence of small particles. The virus progeny from the cells inoculated with such particles consisted exclusively of large particles. The cells infected with a mixture of equal proportions of small and large particles gave progeny consisting of the two types of particles in a 1:1 ratio.

The preparations of large TNV particles were usually contaminated by small particles. Apparently, separation by density gradient centrifugation was not complete, as shown by electron microscopic examination of these fractions (Kassanis and Nixon, 1960). The bottom fraction contained almost exclusively small noninfective particles arranged as aggregates of 12 particles and exhibiting an icosahedral symmetry. Because of the presence of such aggregates of small particles, the complete separation and purification of the large TNV particles by centrifugation are difficult. Isolation of TNV free from STNV is complicated also because of the presence of TNV in many apparently healthy plants.

After it was found that the small and large particles corresponded to two unrelated viruses, one of which (the small) depended on the other for its multiplication, Kassanis (1962) proposed to designate the large virus as TNV and the small one as a satellite of TNV (STNV). We shall use these terms in the following discussion.

Once freed from STNV, TNV isolates remained pure during the course of many subcultures in plants which did not contain satellite virus (Kassanis, 1964; Kassanis and Phillips, 1970; Uyemoto *et al.*, 1968). Thus there is no reason to assume that STNV is necessary for normal TNV multiplication or that it is produced continuously upon replication of the latter.

Replication of STNV in the presence of TNV helper is, in its turn, based on a type of complementation interaction in which the antigenic properties of the satellite are quite unrelated to those of TNV and are fully determined by the genome of STNV itself (Kassanis, 1966). Thus the TNV plus STNV mixture produces two bands in gel diffusion tests in reaction with antisera to the total preparation consisting of large and small particles. Such antisera absorbed with TNV retained fully their ability to react with STNV (Kassanis and Nixon, 1961).

These results were of basic importance since it was the first description of a classical example of viral satellitism. Virus satellite is noninfective by itself since the genetic information it possesses is insufficient to perform all the functions involved in its replication. The missing functions are performed by the products coded by TNV, which "neither needs nor directly produces STNV" (Kassanis and Nixon, 1961).

While discussing the phenomenon of satellitism in plant viruses as exemplified by the TNV-STNV system, it would be pertinent to remember the relationship between certain DNA-containing animal viruses (adenovirus, herpesvirus) and so-called adenovirus-associated virus (AAV), a small parvovirus not infective by itself but replicating in the infected cell in the presence of adenovirus. Herpesvirus also induces the synthesis of AAV DNA, RNA, and protein, but, unlike adenovirus, does not induce mature AAV particles. Therefore, it can be regarded as partial helper. Both types of helper viruses contain double-stranded DNA, whereas AAV DNA is single stranded. A peculiarity of AAV is that different AAV virions contain either "plus" or "minus" strands of DNA. It must be noted, however, that AAV DNA is much larger than STNV RNA.

It was shown that AAV could enter the host cell and that uncoating of DNA took place, hence the helper functions of adenovirus include some steps at the level of DNA replication, RNA and protein biosynthesis, and possibly virus particle assembly.

It should be mentioned that the similarity of the interaction of AAV with adenovirus and TNV with STNV also extends to the fact that both types of satellites induce interference with the replication of their helper viruses (for details, see Chapter 1 in Volume 3 of this series).

3.2. Strains of TNV and STNV

Several strains of TNV derived from different sources were divided into two distinctive groups (serotypes) designated as A and D (Babos and Kassanis, 1963; Kassanis and Phillips, 1970). The term "serotype" was proposed for the strains prominently distinct in their antigenicity.

The strains within each serotype could be distinguished by their antigenic properties and/or by the symptoms they induce in the host plants. Moreover, certain strains differed in their stability, rate of multiplication, infectivity, and crystallizability (Babos and Kassanis, 1963; Kassanis and Phillips, 1970).

Serotype A included strains A, B, C, F, and S; serotype D included strains D, AC-36, GV, A-3, and CT. Strain A was isolated from roots of tobacco plants naturally infected with TNV (Kassanis, 1960); strain B was derived from the Rothamsted culture of TNV. Strain D was isolated from apparently healthy *Datura tatula* L. plants; strain C was an isolate of cucumber necrosis virus from Holland; S was bean stripple-streak virus producing systemic symptoms in bean. GV strain was isolated from grapevine; it was noninfective for tobacco and of low infectivity for beans. CT strain was isolated from citrus trees.

Comparative serological analysis of TNV strains (cross-absorption, immunodiffusion) showed that antigenic differences between the strains of one serotype, if present, are not as prominent as between strains of different serotypes. Some strains within a serotype were serologically similar and differed in other properties. For example, strains A and C are antigenically identical but can be distinguished because strain C (Dutch cucumber necrosis virus) produces a systemic reaction in young cucumber plants (Babos and Kassanis, 1963). In immunodiffusion tests, the strains belonging to the same serotype produce with antiserum to one of the strains either a small spur or no spur at all. By contrast, strains of different serotypes produce large, well-developed reactions of partial intersection (Kassanis and Phillips, 1970).

Several STNV strains were isolated and compared antigenically and for their ability to be activated by different TNV strains (Uyemoto *et al.*, 1968; Rees *et al.*, 1970; Grogan and Uyemoto, 1967; Kassanis and Phillips, 1970). Uyemoto *et al.* (1968) in the United States described three serologically distinct STNV strains designated as A, B, and C. Rees *et al.* (1970) distinguished three STNV strains in Rothamsted which they designated as SV_1, SV_2, and SV_3. Isolates A and B were found to be antigenically identical to SV_1 and SV_2, respectively. On the other hand, STNV C was antigenically related but not identical to the English strains (Kassanis and Phillips, 1970).

When the English STNV strains were compared, it turned out that each of them (SV_1, SV_2, and SV_3) possessed antigenic determinants lacking in other strains. All these strains had common antigenic determinants but were distinctly different serologically (Rees *et al.*, 1970).

3.3. Physicochemical Properties and Structure of TNV and STNV

Concentrated solutions of TNV produce small rhombic crystals of variable thickness upon ultracentrifugation and upon addition of saturated ammonium sulphate to the virus solution (Babos and Kassanis, 1963). Under similar conditions, STNV also crystallizes into different forms (Rees *et al.*, 1970). Cells infected with a TNV plus STNV mixture were found to yield STNV crystalline arrays and rhombic plates (Kassanis *et al.*, 1970).

Sedimentation coefficients reported by different authors for TNV strains varied in the range of 112–133 S (Pirie *et al.*, 1938; Bawden and Pirie, 1942, 1945; Kassanis and Nixon, 1961; Uyemoto and Grogan, 1969). The particle size of TNV is about 6.5×10^5 daltons.

The purified preparations of TNV show a maximum extinction at 260–262 nm and a minimum at 242–244 nm. The A_{max}/A_{min} ratio for different TNV preparations is about 1.3 (not corrected for light scattering); the A_{260}/A_{280} ratio is 1.5 (Babos and Kassanis, 1963; Uyemoto and Grogan, 1969). TNV contains about 20% RNA (Kassanis, 1962; Uyemoto and Grogan, 1969).

The isoelectric point of TNV is about pH 4.5 (for B strain), while STNV is isoelectric about pH 7.0. The differences in the isoelectric values may be utilized for the separation of STNV from the mixture with TNV (Rees *et al.*, 1970). TNV contains single-stranded RNA of molecular weight about 1.3×10^6 ($s_{20,w}$ = 24.1 S) (Uyemoto and Grogan, 1969). It can be concluded from these data that there are approximately 4000 nucleotides in the TNV RNA molecule. Uyemoto and Grogan (1969) and others analyzed the composition of the coat protein and RNA of several TNV strains. The general consensus is that the protein has a molecular weight of about 30,000.

The particle size of STNV was determined by different authors as 1.85×10^6 daltons (Bawden and Pirie, 1945; Kassanis, 1962; Reichmann *et al.*, 1962). The sedimentation constant of STNV reported in the literature varies somewhat but averages about 50 S (Kassanis and Nixon, 1961; Reichmann *et al.*, 1962; Uyemoto and Grogan, 1969).

The molecular weight of the STNV coat protein subunit has been estimated as 20,000–27,000 (Lesnaw and Reichmann, 1970*a*; Rees *et al.*, 1970; Rice, 1974), with the lower value being probably close to correct. Two protein components were revealed in the electropherograms of STNV protein (Rice, 1974). The major component had a molecular weight of about 21,000–22,000, while the minor was 44,000 (2–7% of the total protein preparation). It was suggested that the large component is a dimer of the small component subunits. The chemical nature of bonding and the functional significance of subunit dimerization are obscure. Uyemoto and Grogan (1969) reported that the coat protein molecule of STNV C strain contained 209 amino acids (molecular weight 25,000) with a leucine residue in the *C*-terminal position. Neither TNV nor STNV protein contained free *N*-terminal amino acid resudies.

The purified STNV preparations contain about 20% RNA (Reichmann, 1964; Uyemoto and Grogan, 1969). A study undertaken in Markham's laboratory (Reichmann *et al.*, 1962) showed that STNV contained an unusually short RNA chain. The sedimentation coefficient values of STNV RNA reported in the literature were in the range of 13–14.2 S, which corresponds to a molecular weight of $4–4.5 \times 10^5$ (Reichmann *et al.*, 1962; Reichmann, 1964; Uyemoto and Grogan, 1969). Thus the polynucleotide chain of STNV RNA contains about 1200–1300 residues. Horst *et al.* (1971) showed that the 3′-terminal sequences of STNV RNA were -GACUACCC and -GACUACCCp, occurring in approximately equal amounts. The role or origin of the 3′-phosphorylated sequence is not clear. The 5′ terminus of TNV and STNV RNAs was determined as ppApGpUp (Wimmer *et al.*, 1968; Lesnaw and Reichmann, 1970*a*). In STNV RNA, the 5′-terminal AGU was found to be present in the 5′-diphosphorylated (ppApGpUp) and triphosphorylated (pppApGpUp) form (Horst *et al.*, 1971).

There is circumstantial evidence in favor of TNV and STNV being icosahedral viruses. In electron micrographs, the TNV and STNV particles appear as polyhedral and hexagonal in outline; the detailed structure of these particles, however, remains undetermined (Kassanis, 1964; Reichmann, 1964; Kassanis and Woods, 1968; Uyemoto and Grogan, 1969).

3.4. Specificity of STNV Activation by TNV

The STNV–TNV interaction is highly specific. Satellite virus can be activated by TNV only: none of the other plant viruses tested so far (including TMV, alfalfa mosaic, carnation ringspot, and tomato bushy stunt viruses) was capable of complementing STNV and effecting its replication upon mixed inoculation (Kassanis and Nixon, 1961).

It is clear now that activation occurs because of a very specific match between TNV and STNV. This match is manifested even at the level of TNV and STNV strains. The SV_1 and SV_2 strains of STNV were shown to be activated by different TNV strains, including A, B, S, and E, but not D (Table 4). However, STNV strain C could be complemented by this virus as well as by TNV strains AC-38, AC-36, and NZ (Uyemoto *et al.*, 1968). In contrast, TNV strains which activated STNV strain C (Table 4) were not capable of activating STNV-A or -B. On the whole, it appeared that TNV strains capable of activating STNV-A or -B were incapable of activating STNV-C, and *vice versa* (Uyemoto *et al.*, 1968; Kassanis and Phillips, 1970).

TABLE 4
Activation of Three STNV Strains by Different Strains of TNV[a]

Strain of TNV used for activation	Titers of STNV[b]			Titers of TNV in mixture and when inoculated alone			
	SV_1	SV_2	SV_c	$+SV_1$	$+SV_2$	$+SV_c$	Alone
A	32	32	0	2	4	32	32
B	64	64	0	8	8	32	32
S	32	32	0	8	8	64	64
E	32	32	0	8	8	32	64
AC-43	64	32	0	4	16	64	64
CT	64	16	0	16	16	32	32
D	0	0	16	32	32	16	32
AC-36	0	0	64	32	32	32	64
GV	0	0	64	32	32	32	64

[a] From Kassanis and Phillips (1970).
[b] Serological titers are presented as reciprocal of the dilution end point.

Both groups of authors arrived at the conclusion that ability or inability of different TNV strains to activate a certain STNV strain was not correlated with the antigenic specificity of the helper virus but reflected some "intrinsic" properties of the virus and satellite.

It is noteworthy that the ability of a TNV strain to activate STNV strain C seems to be correlated with its host-range specificity. Thus all TNV strains capable of activating STNV-C (D, AC-36, and GV) were low or noninfective for tobacco and French bean (Kassanis and Phillips, 1970). It is most likely that the congruence between appropriate TNV and STNV is determined by the functional competence of definite TNV-coded (or TNV-induced) proteins in STNV RNA replication in the mixedly infected cell (see below).

It was shown by Teakle (1962) that TNV can be transmitted to the roots of host plants by the zoospores of the fungus *Olpidium brassicae* (Wor.) Dang. The process of TNV transmission by the fungus is rather complicated, and for effective transmission a definite combination of the virus strain, fungus isolate, and host species is required (Kassanis and MacFarlane, 1968). This system is made still more complicated by the inclusion of the additional component, STNV: it turned out that *O. brassicae* can transmit both TNV and STNV present in the mixture. The specificity of transmission of different STNV strains by *O. brassicae* was studied by Kassanis and MacFarlane (1968). The authors failed to transmit strain SV_1 by the fungus, while two other strains (SV_2 and SV_3) could be transmitted by certain peculiar strains of *O. brassicae*.

Activation of STNV can occur in different plant species, and the interaction between the helper and satellite seems to differ somewhat in different hosts. For example, TNV increases more actively in tobacco than in beans, whereas STNV multiplies more effectively and reaches higher concentrations in bean than in tobacco plants mixedly infected by TNV and STNV (Kassanis, 1962). SV_3 multiplies poorly in tobacco and French bean leaves, whereas SV_1 and SV_2 increase readily in the leaves of these plants inoculated mechanically. However, SV_3 reproduces better in tobacco roots infected in a liquid medium containing zoospores of *O. brassicae,* TNV, and STNV. It is not clear why SV_3 reaches a higher concentration in roots than in leaves of tobacco. However, this observation once more points to the complexity of the system of interactions among the host, TNV, and STNV. The facts mentioned above suggest that the process of TNV–STNV interaction not only is controlled by the matching between the appropriate products coded by helper and satellite but also depends on some host cell-coded products yet unknown.

3.5. Interference between TNV and STNV

TNV multiplies most efficiently alone (Table 4). Addition of STNV and a progressive increase of its concentration in the inoculum result in a suppression of the TNV reproduction. With a large excess of STNV in the mixed inoculum, the multiplication of TNV is inhibited to such an extent that its presence in the inoculated plants is difficult to detect serologically (Kassanis, 1962). The extent to which STNV inhibits TNV replication in mixedly infected cells depends on the given combination of TNV and STNV strains (Kassanis and Phillips, 1970).

Kassanis and Nixon (1960, 1961) noted that the size of lesions produced by TNV in bean and tobacco plants depended on the composition of the inoculum. TNV produced large uniform-sized lesions. The size of lesions decreased when STNV particles were present in the mixed (TNV plus STNV) inoculum. On addition of a large excess of STNV, practically no large lesions formed (Kassanis and Nixon, 1960). At a sufficient concentration of STNV, when all or almost all the lesions were small, the total number of lesions decreased.

The decrease in lesion size produced by TNV can occur not only when TNV and STNV are inoculated in mixed inocula but also when these viruses are inoculated at different times. For example, only small lesions were produced when French bean plants were inoculated with TNV even 5 days after STNV inoculation. On the other hand, the ability of STNV to reduce the size of lesions was strongly dependent on the time interval between the first and second inoculations, provided that TNV was inoculated first. It was shown by Kassanis (1962) that the number of small lesions decreased progressively as the interval between inoculations increased from 30 min to 5 h, and all the lesions were large at a 1-day interval. It is important to note that STNV was capable of being replicated even when inoculated a day after TNV, and all the lesions were large.

The data on the extent of inhibition of different TNV strains in mixed infection with different STNV strains were reported by Kassanis and Phillips (1970). It can be seen from Table 4 that inhibition of the replication of TNV strains A, B, S, E, AC-43, and CT occurs only when they are in combination with STNV strains activated by them (i.e., SV_1 and SV_2). No inhibition took place when these TNV strains were mixed with STNV strain SV_c. Interference can occur not only between TNV and STNV but also between different STNV strains. In fact, the STNV strains interfered with each other when one of them was present in the mixture in great excess. The replication of the STNV strain which was in minority was depressed greatly. Kassanis and White

(1972) suggest that interference occurs only between the STNV strains activated by the same helper and is due to the competition between such satellite viruses "for a metabolite that is probably coded by TNV." Thus, although STNV is activated by TNV, a marked competition occurs between TNV and its satellite in the course of lesion formation and virus replication. The mechanism responsible for the interference between TNV and STNV remains unknown. However, according to the data of Jones and Reichmann (1973), this interference consists of the inhibition of TNV both at the level of translation and viral RNA replication.

3.6.   Coding Properties of STNV Genome

3.6.1.   Speculations

The STNV particles contain a RNA molecule composed of about 1200–1300 nucleotide residues. A part of these nucleotides is engaged in coding for the STNV coat protein. It is possible to estimate the size of the coat protein gene from the molecular weight of the STNV structural protein. The molecular weight of the STNV coat protein was first reported as 38,000–39,000 (Reichmann, 1964). This seemed to support the concept that the coding capacity of the STNV genome corresponded to the size of the coat protein. The conclusion that STNV RNA codes for a single structural protein is, however, equivocal, since the molecular weight of this protein proved to be markedly lower than expected, amounting to a little more than 20,000 (see above). About 600 nucleotide residues are necessary to code for such a polypeptide chain, which accounts for one-half of the genetic information contained in STNV RNA. The rest of the STNV RNA molecule might have the potential for coding for one more virus-specific protein. Thus, on the basis of the triplet code, it is apparent that the STNV genome codes for not more than one protein besides the coat protein. This distinguishes STNV from all known viruses, since even the genomes of the simplest RNA viruses (bacteriophages) contain three genes and threefold more RNA.

It is generally believed that any complete RNA-containing virus is capable of coding for part or all of a virus-specific enzyme, RNA-dependent RNA polymerase. Since STNV seems to depend on TNV for all functions concerned with the synthesis of viral RNA, it appears possible that the TNV-specific RNA polymerase is responsible for replication of the RNA of both viruses.

It is well known that prokaryotic RNA replicases are distinguished for their high template specificity and ability to recognize only definite nucleotide sequences. If both TNV and STNV employ the same TNV-coded RNA replicase, it may be assumed that both types of RNA will possess identical or similar nucleotide sequences recognized by the enzyme. Klein and Reichmann (1970) reported that at least 10% of the STNV RNA molecule was homologous with that of TNV. However, this was questioned more recently by Shoulder et al. (1974), who failed to find any significant homology between the genomes of TNV and STNV (homology was negligible, if any, and existed between not more than 30 nucleotides). It may be concluded from these data that TNV and STNV genomes, for the most part, contain different genetic information. However, both TNV and STNV RNAs may contain similar short oligonucleotide sequences serving as a signal for initiating the activity of the TNV-specific polymerase.

While discussing the nature of the "help" rendered by TNV to STNV, it cannot be ruled out that TNV-coded RNA replicase is not involved at all in this interaction. It is possible that the STNV genome carries, besides the coat protein gene, a gene for a protein component of the STNV-specific RNA replicase system. On the other hand, it may also be assumed that this part of the genome codes not for a RNA replicase component but for some other protein, or that it does not contain any translated nucleotide sequences at all.

We know nothing of the properties and functions of the products required by STNV upon mixed infection with TNV. Therefore, we cannot exclude that by their nature such products are virus-induced (i.e., cell-coded). It might also be assumed that hypothetical virus-induced products can be induced by TNV but not by other viruses incapable of performing the role of STNV activators. Moreover, it appears possible that under certain environmental conditions or in some other plant species such products may arise even in a healthy plant, and that therefore replication of STNV might be possible even in the absence of TNV.

It is worthwhile to dwell on one more aspect of interaction of TNV and STNV. It was reported by Kassanis (1962, 1963, 1964, 1966) that STNV particles can be activated by TNV even if introduced into the leaf 5 days before the helper virus. This observation suggests that the STNV genome is somehow conserved in the infected cell in the absence of TNV helper. It could be that STNV particles penetrate into the cell but cannot uncoat their RNA in the absence of helper-virus. However, it does not seem very likely that the helper functions of TNV resides in its capacity to induce in the infected cell some mechanism for the uncoating of STNV particles which is not induced by any other viruses. Unfortunately, the fate of parental STNV particles at the initial stages of infection has not been followed in the infected cells. We do not know whether STNV RNA is uncoated completely or partially, and whether it is translated in the absence of activator.

3.6.2. Translation of STNV RNA *in Vitro* and *in Vivo*

One of the beneficial approaches to estimation of the number of proteins coded by STNV RNA may be a study of the translation products of this RNA *in vitro* in a cell-free protein-synthesizing system and *in vivo* in the infected cell.

The products coded by STNV RNA were studied with the *in vitro* protein-synthesizing systems from *Escherichia coli* and wheat embryo. Thus Clark *et al.* (1965) showed that STNV RNA could be translated in a cell-free system from *E. coli*, producing STNV protein similar to the authentic viral coat protein. Later it was shown that the product of STNV RNA translation in *E. coli* as well as in the wheat germ cell-free system is a protein very similar or identical to STNV coat protein in amino acid sequence. However, it was noted that the *in vitro* product was slightly smaller in size than authentic STNV coat protein (Klein *et al.*, 1972), which may suggest that the translation of the coat protein gene was incomplete or that the *in vitro* translation product was shortened due to the action of *C*-terminal proteases.

More recently, it was found by Rice and Fraenkel-Conrat (1973) that only a negligible part (about 5%) of the translation products synthesized in a *E. coli* cell-free system programmed by STNV RNA is similar in size to the authentic coat protein. The authors concluded that only an insignificant amount of complete STNV coat protein could be produced *in vitro* and that the bulk of the material was of varying smaller sizes. Rice and Fraenkel-Conrat (1973) suggested that "either the translation of STNV-RNA was particularly susceptible to degradative enzyme activities or that *E. coli* ribosomes may have had difficulty in recognizing the proper initiation site(s) on STNV-RNA." The fragmentation of STNV RNA by the endonucleases present in the cell-free *E. coli* system also is not ruled out.

However, all the workers basically agree that the STNV RNA *in vitro* translation products are very similar or identical to the natural STNV coat protein in amino acid sequence (Klein *et al.*, 1972; Lundquist *et al.*, 1972; Rice and Fraenkel-Conrat, 1973; Seal and Marcus, 1973). The correct translation of STNV RNA takes place in both prokaryotic and eukaryotic systems, indicating that the same signal for the proper initiation of translation is recognized by *E. coli* as by wheat germ ribosomes.

The fine structure or localization of this initiator within the STNV RNA molecule is obscure. Yet, as follows from the data of Klein *et al.* (1972), Lundquist *et al.* (1972), and Seal and Marcus (1973), there are an AUG (or GUG) (methionine) codon and two successive codons of alanine and lysine which code for the *N*-terminal sequence of methionine–alanine–lysine of the STNV coat protein. The originally synthesized coat protein later loses its *N*-terminal methionine (Lundquist *et al.*, 1972).*

All studies concerning *in vitro* translation of STNV RNA failed to reveal any polypeptide besides the coat protein among the translation products, supporting the view that STNV RNA is monocistronic. Although the coat protein is the only protein formed upon STNV RNA translation *in vitro*, it must be emphasized once again that the coat protein gene is likely to represent only about one-half of the whole RNA molecule. Presumably, the rest of STNV RNA does not contain translated genetic information; however, it is not excluded that it may correspond to a second gene partially repressed by some regulatory mechanism. It is well known, for example, that the coat protein gene of RNA bacteriophages is translated much more effectively than the A-protein gene (see Chapter 1 in Volume 2 of *Comprehensive Virology*).

The regulation at the level of translation is a known phenomenon for some plant viruses. In particular, it was reported by Shih and Kaesberg (1973) that the coat protein was the only product of translation when the total mixture of four brome mosaic virus (virus with divided genome) RNAs was translated in the cell-free system from wheat embryo. Under these conditions, the translation of three other messengers (fragments 1, 2, and 3 of BMV RNA) was repressed, and only fragment 4 (the monocistronic mRNA coding for BMV coat protein) was actively translated. It may therefore be assumed that a similar regulatory phenomenon may occur also upon STNV RNA translation.

It was especially important to compare the products of the *in vitro* STNV RNA translation with those produced in virus-infected cells. Such an attempt was made by Jones and Reichmann (1973). The authors found that several proteins appeared after infection with TNV alone, and only one additional protein (STNV coat protein) appeared in plants coinfected with TNV and STNV.

---

* *Editor's comment:* See Chapter 4 for more recent data on STNV translation and RNA replicases.

On the whole, it seems reasonable to suggest that STNV RNA actually serves as a monocistronic message for the coat protein. No information, however, is available on the significance of the remaining half of the STNV RNA molecule or the nature of the functions performed by the TNV helper.

4. CONCLUDING REMARKS

By the term "defective viruses" is meant, in a general sense, viruses that lack part of the functional proteins or produce nonfunctional virus-specific protein(s) essential for virus replication. The tentative nature of any subdivision of viruses into "normal," "defective," "deficient," and "satellite" has been discussed.

Defectiveness of a virus may be manifested as interruption of its reproduction at some phase of the infection cycle, as decreased productivity of virus multiplication as compared to the normal virus, or as low specific infectivity of the virus progeny. An attempt has been made to describe the functions for virus replication which, if lacking, may render it defective.

Different examples of defectiveness of the coat protein have been discussed. In the absence of active coat protein, the RNA of many viruses can replicate, yielding infective progeny RNA molecules. This type of infectious agent remains unprotected by any coat protein against the action of RNases in the cell sap, and becomes inactivated by the usual virus extraction methods.

One of the examples of defectiveness in viruses is conditional defectiveness, when the virus-coded product becomes nonfunctional only under certain conditions (e.g., at elevated temperature). Two classes of *ts* TMV mutants have been discussed: class I *ts* mutants, which contain the *ts* mutation in the coat protein gene, and class II *ts* mutants, which contain the mutation in one of the non-coat protein genes. Under nonpermissive conditions, infectious viral RNA not protected by the protein accumulates in cells infected by *ts* I mutants. Phenomenologically similar is the result of infection by the large component of multicomponent viruses, which lacks the coat protein gene.

The phenomenon of satellitism in viruses has been considered as an example of the more general phenomenon—complementation between viruses. An association between TNV and STNV has been discussed in detail as a classical example of satellitism in viruses. It seems reasonable to suggest that, upon TNV–STNV interaction, STNV RNA serves as a monocistronic message for the coat protein and STNV depends on TNV for all the functions concerned with the synthesis of viral RNA. Unfortunately, no information is available concerning the significance of the remaining part of the STNV RNA molecule (besides the coat protein gene) or on the nature of the functions performed by TNV helper.

5. REFERENCES

Atabekov, J. G., 1975, Host-specificity of plant viruses, *Annu. Rev. Phytopathol.* **13**:127.

Atabekov, J. G., and Novikov, V. K., 1966, Some properties of barley stripe mosaic virus nucleoprotein and its substructural components, *Biokhimya (USSR)* **31**:157.

Atabekov, J. G., and Novikov, V. K., 1971, Barley stripe mosaic virus, C.M.I./A.A.B. Descriptions of Plant Viruses No. 68.

Atabekov, J. G., Popova, G. A., Kiselev, N. A., and Kaftanova, A. S., and Petrovsky, G. V., 1968, *In vitro* polymerization of winter wheat mosaic virus antigen, *Virology* **35**:458.

Atabekov, J. G., Schaskolskaya, N. D., Atabekova, T. I., and Sacharovskaya, G. N., 1970, Reproduction of temperature-sensitive strains of TMV under restrictive conditions in the presence of temperature-resistant helper strain, *Virology* **41**:397.

Atabekova, T. I., Taliansky, M. E., and Atabekov, J. G., 1975, Specificity of protein-RNA and protein-protein interaction upon assembly of TMV *in vivo* and *in vitro*, *Virology* **67**:1.

Babos, P., and Kassanis, B., 1962, Unstable variants of tobacco necrosis virus, *Virology* **18**:206.

Babos, P., and Kassanis, B., 1963, Serological relationships and some properties of tobacco necrosis virus strains, *J. Gen. Microbiol.* **32**:135.

Bald, J. G., 1964, Symptoms and cytology of living cells infected with defective mutants of tobacco mosaic virus, *Virology* **22**:388.

Bald, J. G., Gumpf, D. J., and Heick, J., 1974, Transition from common tobacco mosaic virus to the *Nicotiana glauca* form, *Virology* **59**:467.

Ball, L. A., Minson, A. C., and Shih, D. S., 1973, Synthesis of plant virus coat proteins in an animal cell-free system, *Nature (London)* New Biol. **246**:206.

Bawden, F. C., 1941, The serological reactions of viruses causing tobacco necrosis, *Br. J. Exp. Pathol.* **22**:59.

Bawden, F. C., and Pirie, N. W., 1942, A preliminary description of preparations of some of the viruses causing tobacco necrosis, *Br. J. Exp. Pathol.* **23**:314.

Bawden, F. C., and Pirie, N. W., 1945, Further studies on the purification and properties of a virus causing tobacco necrosis, *Br. J. Exp. Pathol.* **26**:277.

Bawden, F. C., and Pirie, N. W., 1950, Some fractions affecting the activation of virus preparations made from tobacco leaves infected with a tobacco necrosis virus, *J. Gen. Microbiol.* **4**:464.

Bawden, F. C., and Pirie, N. W., 1956, Observations on the anomalous proteins occurring in extracts of plants infected with strains of tobacco mosaic virus, *J. Gen. Microbiol.* **14**:460.

Bhalla, R. B., and Sehgal, O. P., 1973, Host range and purification of the nucleic acid of a defective mutant of tobacco mosaic virus, *Phytopathology* **63**:906.

Bos, L., and van der Want, J. P. H., 1962, Early browning of pea, a disease caused by soil- and seed-borne virus, *Tijdschr. Plantenziekten* **68**:368.

Bosch, F. X., and Jockusch, H., 1972, Temperature-sensitive mutants of TMV: Behaviour of a non-coat protein mutant in isolated tobacco cells, *Mol. Gen. Genet.* **116**:95.

Bruening, G., Beachy, R. N., Scalla, R., and Zaitlin, M., 1976, *In vitro* and *in vivo* translation of the ribonucleic acids of a cowpea strain of tobacco mosaic virus, *Virology* **71**:498.

Butler, P. J. G., and Durham, A. C. H., 1972, Structures and roles of the polymorphic forms of tobacco mosaic virus. V. Conservation of the abnormally titrating groups in tobacco mosaic virus, *J. Mol. Biol.* **72**:19.

Butler, P. J. G., Durham, A. C. K., and Klug, A., 1972, Structures and functions of the polymorphic forms of tobacco mosaic virus protein. IV. Control of mode of aggregation of tobacco mosaic virus protein by proton binding. *J. Mol. Biol.* **72**:1.

Cadman, C. H., 1962, Evidence for association of tobacco rattle virus nucleic acid with a cell component, *Nature (London)* **193**:49.

Caspar, D. L. D., 1963, Assembly and stability of the tobacco mosaic virus particle, *Adv. Protein Chem.* **18**:37.

Clark, J. M., Chang, A. Y., Spiegelman, S., and Reichmann, M. E., 1965, The *in vitro* translation of a monocistronic message, *Proc. Natl. Acad. Sci. USA* **54**:1193.

Cole, C. H., and Baltimore, D., 1973a, Defective interfering particles of poliovirus. II. Nature of the defect, *J. Mol. Biol.* **76**:325.

Cole, C. H., and Baltimore, D., 1973b, Defective interfering particles of poliovirus. III. Interference and enrichment, *J. Mol. Biol.* **76**:345.

Cole, C. H., Smoler, D., Wimmer, E., and Baltimore, D., 1971, Defective interfering particles of poliovirus. I. Isolation and physical properties, *J. Virol.* **7**:478.

Diener, T. O., and Schneider, I., 1966, The two components of tobacco ringspot virus nucleic acid: Origin and properties, *Virology* **29**:100.

Diener, T. O., and Smith, D. R., 1973, Potato spindle tuber viroid. IX. Molecular weight determination by gel electrophoresis of formylated RNA. *Virology* **53**:359.

Dodds, J. A., and Hamilton, R. I., 1972, The influence of barley stripe mosaic virus on the replication of tobacco mosaic virus in *Hordeum vulgare* L., *Virology* **50**:404.

Fraenkel-Conrat, H., 1969, *The Chemistry and Biology of Viruses,* Academic Press, New York.

Fraenkel-Conrat, H., and Singer, B., 1957, Virus reconstitution. II. Combination of protein and nucleic acid from different strains. *Biochim. Biophys. Acta* **24**:540.

Francki, R. I. B., 1966, Some factors affecting particle length distribution in tobacco mosaic virus preparations, *Virology* **30**:388.

Funatsu, G., and Fraenkel-Conrat, H., 1964, Location of amino acid exchanges in chemically evoked mutants of tobacco mosaic virus, *Biochemistry* **3**:1356.

Gibbs, A. J., and Harrison, B. D., 1964, A form of pea early-browning virus found in Britain, *Ann. Appl. Biol.* **54**:1.

Grogan, R. G., and Uyemoto, J. K., 1967, A D-serotype of satellite virus specifically associated with a D-serotype of tobacco necrosis virus, *Nature (London)* **213**:705.

Hamilton, R. I., and Dodds, J. A., 1970, Infection of barley by tobacco mosaic virus in single and mixed infection, *Virology* **42**:266.

Hariharasubramanian, V., and Siegel, A., 1967, Studies on a new defective strain of tobacco mosaic virus, *Phytopathology* **57**:814.

Hariharasubramanian, V., and Siegel, A., 1969, Characterization of a new defective strain of TMV, *Virology* **37**:203.

Hariharasubramanian, V., and Zaitlin, M., 1968, Temperature-induced insoluble coat protein in TMV-infected plants, *Virology* **36**:521.

Hariharasubramanian, V., Zaitlin, M., and Siegel, A., 1970, A temperature-sensitive mutant of TMV with unstable coat protein, *Virology* **40**:579.

Hariharasubramanian, V., Smith, R. C., and Zaitlin, M., 1973, Insoluble coat protein mutants of TMV: Their origin, and characterization of the defective coat proteins, *Virology* **55**:202.

Harrison, B. D., 1966, Further studies on British form of pea early browning virus, *Ann. Appl. Biol.* **57**:121.

Harrison, B. D., 1970, Tobacco rattle virus, C.M.T./AAB Descriptions of Plant Viruses No. 12.

Harrison, B. D., and Jones, R. A. V., 1970, Host range and some properties of potato mop-top virus, *Ann. Appl. Biol.* **65**:393.

Harrison, B. D., Murant, A. F., and Mayo, M. A., 1973, Evidence for two functional RNA species in raspberry ringspot virus, *J. Gen. Virol.* **16**:339.

Horst, J., Fraenkel-Conrat, H., and Mandeles, S., 1971, Terminal heterogeneity of both ends of the satellite tobacco necrosis virus ribonucleic acid, *Biochemistry* **10**:4748.

Huang, A. S., and Baltimore, D., 1970, Defective viral particles and viral disease processes, *Nature (London)* **226**:325.

Hubert, J. J., and Zaitlin, M., 1972, A strain of tobacco mosaic virus with defective coat protein and its reversion to a functional form, *Phytopathology* **62**:766 (abst.).

Hulett, H. R., and Loring, M. S., 1965, Effect of particle length distribution on infectivity of tobacco mosaic virus, *Virology* **25**:418.

Huttinga, H., 1969, Interaction between components of pea early-browning virus, *Neth. J. Plant pathol.* **75**:338.

Jockusch, H., 1964, *In vivo* and *in vitro* Verhalten temperatursensitiver Mutanten des Tabakmosaikvirus, *Z. Vererbungsl.* **95**:379.

Jockusch, H., 1966a, Relations between temperature sensitivity, amino acid replacements and quaternary structure of mutant proteins, *Biochem. Biophys. Res. Commun.* **24**:577.

Jockusch, H., 1966b, Temperatursensitive Mutanten des Tabakmosaikvirus. I. *In vivo*-verhalten, *Z. Vererbungsl.* **98**:320.

Jockusch, J., 1966c, Temperatursensitive Mutanten des Tabakmosaikvirus. II. *In vitro*-verhalten, *Z. Vererbungsl.* **98**:344.

Jockusch, H., 1968a, Stability and genetic variation of a structural protein, *Naturwissenschaften* **55**:514.

Jockusch, H., 1968b, Two mutants of tobacco mosaic virus temperature-sensitive in two different functions, *Virology* **35**:94.

Jones, I. M., and Reichmann, M. E., 1973, The proteins synthesized in tobacco leaves infected with tobacco necrosis virus and satellite tobacco necrosis virus, *Virology* **52**:49.

Kado, C. I., and Knight, C. A., 1966, Location of a local lesion gene in tobacco mosaic virus RNA, *Proc. Natl. Acad. Sci. USA* **55**:1276.

Kapitsa, O. S., Andreeva, E. N., and Vostrova, N. G., 1969a, Defective mutant of a thermotolerant strain of tobacco mosaic virus. I. Isolation and properties, *Vopr. Virusol. (USSR)* **14**:397.

Kapitsa, O. S., Andreeva, E. N., Tkalenko, L. V., and Vostrova, N. G., 1969b, Defective mutant of thermotolerant strain of tobacco mosaic virus. III. Detection of the nonfunctional structural protein of the defective mutant and some of its properties, *Biol. Nauki (USSR)* **12**:117.

Kapitsa, O. S., Vostrova, N. G., and Andreeva, E. N., 1969c, Defective mutant of thermotolerant strain of TMV. II. Spread of the virus in plant. Instability. Reversion and reconstitution *in vivo, Vopr. Virusol. (USSR)* **5**:623.

Kapitsa, O. S., Vostrova, N. G., and Andreeva, E. N., 1970, Defective mutant of termotolerant strain of tobacco mosaic virus. V. Complementation between defective mutant and thermotolerant strain at high temperature, *Biol. Nauki (USSR)* **3**:107.

Kassanis, B., 1960, Comparison of the early stages of infection by intact and phenol-disrupted tobacco necrosis virus, *Virology* **10**:353.

Kassanis, B., 1962, Properties and behaviour of a virus depending for its multiplication on another, *J. Gen. Microbiol.* **27**:477.

Kassanis, B., 1963, Interactions of viruses in plants, *Adv. Virus Res.* **10**:219.

Kassanis, B., 1964, Properties of tobacco necrosis virus and its association with satellite virus, *Ann. Inst. Phytopathol. Benaki* **6**:7.

Kassanis, B., 1966, Satellite virus and its interaction with tobacco necrosis virus. *Bull. Soc. Fr. Physiol. Veg.* **12**:257.

Kassanis, B., 1967, Tobacco necrosis virus and its satellite virus, *Nature (London)* **214**:178.

Kassanis, B., 1968, Satellitism and related phenomena in plant and animal viruses, *Adv. Virus Res.* **13**:147.

Kassanis, B., and Bastow, C., 1971a, *In vivo* phenotypic mixing between two strains of tobacco mosaic virus, *J. Gen. Virol.* **10**:95.

Kassanis, B., and Bastow, C., 1971b, Phenotypic mixing between strains of tobacco mosaic virus, *J. Gen. Virol.* **11**:171.

Kassanis, B., and Bastow, C., 1971c, The relative concentration of infective intact virus and RNA of four strains of tobacco mosaic virus as influenced by temperature, *J. Gen. Virol.* **11**:157.

Kassanis, B., and Conti, M., 1971, Defective strains and phenotypic mixing, *J. Gen. Virol.* **13**:361.

Kassanis, B., and McCarthy, D., 1967, The quality of virus as affected by the ambient temperature. *J. Gen. Virol.* **1**:425.

Kassanis, B., and MacFarlane, I., 1968, The transmission of satellite viruses of tobacco necrosis virus by *Olpidium brassicae, J. Gen. Virol.* **3**:227.

Kassanis, B., and Nixon, H. L., 1960, Activation of one plant virus by another, *Nature (London)* **187**:713.

Kassanis, B., and Nixon, H. L., 1961, Activation of one virus by another, *J. Gen. Microbiol.* **25**:459.

Kassanis, B., and Phillips, M. P., 1970, Serological relationship of strains of tobacco necrosis virus and their ability to activate strains of satellite virus, *J. Gen. Virol.* **90**:119.

Kassanis, B., and Turner, R. H., 1972, Virus inclusions formed by the PM$_2$ mutant of TMV, *J. Gen. Virol.* **14**:119.

Kassanis, B., and Welkie, G. W., 1963, The nature and behaviour of unstable variants of tobacco necrosis virus, *Virology* **21**:540.

Kassanis, B., and White, R. F., 1972, Interference between two satellite viruses of tobacco necrosis virus. *J. Gen. Virol.* **17**:177.

Kassanis, B., and Woods, R. D., 1968, Aggregated forms of the satellite of tobacco necrosis virus, *J. Gen. Virol.* **2**:395.

Kassanis, B., and Woods, R. D., 1969, Properties of some defective strains of tobacco mosaic virus and their behaviour as affected by inhibitors during storage in sap, *Ann. Appl. Biol.* **64**:213.

Kassanis, B., Vinee, D. A., and Woods, R. D., 1970, Light and electron microscopy of cells infected with tobacco necrosis and satellite viruses, *J. Gen. Virol.* **7**:143.

Klein, A., and Reichmann, M. E., 1970, Isolation and characterization of two species of double-stranded RNA from tobacco leaves doubly infected with tobacco necrosis and satellite tobacco necrosis viruses, *Virology* **42**:269.

Klein, W. H., Nolan, C., Lazar, J. M., and Clark, J. M., 1972, Translation of satellite tobacco necrosis virus ribonucleic acid. I. Characterization of *in vitro* procariotic and eucariotic translation products, *Biochemistry* **11**:2009.

Lebeurier, G., and Hirth, L., 1966, Effect of elevated temperatures on the development of two strains of tobacco mosaic virus, *Virology* **29**:385.

Lebeurier, G., and Wurtz, M., 1968, Properties d'un clone isolate a partir d'une souche thermophile du virus de le mosaique du tabac, *C. R. Hebd. Seances Acad. Sci.* **267**:871.

Lesnaw, J. A., and Reichmann, M. E., 1970*a*, Identity of the 5′-terminal RNA nucleotide sequence of the satellite tobacco necrosis virus and its helper virus: Possible role of the 5′-terminus in the recognition by virus-specific RNA replicase, *Proc. Natl. Acad. Sci. USA* **66**:140.

Lesnaw, J. A., and Reichmann, M. E., 1970*b*, Determination of molecular weights of plant virus subunits by polyacrylamide gel electrophoresis, *Virology* **42**:724.

Lister, R. M., 1966, Possible relationships of virus-specific products of tobacco rattle virus infections, *Virology* **28**:350.

Lister, R. M., 1967, A symptomatological difference between some unstable and stable variants of pea early browning virus, *Virology* **31**:739.

Lister, R. M., 1969, Tobacco rattle, NETU, viruses in relation to functional heterogeneity in plant viruses, *Fed. Proc. Am. Soc. Exp. Biol.* **28**:1875.

Lundquist, R. E., Lazar, J. M., Klein, W. H., and Clark, J. M., 1972, Translation of satellite tobacco necrosis virus ribonucleic acid. II. Initiation of *in vitro* translation in procaryotic and eucaryotic systems, *Biochemistry* **11**:2014.

Matthews, R. E. F., 1970, *Plant Virology,* Academic Press, New York.

Matthews, R. E. F., and Ralph, R. K., 1966, Turnip yellow mosaic virus, *Adv. Virus Res.* **12**:273.

McKinney, H. H., and Greeley, L. W., 1965, Biological characteristics of barley stripe mosaic strains and their evolution, *U.S. Dep. Agr. Tech. Bull.* **118**:1.

Morris, T. J., 1974, Two nucleoprotein components associated with the cowpea strain of TMV, *Proc. Am. Phytopathol. Soc.* **1**:83.

Nagaraj, A. N., 1965, Immunofluorescence studies on synthesis and distribution of tobacco mosaic virus antigen in tobacco, *Virology* **25**:133.

Parish, C. L., and Zaitlin, M., 1966, Defective tobacco mosaic virus strains: Identification of the protein of strain PM1 in leaf homogenates, *Virology* **30**:297.

Pirie, N. W., Smith, R. M., Spooner, E. T. C., and McClement, W. D., 1938, Purified preparations of tobacco necrosis virus (*Nicotiana* virus II), *Parasitology* **30**:543.

Rappaport, I., 1965, The antigenic structure of tobacco mosaic virus, *Adv. Virus Res.* **11**:223.

Rappaport, I., and Zaitlin, M., 1967, Antigenic study of the protein from a defective strain of tobacco mosaic virus, *Science* **157**:207.

Rappaport, I., Siegel, A., and Zaitlin, M., 1964, Unpublished data cited by I. Rappaport, 1965.

Razvjazkina, G. M., Poljakova, G. P., Stein-Margolina, V. A., and Cherny, N. E., 1968, Electron microscopic studies of plant viruses in cells of plants and vectors, *First Int. Congr. Plant Pathol., London*, p. 162.

Rees, M. W., Short, M. N., and Kassanis, B., 1970, The amino acid composition, antigenicity, and other characteristics of the satellite viruses of tobacco necrosis virus, *Virology* **40**:448.

Reichmann, M. E., 1964, The satellite tobacco necrosis virus: A single protein and its genetic code, *Proc. Natl. Acad. Sci. USA* **52**:1009.

Reichmann, M. E., Rees, M. W., Symons, R. H., and Markham, R., 1962, Experimental evidence for the degeneracy of the nucleotide triplet code, *Nature (London)* **195**:999.

Rezaian, M. A., and Francki, R. I. B., 1974, Replication of tobacco ringspot virus. II. Differences in nucleotide sequence between the viral RNA components, *Virology* **59**:275.

Rice, R. H., 1974, Minor protein components in cowpea chlorotic mottle virus and satellite of tobacco necrosis virus, *Virology* **61**:249.

Rice, R., and Fraenkel-Conrat, H., 1973, Fidelity of translation of satellite tobacco necrosis virus ribonucleic acid in a cell-free *Escherichia coli* system, *Biochemistry* **12**:181.

Rochow, W. F., 1970, Barley yellow dwarf virus, C.M.I./A.A.B. Descriptions of Plant Viruses No. 32.

Roy, D., Fraenkel-Conrat, H., Lesnaw, J., and Reichmann, M. E., 1969, The protein subunit of the satellite tobacco necrosis virus, *Virology* **38**:368.

Samuel, G., 1931, Some experiments on inoculating methods with plant viruses and on local lesions, *Ann. Appl. Biol.* **18**:494.

Sarkar, S., 1967, Characterization and measurement of virus-specific nucleic acids during early stages of infection by tobacco mosaic virus, *Plant Disease Problems, Proc. 1st Int. Symp. Plant pathol. Indian Agr. Res. Inst. New Delhi*, p. 772.

Sarkar, S., 1969, Evidence of phenotypic mixing between two strains of tobacco mosaic virus, *Mol. Gen. Genet.* **105**:87.

Sarkar, S., and Jockusch, H., 1968, Wild type and defective coat proteins of tobacco mosaic virus: Electrophoretic analysis of plant extracts in polyacrylamide gels, *Biochim. Biophys. Acta* **106**:259.

Schaskolskaya, N. D., Atabekov, J. G., Sacharovskaya, G. N., and Javachia, V. G., 1968, Replication of temperature-sensitive strain of tobacco mosaic virus under nonpermissive conditions in the presence of helper strain, *Biol. Sci. (USSR)* **8**:101.

Schneider, I. R., 1969, Satellite-like particle of tobacco rinspot virus that resembles tobacco ringspot virus, *Science* **166**:1627.

Schneider, I. R., 1971, Characteristics of a satellite-like virus of tobacco ringspot virus, *Virology* **45**:108.

Schneider, I. R., 1972, TRSV codes for the coat protein of its satellite, *Phytopathology* **62**:788 (*abst.*)

Schneider, I. R., and Diener, T. O., 1966, The correlation between the proportions of virus-related products and the infectious component during the synthesis of tobacco ringspot virus, *Virology* **29**:92.

Schneider, I. R., and White R. M., 1976, Tobacco ringspot virus codes for the coat protein of its satellite, *Virology* **70**:244.

Schneider, I. R., Hull, R., and Markham, R., 1972a, Multidense satellite of tobacco ringspot virus: A regular series of components of different densities, *Virology* **47**:320.

Schneider, I. R., White, R. M., and Gooding, G. V., 1972b, Two new isolates of the satellite of tobacco ringspot virus, *Virology* **50**:902.

Schuster, H., and Schramm, G., 1958, Bestimmung der biologisch wirksamen Einheit in der Ribosenucleinsäure des Tabakmosaikvirus auf chemischen Wege, *Z. Naturforsch.* **13b**:697.

Seal, S. N., and Marcus, A., 1973, Translation of the initial codons of satellite tobacco necrosis virus ribonucleic acid in a cell-free system from wheat embryo, *J. Biol. Chem.* **248**:6577.

Sehgal, O. P., 1973, Biological and physico-chemical properties of an atypical mutant of tobacco mosaic virus, *Mol. Gen. Genet.* **121**:15.

Shih, D. S., and Kaesberg, P., 1973, Translation of brome mosaic viral ribonucleic acid in a cell-free system derived from wheat embryo, *Proc. Natl. Acad. Sci. USA* **70**:1799.

Shoulder, A., Darby, G., and Minson, T., 1974, RNA-DNA hybridisation using I[125]-labelled RNA from tobacco necrosis virus and its satellite, *Nature (London)* **251**:733.

Siegel, A., 1965, Artificial production of mutants of tobacco mosaic virus, *Adv. Virus Res.* **11**:25.

Siegel, A., Zaitlin, M., and Sehgal, O. P., 1962, The isolation of defective tobacco mosaic virus strains. *Proc. Natl. Acad. Sci. USA* **48**:1845.

Siegel, A., Hills, G. J., and Markham, R., 1966, *In vitro* and *in vivo* aggregation of the defective PM2 TMV protein, *J. Mol. Biol.* **19**:140.

Singer, B., and Fraenkel-Conrat, H., 1974, Correlation between amino acid exchanges in coat protein of TMV mutants and the nature of the mutagenesis, *Virology* **60**:485.

Smith, , and Bald, , 1935,

Smith, K., and Bald, J., A description of a necrotic virus disease affecting tobacco and other plants, *Parasitology* **27**:231.

Sogo, J. M., Schneider, I. R., and Koller, T., 1974, Size determination by electron microscopy of the RNA of tobacco ringspot satellite virus, *Virology* **57**:459.

Stace-Smith, R., Reichmann, M. E., and Wright, N. S., 1965, Purification and properties of tobacco ringspot virus and two RNA-deficient components, *Virology* **25**:487.

Suckov, R. S., 1943, Purification of crystal preparation of winter wheat mosaic virus, *Dokl. Acad. Nauk SSSR* **39**:72.

Teakle, D. S., 1962, Transmission of tobacco necrosis virus by a fungus, *Olpidium brassicae*, *Virology* **18**:224.

Tsugita, A., and Fraenkel-Conrat, H., 1962, The composition of proteins of chemically evoked mutants of TMV-RNA, *J. Mol. Biol.* **4**:73.

Uyemoto, J. K., and Grogan, R. G., 1969, Chemical characterization of tobacco necrosis and satellite viruses, *Virology* **39**:79.

Uyemoto, J. K., Grogan, R. G., and Wakeman, J. R., 1968, Selective activation of satellite virus strains by strains of tobacco necrosis virus, *Virology* **34**:410.

van Kammen, A., 1972, Plant viruses with a divided genome, *Ann. Rev. Phytopathol.* **10**:125.

Veldee, S., and Fraenkel-Conrat, H., 1962, The characterization of tobacco mosaic virus strains by their productivity, *Virology* **18**:56.

Wimmer, E., Chang, A. Y., Clark, J. M., and Reichmann, M. E., 1968, Sequence studies of satellite tobacco necrosis virus RNA. Isolation and characterization of a 5′-terminal trinucleotide, *J. Mol. Biol.* **38**:73.

Wittmann, H. G., 1964, Proteinanalysen von chimisch induzierten Mutanten des Tabakmosaikvirus, *Z. Vererbungsl.* **95**:333.

Wittmann, H. G., 1965, Die Proteinstruktur der Defektmutante PM2 des Tabakmosaikvirus, *Z. Vererbungsl.* **97**:297.

Wittmann, H. G., and Wittmann-Liebold, B., 1966, Protein chemical studies of two RNA viruses and their mutants, *Cold Spring Harbor Symp. Quant. Biol.* **31**:163.

Wittmann-Liebold, B., Jauregui-Adell, J., and Wittmann, H., 1965, Die primare Proteinstruktur temperatursensitiver Mutanten des Tabakmosaikvirus. II. Chemisch induzierte Mutanten, *Z. Naturforsch.* **206**:1235.

Zaitlin, M., and Ferris, W. R. 1964, Unusual aggregation of a nonfunctional tobacco mosaic virus protein, *Science* **143**:1451.

Zaitlin, M., and Hariharasubramanian, V., 1968, The purification of insoluble coat proteins from defective mutants of tobacco mosaic virus (TMV), *Phytopathology* **58**:1074 (abst.).

Zaitlin, M., and Keswani, C. L., 1964, Relative infectivities of tissues containing a defective tobacco mosaic virus strain, *Virology* **24**:495.

Zaitlin, M., and McCaughey, W. F., 1965, Amino acid composition of a nonfunctional tobacco mosaic virus protein, *Virology* **26**:500.

Zashurilo, V. K., and Sitnikova, G. M., 1939, Winter wheat mosaik, *Dokl. Akad. Nauk SSSR* **25**:9.

The Translation of Large Plant Viral RNAs

H. Fraenkel-Conrat and M. Salvato
Department of Molecular Biology and Virus Laboratory
University of California
Berkeley, California 94720

and

L. Hirth
Institut de Biologie Moleculaire et Cellulaire du C.N.R.S.
Strasbourg, France

1. HISTORICAL INTRODUCTION

The following overview of plant viral translation will center on the viruses with large, presumably multigenic RNAs (molecular weight over 10^6). This includes both the classical homodisperse viruses like TMV, and the large components of the multicomponent viruses like the bromoviridae.* Such viruses have lent themselves well to biochemical analyses and *in vitro* studies, but the mode of gene expression *in vivo* has proven difficult to elucidate.

The first identification of a mRNA in terms of its product was that poly(U) coded for polyphenylalanine (Nirenberg and Matthaei, 1961). Prior to that, Nirenberg had developed the preincubated *Escherichia coli* cell-free system and found TMV RNA to greatly stimulate

---

* The translation of the small components of the three-component viruses is discussed in detail by Van Vloten-Doting and Jaspars in Chapter 1.

amino acid incorporation by this system. This RNA, already known to be infective (Fraenkel-Conrat, 1956; Gierer and Schramm, 1956), was also a likely messenger, and it thus seemed logical for Nirenberg to initiate collaboration with Tsugita and Fraenkel-Conrat in hopes of quickly identifying the only known TMV gene product, the viral coat protein. This effort seemed at first successful since radioactive amino acids, presumably in TMV coat protein, appeared to reconstitute with TMV RNA to form virus (Tsugita *et al.,* 1962). However, as the difficulties in removing the last traces of radioactive amino acids from proteins and protein aggregates became more fully appreciated, and with improved techniques, it became apparent that most of the amino acids polymerized by the *E. coli* system upon addition of TMV RNA were not associated with TMV coat protein. This negative conclusion was arrived at on different grounds by Nathans *et al.* (1962), Aach *et al.* (1964), Schwartz (1967), and later Rice (1972).

Since in the meantime the same *E. coli in vitro* system had been found to synthesize two of the three known gene products of RNA phages, it was thought that the failure to obtain TMV protein *in vitro* might be due to differences in the mode of translation of eukaryotic mRNAs by prokaryotic systems. In particular, it seemed possible that eukaryotic messengers might possess initiation and termination signals which were not recognized by prokaryotic ribosomes. This explanation became dubious when evidence was adduced that several particularly small plant viral RNAs of molecular weights below 0.5×10^6 were translated with more or less fidelity into coat protein sequences by the *E. coli* system. This was the case for the smallest components of several coviruses (van Ravensway Claasen *et al.,* 1967; Stubbs and Kaesberg, 1967) as well as tobacco necrosis satellite virus (STNV) (Clark *et al.,* 1965; Rice, 1972; Klein *et al.,* 1972; Rice and Fraenkel-Conrat, 1973). These studies established the ability of plant viral RNA to serve directly as messenger, but the number and mode of translation of multiple genes on typical plant viral RNAs of $1-2 \times 10^6$ molecular weight remained unknown.

The next advance came with the development of effective cell-free amino acid incorporation systems from several eukaryotic cells such as wheat germ, ascites cells, and reticulocytes. Although the first reported product of *in vitro* translation of a plant gene by the wheat germ system, that of the STNV coat protein, was not identical in size to that protein (Klein *et al.,* 1972), unequivocal evidence for complete translation of the other small viral RNAs quickly established the usefulness of this system (Shih and Kaesberg, 1973; Davies and Kaesberg, 1974;

Schwinghamer and Symons, 1975). Yet with TMV RNA as messenger some of the multiple products were quite large, adding up in molecular weight to considerably more than the genome's capacity, while very little coat protein-sized product was seen.

It had in the meantime become evident that the picornaviridae, as exemplified by poliovirus, contained, like the RNA phages and most plant viruses, infective and thus directly messenger-active RNA, now termed "plus-strand RNA." The *in vivo* translation of the RNA of these viruses, however, differed from that of the then thoroughly studied phages in that multiple large products appeared, which showed under some conditions molecular weights greater than 0.2×10^6 and thus corresponded to almost the entire genome's length of 2.6×10^6 (Jacobson and Baltimore, 1968). The four coat proteins of the picornaviruses as well as other virus-coded proteins were actually shown to result from posttranslational cleavage of a large primary gene product. The question thus arose whether the same mechanism of secondary formation of gene products by proteolytic cleavage of a primary large translation product was also operative in plants, and whether this could account for the ambiguous results obtained in the studies of the translation of large plant viral RNAs. Although research in this area is still in an early stage and no clear general answers are at hand, it now appears that posttranslational cleavage is not the preferred strategy of plant viral translation. Instead, multigenic plant viral RNAs appear to be more frequently subjected to pretranslational processing, and most of the large proteins that are being made appear to be the ultimate products.

2. METHODOLOGY

Plant viral protein synthesis has been studied *in vivo* and *in vitro* in infected host plants, host protoplasts, frog oocytes, and various eukaryotic cell-free systems. We will discuss these studies in this order.

In general, plant protein synthesis is not markedly affected by virus infection, and thus the search for virus-coded proteins must be carried out with a background of high host-specific protein synthesis. This is particularly a problem for whole plants and protoplasts, but much less for oocytes and *in vitro* systems. Chloramphenicol treatment, and UV irradiation in the hands of some investigators, shows some selectivity in repressing synthesis of host proteins more than that of viral proteins.

Two techniques have been used to detect virus-coded proteins in plant cells. Earlier studies used double labeling: the infected and uninfected plants were given the same amino acid with ^{3}H or ^{14}C label, respectively; the plot of the ratios of these isotopes in polyacrylamide gel slices revealed protein peaks resulting from virus infection. The other technique relied on the high resolving power of slab gels and autoradiography or more recently fluorography (Bonner and Laskey, 1974) of singly labeled proteins: the appearance of new or denser bands as a result of infection was regarded as indicative of new viral proteins. The problem with both methods is that they do not distinguish between virus-coded proteins and host proteins induced by viral infection. It actually became evident in the course of such studies that induction as well as repression of individual host proteins was indeed a frequent occurrence (van Loon and van Kammen, 1970; Singer and Condit, 1974).

The oocyte system requires special techniques but affords an advantage in that protein synthesis from an injected message can continue over 24 h against a very low background (Gurdon *et al.*, 1971). So far, TMV appears to be the only plant virus whose RNA has been successfully injected and translated, although positive results have also been described for AMV by Marbaix (see Chapter 1, Section 5.2.2). The lack of more reports on plant viral translation in this system is probably due to technical problems such as keeping RNA intact during the injection procedure.

Among the cell-free incorporation systems, the wheat germ system has been most widely used. Mammalian systems such as derived from Krebs ascites or HeLa cells, as well as reticulocyte lysates, also respond well to plant viral RNA. In particular, the rabbit reticulocyte system is relatively RNase free and hence translates the high molecular weight products more faithfully than other *in vitro* systems, although its high endogenous mRNA activity can represent a problem. However, it has recently been reported that the endogenous messenger activity of this system can be considerably reduced by preincubating the reticulocyte lysate in the presence of micrococcal nuclease which is then inactivated by chelating the required Ca^{2+} (Pelham and Jackson, 1976; Pelham and Stuick, 1976). Under these conditions, the reticulocyte system may be a very suitable system for viral RNA translation.

The characterization of cell-free gene products uses the same methods as that of the *in vivo* products. Polyacrylamide gel (PAG) electrophoresis of denatured peptide chains obtained by treatment with 1% or 2% sodium dodecylsulfate (SDS) at 100°C for 5 min is now usually the primary tool. Additional evidence for the identification of gene products is frequently obtained by serology, CNBr or tryptic peptide mapping analysis, isoelectric precipitation, carboxy- and *N*-terminal analyses, etc. In the case of TMV and TRV coat proteins, the functional test of reconstitutability has also frequently been applied. A more detailed discussion of the various translation systems and their advantages can be found in the chapter by Shatkin *et al.* on translation of animal virus RNAs *in vitro* in Volume 10 of *Comprehensive Virology*.

3. TRANSLATION OF TMV RNA

3.1. *In Vivo* (Table 1)

3.1.1. In *Nicotiana tabacum*

TMV-infected leaf tissue was analyzed for virus-specific proteins by the double-label technique simultaneously in two laboratories. One very predominant band was found which coelectrophoresed with TMV coat protein (Singer, 1971; Zaitlin and Hariharasubramanian, 1970, 1972) and, like TMV coat protein, was deficient in histidine and methionine. In addition, Zaitlin and Hariharasubramanian (1972) found lesser amounts of proteins ranging from 245,000 to 37,000 daltons, particularly in two subcellular fractions ("mitochondria" and "nuclear"); the presence of small amounts of large proteins could be confirmed by Singer only when she used the same technique of vacuum-imbibing the radioactive amino acids. This procedure may be more traumatic to the leaf tissue and may induce artifactual appearance of new proteins; on the other hand, it may achieve higher specific activities, thus allowing better resolution on gels such that minor products become detectable.

The data obtained later with other techniques and to be discussed below suggest that at least one of the large proteins, said to be of molecular weight 155,000, might represent a genuine viral gene product now believed to be closer to 140,000 molecular weight. However, regardless of the nature of the large protein product(s), the disproportion in amounts between coat and other products at all stages of infection seemed to rule out the hypothesis that these viral proteins might result from posttranslational cleavage of a primary complete genome translation product (Singer, 1971).

It appears of interest that the nascent TMV coat protein carries the terminal acetyl group by the time the peptide chain is 30 residues

TABLE 1

Translation Products of TMV *vulgare in Vivo* and *in Vitro*

mRNA	Products ($\times 10^{-3}$ daltons) detected in various systems[a]				
	Plants (tobacco)[b]	Protoplasts[b]	Oocytes	Wheat	Reticulocytes
Virion RNA (2.1×10^6 daltons)	245,195 (1)[c] 155 (1) 150 (2) 130 (2) 37 (1)	180 (4) 165 (5) 140 (4) 135 (5)	165 (6,7) 140 (6,7)	140–10, (mainly 50–20, 12) (7, 8)	165 (7) 140 (7)
	18 (CP)(1,3)	18 (CP)(4,5)			
LMC (0.35×10^6 daltons) (from infected plants)			18 (CP)(7)	18 (CP)(7)	18 (CP)(7)

[a] Numbers in parentheses refer to references listed below; CP stands for "coat protein"; of the large proteins, that of 135 or 140×10^3 daltons predominated always.

[b] Tobacco plants and protoplasts were usually infected with the whole virus rather than with the RNA.

[c] References: 1, Zaitlin and Hariharasubramanian (1972); 2, Scalla et al. (1976); 3, Singer (1971); 4, Sakai and Takebe (1974); 5, Paterson (1974); 6, Knowland (1974); 7, Knowland et al. (1975); 8, Roberts et al. (1973, 1974).

long. Whether acetylation occurs at the level of initiation or soon thereafter, possibly after cleavage of a leader peptide, remains unknown (Filner and Marcus, 1974). This finding can be correlated with the observation of Shih and Kaesberg (1973) that nascent BMV coat protein became terminally acetylated by the wheat system when acetyl CoA was present but that this probably did not involve the initiation step.

3.1.2. In Tobacco Protoplasts

The use of protoplasts in the study of virus replication is dealt with in detail by Takebe in Chapter 5. Therefore, in this chapter we will describe only the results of protein synthesis analyses as they relate to those obtained with other techniques. A beautiful analysis of the protein products observed to be synthesized in *Nicotiana tabacum* protoplasts as a consequence of TMV infection was reported by Paterson (1974) and Paterson and Knight (1975). These data showed, besides the by far predominating and progressive coat protein synthesis, the appearance particularly early during infection of small amounts of a 135,000-dalton and yet less of a 165,000-dalton protein. These findings and similar conclusions reached also in Takebe's laboratory (Sakai and Takebe, 1974) are in general accord with those obtained with infected plants in that coat protein production greatly exceeds that of one or two large probably virus-coded proteins. The advantage of protoplasts is that they, unlike whole plants, can be synchronously infected, and additional information can be obtained from the kinetics of appearance of virus-specific proteins. The two larger virus-coded proteins can be detected as early as 9–12 h postinfection. Since the synthesis of these proteins declines after about 24 h, while coat protein production continues, usually at increasingly high levels, for at least 72 h, we have further evidence that there is no precursor–product relationship between the large proteins and the coat protein. The presumed role of these "early" proteins will be discussed later.

3.1.3. In Frog Oocytes

When TMV RNA was injected into frog oocytes, small amounts of two large proteins, one in minimal amounts, were detected (Knowland, 1974). These corresponded approximately to the two large proteins seen in infected protoplasts in both molecular weight and proportion. In these experiments, the gel electrophoretic patterns were strikingly different, depending on whether [³⁵S]methionine or [¹⁴C]valine was used. Thus with labeled methionine very much label was introduced into very many products smaller than 140,000 daltons, covering the entire lower two-thirds of the gel, whereas with labeled valine the pattern showed only quite faint bands closely below the 140,000 band, and the absence of bands in the area corresponding to coat protein was very evident. The conclusion of the author, based also on further analyses of degradation products of the 140,000-dalton peptide, was that coat protein was not directly translated, nor did it represent part of the large peptide. The significance of the large peptide forming dual valine-labeled bands, particularly evident on 18% gels, was not understood. The similarity of the large translation products of TMV RNA in plant cells and protoplasts as well as in frog oocytes suggests that there is nothing fundamentally different in the translation systems of plants and animals. Yet a mechanism exists in plant cells, and is absent from this animal cell, which is able to reveal or activate a highly efficient coat protein gene. Further studies to be reported (Sections 3.3 and 3.4) have thrown some light on this paradox.

3.2. In Cell-Free Systems (Table 1)

3.2.1. Prokaryotic Systems

When TMV RNA was added to an *E. coli* protein-synthesizing system which is able to translate MS2 RNA, various techniques failed to reveal detectable amounts of TMV coat protein (Nathans *et al.,* 1962; Aach *et al.,* 1964; Schwartz, 1967; Rice, 1972). The products as studied by PAG electrophoresis are multiple, ranging from about 30,000 to less than 10,000 in molecular weight; most of the counts are usually associated with smaller peptides (< 15,000 daltons), and there is very little radioactivity, not forming a peak but rather a minimum, at the position of a TMV coat protein marker. This finding confirms earlier conclusions, but is nevertheless difficult to understand in view of the fact that in plant cells the predominant product is always the coat protein by far.

3.2.2. Eukaryotic Systems

When TMV RNA is added to the wheat germ protein-synthesizing system [which translates unfractionated BMV RNA, and particularly its component 4, into pure BMV coat protein (Shih and Kaesberg, 1973; Davies and Kaesberg, 1974; see also Chapter 1)], the PAG electrophoretic pattern shows proteins ranging from about 140,000 to 10,000 daltons and also in this case little radioactivity is associated with the TMV coat protein marker (Roberts *et al.*, 1973; Davies and Kaesberg, 1974; Salvato, 1977).

However, by comparing the protein products obtained with wild-type TMV RNA and those directed by the RNA of a TMV mutant which contains one methionine residue in the coat protein, evidence was adduced that a specific peptide, "mutated" to contain the [^{35}S]methionine, could be detected in a tryptic digest of the unfractionated products (Roberts *et al.*, 1973). In a subsequent paper, the authors claimed that incubation of the translation products with tobacco plant extracts, TMV infected or not, caused the appearance of a product of 17,400 daltons, which was suggested to be TMV coat protein resulting from posttranslational cleavage of larger products (Roberts *et al.*, 1974). To test the authenticity of the protein, they resorted, as had most of their predecessors, to the functional test for TMV protein, reconstitution to TMV rods, using unlabeled carrier protein and TMV RNA. They found about 0.7% of the incorporated ^{35}S to be associated with virus particles and diminishing fractions thereof to remain associated with the re-isolated 17,400-dalton coat protein and the specific methionine-containing mutant peptide. While this represented the first evidence for cell-free synthesis of TMV coat protein, the low yield as contrasted to the great amount of *in vivo* coat protein production suggests that the system does not translate TMV RNA properly. That that protein was not detected by Aach *et al.* when they used reconstitution to isolate functional biosynthesized TMV coat protein in 1964 is probably due to its production being below the threshold of detection by the methods then available. Evidence has also been presented for the limited production of coat protein without a posttranslational cleavage step (Efron and Marcus, 1973). Here, too, tryptic peptide patterns resembling those of TMV coat protein represented only a small fraction of the total protein synthesis.

The translation of TMV RNA in the reticulocyte lysate system was shown as a control to the oocyte system (Knowland, 1974), but it was not described in detail or discussed. In this system also there was no evidence for coat protein translation. The only definitive products were said to be of 140,000, and less of 165,000 daltons, similar to the two minor products seen in infected plants and protoplasts, and to the only products detected in frog oocytes.

3.3. Isolation and Translation of TMV LMC (Table 1)

The turning point in the search for the coat protein gene came when attention was turned to some earlier findings (Babos, 1971) of low molecular weight, rapidly labeled RNA (RL) associated with polysomes in TMV-infected cells. This was confirmed and the RNA was further studied by Jackson *et al.* (1972) and Siegel *et al.* (1973), who termed it "LMC" (low molecular component) and gave its molecular weight as 350,000. It was suggested in the course of these studies and a subsequent one by Beachy and Zaitlin (1975) that the RL, alias LMC RNA (and possibly other somewhat larger RNAs), might play mRNA roles in TMV biogenesis. To test this possibility, Knowland *et al.* (1975) added various molecular weight fractions of RNA from TMV-infected tobacco leaves to the wheat embryo cell-free system. When the 18 S and < 18 S RNA fractions from infected leaves were used as messenger, these authors actually found marked or predominant production of a protein resembling TMV coat protein. TMV coat protein was also produced in frog oocytes when the LMC-containing RNA from infected cells, rather than typical TMV RNA, was used as messenger. Subsequent refinements not yet reported in detail were the use of purified LMC and the identification of the product by the functional test of reconstitution and by peptide map analyses (Hunter *et al.*, 1976). It thus seemed established that systems which were unable to synthesize detectable amounts of coat protein when viral TMV RNA was added produced mainly coat protein, or something very similar to it, when the LMC RNA fraction from TMV-infected plants was used (Siegel *et al.*, 1976). Whether that effective messenger RNA arises through intracellular cleavage from the infecting 30 S viral RNA and/ or its plus-strand progeny, or whether it is selectively transcribed from the minus strand, remains to be established. The finding by Beachy and Zaitlin (1975) that replicative intermediate RNA (RI) tends to be associated with the LMC-containing polysomes seems to favor the latter possibility.

In the light of present knowledge concerning the secondary appearance of an effective coat protein messenger in TMV-infected plants, one may assume that the earlier detection of traces of TMV coat protein synthesis by the wheat system under the direction of whole TMV RNA was due to translation of accidental fragments containing LMC with available initiation site (Roberts *et al.*, 1973; Efron and Marcus, 1973). This cannot account for the slight increase in yield upon incubation of the RNA-free products (Roberts *et al.*, 1974); posttranslational cleavage of small amounts of readthrough products of the entire genome would appear at this time the most plausible explanation for that observation, if it can be confirmed.

3.4. Cowpea Strain of TMV; LMC Virions (Table 2)

Recent studies from several laboratories of certain strains of TMV have added a new facet to our understanding of TMV replication. Some of these strains had an unusual history in that they had been reported (Bawden, 1958) as changing their physical and chemical properties reversibly depending on which host (bean vs. tobacco) they were grown on. Later studies suggested that these differences were due to the susceptibility of such strains to carboxypeptidase attack, which differed in different hosts (Rees and Short, 1965, 1972). It also appeared possible that the hosts favored replication of different components of a two-strain mixture, thus causing a selection. This possibility should now be reconsidered in the light of what has recently been learned about these TMV strains.

Two different types of observations stimulated interest in these strains which include the cowpea strain or "bean form" (B-TMV), the dolichos enation mosaic virus, and the sunhemp mosaic virus, all of which may be identical. Earlier studies had shown that preparations of several of these strains contained a high proportion of short rods (Dunn and Hitchborn, 1965; Kassanis and McCarthy, 1967), as more recently confirmed by Morris (1974). About that time, Australian workers observed that the RNA of the cowpea strain of TMV, upon translation by the wheat germ system, yielded what appeared to be viral coat protein (Goodwin and Higgins, 1974). Careful fractionation of B-TMV preparations showed the presence of two main rod lengths (300 and 30–40 nm) as well as lesser amounts of intermediate length. The RNA obtained from the main virus fractions had approximate molecular weights of 2×10^6 and 0.3×10^6 (Whitfeld and Higgins, 1976).

These observations were characteristic for the cowpea strain and could not be duplicated when TMV *vulgare* was subjected to the same separation methods. The appearance of short particles was at first observed with virus grown on its typical hosts, legumes, but could later also be demonstrated with the cowpea strain grown on tobacco, although the virus replicated poorly on this host. When these two rod-size populations were separated and their RNAs tested for their

TABLE 2

Translation Products of Viral RNAs Other Than TMV Vulgare in Various *in Vitro* Systems

Source	RNA used (approximate molecular weight)	Main products (molecular weight $\times 10^{-3}$) detected in various systems[a]		
		Wheat	Reticulocytes	Other
Alfalfa mosaic virus (AMV)	(1) 1.3×10^6	Multiple (10–100) (1)	124 (2)	(Krebs II) 124 (2)
	(2) 1.0×10^6	Multiple (10–100) (1)	100 (2)	100 + smaller (2)
	(3) 0.7×10^6	35 (1)	35 (2)	35 (2)
	(4) 0.34×10^6	25 (CP) (1, 3)	25 (CP) (2)	25 (CP)(2)
	All RNAs	10–120 (many bands) (1)		
Broadbean mottle virus (BBMV)	All RNAs (1.1, 1.03, 0.9, 0.3)	5 peaks; (CP) is minor (3)		
Brome mosaic virus (BMV)	(1) 1.1×10^6	120 (4)		
	(2) 1.0×10^6	110 (4)		
	(3) 0.7×10^6	35 (5)		
	(4) 0.3×10^6	20 (CP) (5)		(Mouse L cell)
	All RNAs	20 (CP) (5)		20 (CP (15)

Virus	RNA	Products	
Cowpea chlorotic mottle virus (CCMV)	(1) 1.15×10^6 }	Many bands (3)	
	(2) 1.07×10^6 }		
	(3) 0.85×10^6	30, 19 (CP) (3)	
	(4) 0.32×10^6	19 (CP) (3)	
	All RNAs[b]	30, 19 (CP) (3)	
Cowpea mosaic virus (CPMV)	(L) 2.4×10^6		220 (7)
	(S) 1.4×10^6		130 (7)
	Both RNAs	6 bands, the 2 largest corresponding to the 2 CPs of CPMV: 49, 27 (3)	220, 130 (7)
Cucumber mosaic virus (CMV)	(1) 1.35×10^6 }	13–90 (many bands) (6)	
	(2) 1.16×10^6 }		
	(3) 0.85×10^6	27, 24 (CP) (6)	
	(4) 0.35×0^6	24 (CP) (6)	
	All RNAs[c]	24 (CP) + 2 faint larger peaks (3) 24 (CP) (6)	
Eggplant mosaic virus (EMV)	2×10^6	180, 100, 35, 24; no (CP) (8)	150 (poor incorporation) (8)
Tobacco mosaic virus (TMV), B or cowpea strain	(L) 2.1×10^6	10–130 (9, 10) in high KCl: 150, 130 (9, 10)	
	(I) 1.4×10^6	No mRNA activity (10)	
	(S₁) 0.65×10^6	30 (10)	
	(S₂) 0.23×10^6	18 (CP) (9, 10)	
	All RNAs	150, 130, 18 (CP) (9, 10)	
Tobacco necrosis virus (TNV)[d]	1.3×10^6	30 (CP) + 2 faint larger peaks (11)	
TNV satellite (STNV)	0.4×10^6	22 (CP) (11)	

(continued)

TABLE 2 (Continued)

Source	RNA used (approximate molecular weight)	Main products (molecular weight $\times 10^{-3}$) detected in various systems[a]		
		Wheat	Reticulocytes	Other
Tobacco rattle virus (HSN or PRN strains)	(1) 2.5×10^6	10–100 (13) With spermine: 170, 140 (14)	170, 140, (14)	
	(2) 1.0×10^6	32, 29 (CP), 22, 20, 16 (13, 14)		
	Both RNAs	29 (CP) (14)		
(CAM strain)	(1) 2.5×10^6	10–100 (13)		
	(2) 0.7×10^6	29 (CP) (13)		
	Both RNAs	29 (CP) (13)		(Mouse L cell) 29 (CP) (15)
Turnip yellow mosaic virus (TYMV)	(L) 2.0×10^6	200, 150 (8)	200, 150	
	(S) 0.3×10^6	20 (CP) (8)	20 (CP)	
	Both RNAs[e]	5–100 (many bands including 20 (CP) (8)		

[a] Numbers in parentheses refer to references as follows: References: 1, Thang et al. (1976); 2, Mohier et al. (1975, 1976); 3, Davies and Kaesberg (1974); 4, Shih and Kaesberg (1976); 5, Shih and Kaesberg (1973); 6, Schwinghamer and Symons (1975); 7, Pelham and Stuick (1976); 8, Klein et al. (1976); 9, Higgins et al. (1976); 10, Bruening et al. (1976); 11, Salvato and Fraenkel-Conrat (1977); 12, Jones and Reichmann (1973); 13, Mayo et al. (1976); 14, Fritsch et al. (1976); 15, Ball et al. (1973); 16, Dawson et al. (1975); 17, Sakai et al. (1975); 18, Ziemiecki and Wood (1976). CP stands for "coat protein"; frequently only identified by molecular weight estimation on PAG. Minor products are not listed.

[b] Coat protein was detected in cowpeas and tobacco protoplasts as the predominant product (16), with much smaller amounts of the 36 and 100×10^3 protein (17).

[c] In cucumber cotyledon, proteins of 78, 62, 58, 26 (CP), and 24×10^3 were seen (18).

[d] In tobacco plants, proteins of 64, 42, 32 (CP) 23, 15, and 12×10^3 were seen (12).

[e] Upon treatment with EDTA or H-bond-breaking agents, large proteins (165 and 200×10^3 daltons) and the 20×10^3 daltons coat protein predominate in both the wheat and reticulocyte system.

messenger activity in the wheat germ system, the dramatic discovery was made that the small RNA of about 0.3×10^6 daltons induced the synthesis of a protein resembling B-TMV coat protein in most respects, while the large RNA (2×10^6 daltons), like all typical TMV RNA preparations, did not show coat protein messenger activity (Higgins *et al.*, 1976). The specific and definitive identification of the predominant *in vitro* product with the coat protein of this strain of TMV is complicated by the fact that the latter appears to occur naturally in part in a modified form (16,500 rather than almost 18,000 daltons), apparently because of proteolytic cleavage of possibly ten amino acids. In contrast, the *in vitro* product was reported by the Australian authors as slightly larger than the larger natural coat protein component, and also to contain methionine in contrast to the latter. Yet in regard to most tryptic peptides, as well as antigenically and functionally in terms of reconstitutability, the *in vitro* product corresponded to the viral coat protein. Thus there seems to be no question that the cowpea strain of TMV produces and encapsidates, besides the complete genome, a definitive fragment which functionally corresponds to the nonencapsidated LMC of common TMV.

Another independent study of the cowpea strain of TMV and its translation has corroborated, with minor differences, the findings of the Australian group. Besides, Bruening *et al.* (1976) and Zaitlin *et al.* (1976) found that the RNA from an intermediate rod-length species, of about 0.6×10^6 daltons, was translated to protein products of about 30,000 daltons. The two smaller RNAs seem to share sequences with the large RNA, and inoculation of plants with only the latter caused the appearance of the tripartite pattern of virus rods characteristic for this strain. Only the translation of the small RNA component (by the wheat germ system) yielded material that resembled the coat protein electrophoretically, and reconstituted to TMV rods. Although Bruening *et al.* (1976) detected no electrophoretic difference between the *in vitro* and *in vivo* produced protein, they did not exclude the possibility of minor (terminal) differences, and characterized their *in vitro* product as showing "some properties of capsid protein."

3.5. The Genetic Map of TMV

According to Hunter *et al.* (1976), the genes to be mapped are two large and therefore presumably overlapping ones, and the coat protein. According to Zaitlin *et al.* (1976) and Bruening *et al.* (1976), the rod size distribution of the cowpea strain indicates that besides full-length and short rods there exists an intermediate rod species whose RNA is translated into one or two 30,000-dalton products.

As far as arranging these genes on a map, all groups of investigators have relied largely on two features of TMV and its RNA, namely, polar stripping of the rod by alkali or detergents and the capability of the 3′-terminal-GCCCA (Steinschneider and Fraenkel-Conrat, 1966) to become charged with histidine under appropriate conditions (Öberg and Philipson, 1972). Unfortunately, neither of these techniques is unambiguous. Polar stripping with SDS has long been believed, on seemingly sound evidence, to start at the 3′ end (May and Knight, 1965; Kado and Knight, 1968; Mandeles, 1968), but has recently been reported to start at the other end (Wilson *et al.*, 1976). Obviously, this question has to be definitively settled before gene mapping can be based on such data. The capability of TMV RNA to accept amino acids is less dubious in terms of location, but always far from stoichiometric, and it is this aspect which complicates the interpretation of amino acid binding data. To the extent that the recent stripping experiments rely on the aminoacylation as a test for which end is revealed, they are thus dubious. As far as the alkali stripping experiments are concerned (Perham and Wilson, 1976), the end-group characterizations were performed on a very extensively stripped alkali-resistant fragment (< 50 nm long rods). It has not been shown that this alkali-resistant fraction is an indicator of the initial stripping behavior of the entire rod population since neither the stoichiometry nor the intermediate product of its formation have been demonstrated. Also, it is not excluded that the stripping polarity is not absolute, either in statistical or in temporal terms. The polarity of stripping with SDS and alkali has been reinvestigated by Ohno and Okada (1977), and these authors concur that stripping by these agents starts at the 5′ end. Current studies by one of us (H. F.-C.) also find undiminished 3′ terminal (-Gp)CpCpCpA in SDS-stripped TMV-RNA. However, according to Beachy *et al.* (1976), both long and short TMV cowpea strain particles are stripped from the 3′ end on the basis of data on 3′-terminal aminoacylation, which surprisingly attaches valine, not histidine, to this strain of TMV. Also at certain concentrations of dimethylsulfoxide, stripping of TMV vulgare starts at the 3′ end (Nikolaieff *et al.*, 1975).

Oddly enough, without agreement concerning the polarity of stripping, all groups of workers (Hunter *et al.*, 1976; Beachy *et al.*, 1976; Richards *et al.*, 1975) propose that the large genes are located toward the 5′ end, probably followed by the intermediate-size gene (although that was seen only in the cowpea strain), and then the coat protein gene near the 3′ end. The large gene is stated by Hunter *et al.* (1976) to have two initiation sites, but no detailed data have as yet been published on this matter. One would not expect that certain strains of TMV have an additional gene; thus the possibility must be considered that an intermediate mRNA and translation product is produced at too low a level for detection also in common TMV-infected cells. Such a hypothetical product might account for the second initiation site noted by Hunter *et al.* (1976). Recent electron micrographs of partially reconstituted TMV rods with two RNA "tails" protruding from the same end (Leburier *et al.*, 1977; Butler *et al.*, 1977) have led to a more positive visualization of the directionality of the RNA and this opens up the possibility of gene mapping techniques developed for electron microscopy.

4. TRANSLATION OF TURNIP YELLOW MOSAIC VIRUS RNA (TABLE 2)

When TYMV RNA is introduced into the wheat germ cell-free system, many protein bands are observed when the translation products are examined by means of slab gel electrophoresis. The molecular weights of these proteins range from about 5000 to 100,000, and among them is a 20,000-dalton protein which comigrates with the coat protein. Serological precipitation tests suggest strongly that this protein is indeed coat protein. When the viral RNA is subjected to treatment with EDTA or with agents which rupture hydrogen bonds, much more coat protein is translated and the molecular weight of the heaviest protein produced increases to 165,000 (Klein *et al.*, 1976). The same results are obtained with the rabbit reticulocyte system, except that only the two major proteins are observed and the molecular weight of the heavier one is very close to 200,000 (Mohier *et al.*, to be published).

It is known that TYMV RNA can be aminoacylated by valine (Yot *et al.*, 1970). Recently, it was found that if aminoacylation is performed with highly purified valyl-tRNA synthetase from yeast, 1.5 mol of valine is fixed per mole of TYMV RNA on the basis of a molecular weight of 2×10^6 (Giege *et al.*, 1977). This surprising result and the finding that TYMV RNA differs from TMV RNA in that the virion RNA is apparently able to express the protein gene led to a reinvestigation of the structure of the RNA.

When TYMV RNA was heated and treated with SDS or EDTA and then analyzed by column chromatography, two major components were isolated. The heavier one (molecular weight $1.8-2 \times 10^6$), when used as messenger, yielded the large proteins but only a very small amount of the 20,000 molecular weight protein. The smaller component (molecular weight 300,000) translated the coat protein gene very efficiently (as proved by serological precipitation tests and peptide mapping analysis) (Klein *et al.*, 1976). Pleij *et al.* (1976) have obtained very similar results concerning the occurrence of two RNAs in TYM virions and their role in the translation of different viral genes.

Both small and large RNAs are "capped," the cap being $m^7G^{5'}ppp^{5'}Gp$ for the large RNA and a mixture of $m^7G^{5'}ppp^{5'}Ap$ and $m^7G^{5'}ppp^{5'}Gp$ for the small RNA. This rules out the possibility that the small RNA can arise from the large one by degradation during purification of the virus or of the RNA. Both species of RNA are able to be aminoacylated by valine to a comparable extent, thus explaining the unexpectedly high yield of aminoacylation for the whole RNA. There was about 0.5 mol of small RNA per mole of large RNA; this may well be an underestimate and most of the virions may contain both RNAs. In the light of these new findings, the question of particle heterogeneity in TYMV needs to be reinvestigated.

Recently, Briand *et al.* (1977) have sequenced a fragment of 159 nucleotides originating from the 3′ end of (unfractionated) TYMV RNA. This fragment contains the last part of the coat protein cistron and a tRNA-like structure which is presumably responsible for the aminoacylation of the TYMV RNA. But the origin of the sequenced fragment must now be considered an open question in view of the above-noted discovery of two components in TYMV RNA. This raises the interesting question of whether or not the coat protein cistron is present on both RNAs. The fact that both RNAs are able to be aminoacylated by valine under the same conditions suggests that the 3′ end of both RNAs are the same and that the coat protein cistron is redundant. This was recently demonstrated by oligonucleotide mapping (Richards *et al.*, 1977). Thus, the whole genetic information is present on the heavy RNA of TYMV, which is then not a multicomponent virus but rather, like TMV, a genome that is "processed" *in vivo* by cutting or by partial transcription, but as in the cowpea strain of TMV, the protein gene is also encapsidated.

It is worth noting that the RNA of eggplant mosaic virus, although related to TYMV, is translated only into large proteins in both the wheat germ system and the reticulocyte lysate system and that no coat protein was observed. This would seem to suggest that EMV resembles the common strain of TMV in that a hypothetical processed fragment (LMC) is used for translation of the coat protein gene in the cell, but is not coated. Further experiments are in progress in order to substantiate this hypothesis (Fritsch *et al.,* to be published). On the other hand, earlier experiments have shown (Pinck *et al.,* 1974) that this virus carried a noncovalently linked lysine tRNA-like nucleic acid, and it now appears necessary to consider and test any small RNA associated with a virus for mRNA activity.

5. TRANSLATION OF THE RNA OF TOBACCO NECROSIS VIRUS AND ITS SATELLITE

The translation of tobacco necrosis virus (TNV) and its satellite, STNV, has been studied off and on, without very clear insight having been gained into this relationship. One *in vivo* study has reported the detection of six virus-coded (or virus-induced) proteins upon TNV infection of tobacco, and an additional protein upon coinfection with STNV(Jones and Reichmann, 1973); the latter of molecular weight 20,000 and the predominant peak upon TNV infection of 32,000 molecular weight could represent the respective coat proteins of these viruses (see Chapter 3, this volume). The largest product was reported to be 64,000 daltons. However, attempts by C. Stussi to repeat these experiments when at Berkeley were unsuccessful.

A current study in this laboratory (C. Condit, personal communication) of the proteins made in protoplasts upon infection with TNV has not shown any detectable virus-coded (or -induced) proteins above the background of host protein synthesis, except for one strong band corresponding to the TNV coat protein in electrophoretic mobility. However, it appears that up to the present time only one protoplast system, namely tobacco protoplasts infected with TMV or CCMV, has given clear and definitive translation results.

STNV RNA was among the first viral RNAs to be successfully used as an *in vitro* messenger with the *E. coli* system (Clark *et al.,* 1965), and indications were obtained and later confirmed that characteristic STNV coat protein peptides were synthesized. However, initiation or termination was imperfect, most of the products being smaller than the coat protein (Rice, 1972; Rice and Fraenkel-Conrat, 1973). More uniform size distributions, but also a slightly shorter main product, were obtained by Klein *et al.* (1972) upon translation of STNV RNA in both the *E. coli* and the wheat system. Thus the failure of the *in vitro* systems to give the authentic *in vivo* product cannot be attributed to the nature of the prokaryotic as contrasted to the eukaryotic system.

Recently new data on the translation of STNV RNA and TNV RNA using a wheat system optimized with spermine were reported (Salvato and Fraenkel-Conrat, 1977). These indicated that the predominant product with STNV RNA was STNV coat protein by gel sizing. Both this and a minor product of lower molecular weight (about 18,000) were precipitated with STNV antiserum. These findings thus confirm that STNV RNA carries only one gene. Leung *et al.* (1976) in a paper discussing the mechanism of translation of STNV RNA in some detail, state but do not document that the only translation product of STNV RNA is the coat protein.

Concerning TNV RNA translation, the surprising finding was made (Salvato and Fraenkel-Conrat, 1977), that this RNA of 1.4×10^6 daltons also gives a single very predominant protein, of 30,000 molecular weight and corresponding in size, serology and tryptic pattern to the viral coat protein. A smaller product (26,000 daltons) also crossreacts with TNV antiserum and thus appears to be a degradation product of the coat protein.

In view of the recent results concerning TYMV translation (Klein *et al.*, 1976, Pleij *et al.*, 1977) no conclusions concerning the messenger activity of any viral RNA are valid until that RNA has been shown to be homogeneous by most rigorous criteria. In the case of TNV RNA, treatment with and electrophoresis in 10 M urea did not show any small component. Also when the RNA was heated at 65°C for 5 min prior to gradient purification, its ability to be translated into coat protein was not lost.

Two larger proteins of molecular weight 63,000 and 43,000 observed regularly though in very small amounts may represent genuine gene products of TNV RNA translated with very low efficiency. If this is the case, then the total coding potential of TNV RNA would be accounted for by 3 genes. Thus this viral RNA may resemble in its translation strategy the RNA of the phages more than that of typical eukaryotic viruses.

6. COVIRUS GENOME TRANSLATION (TABLE 2)

6.1. Three-Component Coviruses: AMV, BMV

Our beginning understanding of the strategy of RNA virus translation by plants derives in good part from studies of the three-component viruses. We will here limit our discussion to only those aspects that have not been dealt with in detail in Chapter 1 of this volume and that relate to the overall picture sought in the present chapter.

The remarkably similar conclusions derived from the study of the translation of alfalfa mosaic virus and the bromo- and cucumoviruses appears to be as follows (Shih and Kaesberg, 1973; Mohier *et al.*, 1975; Schwinghamer and Symons, 1975). The small RNA component (4) is always monocistronic, coding only for the respective coat protein which requires only about two-thirds of its length. The next larger component (3) carries two genes, that of the coat protein, and a protein of molecular weight 35,000 and possibly representing a (component of) viral RNA polymerase (Hariharasubramanian *et al.*, 1973; Sakai *et al.*, 1975) (see Section 7.3). These two genes correspond to four-fifths of the length of this RNA. However, the concept that this RNA really acts as a bicistronic messenger has been recently modified in the case of both BMV and AMV. It appears that only the first initiation site near the 5′ end of component 3 is actually effectively recognized in the wheat germ and reticulocyte systems, and that this leads to translation of only the 30,000–36,000 dalton protein (Shih and Kaesberg, 1976; Mohier *et al.*, 1976). This may be true also *in vivo.* It now appears probable, although this has not yet been proven, that in the host cell the coat protein gene must be split off from component 3 by pretranslational cleavage, or separately transcribed from the minus strand, before it can become efficiently translated. Whether in the case of alfalfa mosaic virus this cleavage requires the presence of coat protein, or in what other manner that protein can replace RNA 4, is not yet clear. In any case, normally the internal initiation site of the bicistronic RNA 3 of the three-component coviruses is not utilized by the plant cell or cell-free extracts (Gerlinger *et al.*, 1977).

The two large genome components of these viruses of about 10^6 daltons were believed to be polycistronic until it was recently shown both for BMV with the wheat system (Shih and Kaesberg, 1976) and for AMV with the reticulocyte system (Mohier *et al.*, 1975, 1976) that *in vitro* each was translated predominantly as a single protein chain, corresponding to the length of the respective RNA. Thus a single initiation site was found in these, as in the smaller components of AMV. Whether these two comparatively large proteins (about 10^5 daltons) represent ultimate gene products and what biological activities they carry remains to be established; the possibility that they represent precursors which become functional only upon posttranslational processing cannot be excluded.

6.2. Two-Component Coviruses: TRV, CPMV

The study of the *in vitro* translation products has been extended to the typical two-component covirus system, tobacco rattle virus. The translation of the large component of the tobacco rattle virus (RNA-1, molecular weight about 2.5×10^6) (HSN and PRN strains) resembles that of other large RNAs, in that two predominant large gene products are seen which must share a good part of their genome (170,000 and 140,000 daltons) (Fritsch *et al.*, 1976); in the wheat system smaller products are seen under some conditions, while again the reticulocyte system, presumably because it lacks RNase, shows only the large products. It is worth noting that the small RNA of the CAM strain is "capped." The cap is $m^7G^{5'}ppp^{5'}Ap \ldots$, while the large RNA is not capped (Abou Haidar and Hirth, 1977). It is not known whether the large RNA is capped *in vivo* and whether this observation is related to the high rate of translation of the small RNA as compared to the large RNA.

The coding capability of the smaller RNA component 2 is less clear. In earlier studies with the CAM strain (serotype III), component 2 of molecular weight 0.7×10^6 yielded only one major product in both the mouse L cell (Ball *et al.*, 1973) and the wheat system (Mayo *et al.*, 1976) which corresponded to the coat protein (apparent molecular weight 29,000) in various respects; thus over half of that RNA seemed to remain untranslated. In the more recent study (Fritsch *et al.*, 1976) of the strains of serotype I (PRN, HSN), which have a larger component 2 (10^6 daltons), five translation products were seen in both the wheat and reticulocyte system: one larger than coat protein, one similar, and three smaller. The smaller proteins seemed to be related to the coat protein. The largest product seemed to have some tryptic peptides in common with coat protein, but was for the most part a different protein. If both the coat protein and the larger product are translated from the same RNA it would contradict the presently prevailing concept that multiple internal initiation is not favored in eukaryotic cells. However, the total molecular weight of these products exceeds the genome's capacity; it thus appears possible that these five products really represent steps in the processing of two primary products.

The cowpea mosaic virus RNAs have been only cursorily studied in the wheat germ system (Davies and Kaesberg, 1974). The mixture of the two RNAs showed multiple products, as indicated by Bruening in Chapter 2, but no conclusions are possible regarding the strategy of translation or the nature and number of primary gene products. A recent report indicates, however, that in a reticulocyte system freed from endogenous mRNA the two cowpea virus RNAs, singly or together, are translated to two large proteins corresponding approximately to their genetic capacity. Neither of the two coat proteins of the virus was evident (Pelham and Stuick, 1976). This seems to call for posttranslational cleavage as the mechanism of their formation. Since this virus, besides having two coat proteins, is unusual also in regard to its end groups [it has no 5′ cap, but has 3′-terminal poly(A)], one begins to wonder whether it could be evolutionarily related to the animal picornaviruses which it also resembles in its translation strategy.

7. GENERAL ASPECTS OF TRANSLATION OF PLANT VIRAL RNAs

In this chapter, we have dealt with the translation of the most common plant viruses, those with single-stranded, plus-stranded, and presumably multigenic RNAs. Since plants are eukaryotes with long-lived mRNAs as compared to the short-lived mRNAs of bacterial systems, it is reasonable to speculate that the control of plant viral gene expression differs from phage expression in that selection of messages at the translational level is of prime importance. As plants also harbor viruses very similar to such animal virus families as the reoviridae and rhabdoviridae, and as many plant viruses are replicated in their insect vectors, one would expect close similarities in the translational strategies of plant and animal viruses.

However, in contrast to small animal viruses, e.g., picornaviruses, the simple plant viruses discussed here do not generally inhibit or eclipse host translation; instead, they synthesize their proteins in the midst of continuing host protein synthesis. Recognition of plant viral RNA by host ribosomes may therefore require special factors or initiation sites which give a slight translational advantage to the viral RNA. The search for translation-promoting factors has so far been fruitless, but the *in vitro* binding studies of viral RNA to host translation components which are discussed below suggest that the structure of an RNA can greatly affect its translatability.

7.1. Importance of RNA Structure

Several plant viral RNAs have 3′-terminal tRNA-like structures and are able, like tRNA, to bind specific amino acids: TYMV RNA and other members of its group bind valine (Yot *et al.,* 1970), TMV RNA binds histidine (Öberg and Philipson, 1972), and the RNAs of the

BMV group and CMV bind tryosine (Kohl and Hall, 1974). It is unlikely that these aminoacylated viral RNAs replace tRNAs during protein synthesis since only TYMV is capable of donating its amino acid to a growing peptide chain, and even then only 1% as efficiently as Val-tRNA (Haenni *et al.*, 1973). Blocking the aminoacylation of the 3′ end by periodate oxidation does not impair the *in vitro* translatability of BMV RNA (Shih *et al.*, 1974). Nevertheless, the 3′-terminal tRNA-like structures may facilitate the interaction of viral RNA with host polysomes since a preferential binding has been shown between wheat translation factor EFl and aminoacylated as opposed to nonamino-acylated TMV RNA and TYMV RNAs (Litvak *et al.*, 1973).

Capped structures (7-methyl G5′ppp5′G-), which have been dis-covered at the 5′ end of many eukaryotic mRNAs (see Both *et al.* in Vol. 10 of *Comprehensive Virology*), also occur on several plant viral RNAs (Keith and Fraenkel-Conrat, 1975; Keith, 1976; Zimmern, 1975; Pinck, 1975; Dasgupta *et al.*, 1976; Abou Haidar and Hirth, 1977). In the case of BMV, the cap is within ten bases of the initiation codon AUG (Dasgupta *et al.*, 1975), and the removal of the cap results in reduced ribosome binding and translation (Shih *et al.*, 1976). It is not entirely clear whether the cap interacts primarily with ribosomes or whether its function is to protect the initiation site, or make it more available to the ribosomes. The cap could conceivably regulate which initiation site is to be translated when more than one internal site exists. Until data become available that disprove this hypothesis, one may sur-mise that initiation of translation of a multigenic RNA occurs only if the initiation site is near a capped end, as it is the case for BMV. Whether the TMV protein messengers (LMC or cowpea strain S-RNA) are capped remains to be established, as does the exact nature of their primary translation product. The translation strategy of the noncapped TNV RNA (Horst *et al.*, 1971; Keith, 1976) and STNV RNA (Leung *et al.*, 1976) may be radically different, or a capped structure may be added just before translation and again removed prior to packaging of these viruses. This may also be the case for the large RNA of TRV.

The 3′-terminal poly(A) observed on so many animal viruses has been seen on only one plant viral RNA, that of cowpea mosaic virus (El Manna and Bruening, 1973), but it does not seem to confer any translational advantage to that RNA *in vitro*. The role of poly(A) *in vivo* remains to be discovered.

The large RNAs of TMV, TYMV, and BMV yield discrete T_1 RNase partial-digestion products which are consistent with regions of folded secondary structure. TMV RNA has been treated with formaldehyde in order to remove secondary structure, and this treatment results in 1.5 times more ribosome binding (Hashimoto and Okamoto, 1975). However, such disruption of the secondary structure does not seem to reveal hidden cistrons as in the RNA phages, since no difference was detected in *in vitro* protein synthesis after formaldehyde treatment (Salvato, thesis, 1977). But secondary structure as observed *in vitro* is highly sensitive to ionic environment, and its physiological significance is hard to assess. In the case of TYMV, it has been demonstrated that an effective coat protein mRNA is associated in noncovalent manner with the larger genomic RNA. This possibility was considered in the case of TNV RNA, which also effectively translates only the coat protein gene, but no such hidden messengers have so far been detected upon denaturing TNV RNA. Its large RNA retains its coat protein mRNA function (Salvato and Fraenkel-Conrat, 1977). The preferential coat protein translation in this case may be due to conformational inhibition of translation at other sites on the RNA. A similar explanation could be given for the translation of protein 3a on BMV RNA 3 in preference to the coat protein which is encoded on the same messenger. It is likely that secondary structure, tRNA-like structures, and the various nucleotide modifications will prove important to the translational strategy of these plant viruses.

7.2. Translation of Multiple Products from Large RNAs

Unlike the translation of RNA phages, the multicistronic translation of a eukaryotic viral RNA molecule to several proteins has not been incontrovertibly demonstrated. When multiple small translation products are observed they appear often to represent cleavage products or incomplete translations of a single protein. The second translation product of BMV RNA component 3, the coat protein, most probably results from contamination by small amounts of RNA 4. Evidence that a single large TYMV RNA codes for both coat protein and several larger translation products has been discounted by the very recent finding that a small RNA noncovalently linked to the large RNA codes for the coat protein, while the large RNA seems to code for one or two large proteins.

The two large proteins (140,000 to 180,000 daltons) frequently seen after translation of TMV, TYMV, EMV, and TRV are certainly not translated from separate cistrons because their sum exceeds the coding capacity of the respective RNAs. Instead, the smaller of these pairs of proteins may arise by posttranslational processing, or the larger, in analogy to protein A2 of the RNA phage $Q\beta$, from readthrough of a normal termination signal. Whether both products are ever functional has not been demonstrated. Demonstration of multiple ribosome binding sites for one mRNA, as claimed for TMV RNA (Hunter *et al.*, 1976), is also insufficient evidence for multicistronic translation because the second binding site may be internal to a larger cistron, or it may be at the beginning of a cistron which can be initiated but not translated until a cleavage event occurs. Therefore, until a single RNA is shown to remain intact upon translation into multiple products, multicistronic readout cannot be regarded as a proven mechanism of plant virus translation.

Instead, plant viruses seem to achieve monocistronic readout in a variety of ways. The coviruses which carry four separate RNAs translate each of these into a single protein. While RNA component 3 carries two genes, it appears that the coat protein gene becomes translatable only after partial transcription or posttranscriptional processing has yielded component 4. The situation for the smaller component of TRV is not yet clear.

The classical single-component plant viruses as exemplified by TMV and TYMV also seem to produce functionally monocistronic messages. For TMV, it has now been clearly established that its coat protein gene becomes efficiently functional only after release of a subgenomic fragment. Whether this is achieved by cleavage or by separate transcription of this segment of the viral RNA has not been established. This coat protein messenger is separately encapsidated in certain strains of TMV, a situation formally similar to the gene redundancy of covirus components 3 and 4. However, the fact that the full-length TMV RNA carries all the necessary genetic information differentiates it from the coviruses.

The very recent findings regarding TYMV do not yet allow such clear classification. The coat protein gene was in this case found as a separate RNA noncovalently linked to the larger RNA. If both RNAs are unique, TYMV could be classified as a two-component covirus. If the coat protein gene is redundant to information on the large RNA as now seems to be the case, the situation is similar to that for the cowpea strain of TMV (although there the two RNAs are separately encapsidated) or to that for the bromoviridae components 3 and 4 (although these are part of a covirus system). In any case, the discovery of a small monocistronic message in association with a classical single-component genome now throws doubt on the interpretation of the studies of other viral RNAs that yield multiple products in *in vitro* translation, unless such RNAs have been rigorously shown to be homodisperse by electrophoresis under denaturing conditions.

Posttranslational cleavage is the prime mode by which the several functional proteins of the picornaviruses are obtained from a single large gene product (Jacobson and Baltimore, 1968). Posttranslational terminal proteolytic processing occurs more commonly and transforms single precursor proteins to functional entities; this also has been observed to occur with the picornaviridae (Smith, 1973). For most plant viruses, there exists no evidence that RNA translation relies on posttranslational cleavage of a single monster protein to yield the ultimate gene products. In the case of CPMV (Pelham and Stuick, 1976), cleavage of a large initial translation product has been postulated but in no way demonstrated. Minor processing, however, is not excluded. The finding that the translation product of the coat protein mRNA of the cowpea strain of TMV (and possibly others) is slightly larger than the corresponding *in vivo* product may be due to the lack of the proper processing enzymes in the wheat embryo extract. The use of various translation systems should contribute important information as to the role of processing in the biogenesis of plant viral products.

7.3. Identification of Gene Products, with Particular Reference to RNA Replicase

Quantitation and functional identification of plant viral genes has so far been meager. No gene products of the viruses under discussion have been definitively related to such genetic markers as host range and symptoms (see Chapters 1–3). Even the RNA-dependent RNA polymerase, the one gene product that should be clearly defined in functional and molecular terms, has been elusive. For the RNA phages, it has been established that one of the three gene products complexes with three host proteins to form the phage-specific RNA polymerase (Kamen, 1970; Kondo *et al.*, 1970), but as yet no analogous mechanism has been proven to exist in eukaryotic cells. The fact that virus infection leads to increases in the RNA polymerase activity in infected tissues is clear, but doubts have been repeatedly raised as to whether this activity is virus-coded or needs a viral component (Duda *et al.*, 1973; Astier-Manifacier and Cornuet, 1971). Thus it was recently shown that TNV infection induces a much greater increase in polymerase activity than TMV infection, yet comparisons of solubilized and partially purified enzyme from uninfected and TMV- or TNV-

infected tobacco showed no qualitative differences in the properties of
the enzymes from these three sources in regard to sedimentation, electrophoresis, and isoelectric focusing on sucrose gradients (Fraenkel-
Conrat, 1976, and unpublished results). Thus there exists no definitive
evidence that this enzyme represents a viral gene product.

TMV, EMV, TYMV, and TRV all yield two large proteins upon
in vitro translation, and yet have the coding capacity for only one. That
these pairs of proteins, about 170,000 and 140,000 $\pm$ 20,000 daltons,
which presumably share identical amino acid sequences, actually
represent different functional entities appears unlikely, although it has
been postulated that they are both polymerases, perhaps coming into
play at different stages of replication (Knowland *et al.*, 1975). However,
a recent report suggests that the same nucleotide sequence may be read
in two different phases, and thus code for two different proteins (Barrell
et al., 1976). In the case of TMV, the early appearance of the large
products and their subsequent diminished synthesis may be regarded as
suggestive evidence for attributing to them a replicase function
(Paterson, 1974; Sakai and Takebe, 1972; Paterson and Knight, 1975).
The purification and characterization of the enzyme have not
progressed any further with the TMV- than with the TNV-stimulated
enzyme mentioned above, the greatest limitation being the instability of
the enzymatic activity. The sedimentation behavior of the enzyme
extracted from TMV-infected tobacco is in approximate accord with
the molecular weight of the large *in vitro* and *in vivo* translation
products of TMV RNA. But this signifies little, since the sedimentation
behavior of the corresponding enzyme from uninfected plants, as well
as that from TNV-infected plants is also similar, and no proteins of
such size have been detected upon translation of TNV RNA *in vivo* or
in vitro. Among the TNV RNA translation products the largest, of
about 63,000 daltons, may represent a RNA polymerase component
(Salvato and Fraenkel-Conrat, 1977), since a 60,000 dalton protein was
observed in fractions of TNV-infected tobacco which had high
polymerase activity (Fraenkel-Conrat, 1976).

The situation is slightly less ambiguous for the three-component
coviruses. Evidence was obtained in our laboratory that in BMV-
infected barley a protein of molecular weight 35,000, the same as the
translation product of RNA 3, was formed early upon infection
(Hariharasubramanian *et al.*, 1973). This protein reached its maximum
when the increase in RNA replicase activity was maximal, and it was
found in the fractions richest in replicase activity. Indications that gene
product 3 may represent a replicase component were also reported by

others working with other three-component coviruses (Sakai *et al.,* 1977; see also Chapter 1). The observed subunit molecular weight is about one-fourth of that of the active enzyme (Hadidi and Fraenkel-Conrat, 1973). This tentative identification in no way precludes the possibility of other subunits of the active enzyme being derived from the host.

This hypothetical subunit model for BMV (or barley) RNA replicase contrasts with the single-peptide-chain model for TMV (or tobacco) RNA replicase. One must await future experiments to establish which (if not both or neither) is the true nature of the RNA replicases of eukaryotes. Attention might be drawn again to the finding of a possible third gene product in the cowpea strain of TMV, of 30,000 daltons. This protein happens to be of similar size to the presumed BMV RNA replicase subunit.

In conclusion, the identification of plant viral gene products other than the coat proteins and the elucidation of their translational strategies are as yet very incomplete. Continued biochemical analyses of RNA size and structure, binding studies, and comparisons of *in vitro* and *in vivo* products will be necessary to clearly define the mechanism of translational specificity and its role in plant virus infection.

8. REFERENCES

Aach, H. G., Funatsu, G., Nirenberg, M. W., and Fraenkel-Conrat, H., 1964, Further attempts to characterize products of TMV-RNA-directed protein synthesis, *Biochemistry* **3**:1362.

Abou Haidar, M., and Hirth, L., 1977, 5′-terminal structure of tobacco rattle virus RNA: Evidence for polarity of reconstruction, *Virology* **76**:173.

Astier-Manafacier, S., and Cornuet, P., 1971, RNA-dependent RNA polymerase in Chinese cabbage, *Biochim. Biophys. Acta* **232**:484.

Babos, P., 1971, TMV-RNA associated with ribosomes of tobacco leaves infected with TMV, *Virology* **43**:597.

Ball, L. A., Minson, A. C., and Shih, D. S., 1973, Synthesis of plant virus coat proteins in an animal cell-free system, *Nature (London) New Biol.* **246**:206.

Barrell, B. G., Air, G. M., and Hutchison, C. A., 1976, Overlapping genes in bacteriophage ΦX174, *Nature* **264**:34.

Bawden, F. C., 1958, Reversible changes in strains of tobacco mosaic virus from leguminous plants, *J. Gen. Microbiol.* **18**:751.

Beachy, R. N., and Zaitlin, M., 1975, Replication of tobacco mosaic virus. VI. Replicative intermediate and TMV-RNA-related RNAs associated with polyribosomes, *Virology* **63**:84.

Beachy, R. N., Zaitlin, M., Bruening, G., and Israel, H. W., 1976, A genetic map for the cowpea strain of TMV, *Virology* **73**:498.

Bonner, W. M., and Laskey, R. A., 1974, A film detection method for tritium-labeled proteins and nucleic acids in polyacrylamide gels, *Eur. J. Biochem.* **46**:83.

Briand, J. P., Richards, K. E., Bouley, J. P., Witz, J., and Hirth, L., 1976, Structure of the amino-acid accepting 3′-end of high-molecular-weight eggplant mosaic virus RNA, *Proc. Natl. Acad. Sci. USA* **73**:737.

Briand, J. -P., Jonard, G., Guilley, H., Richards, K., and Hirth, L., 1977, Nucleotide sequence (η = 159) of the amino-acid-accepting 3′-OH extremity of turnip-yellow-mosaic-virus RNA and the last portion of its coat-protein cistron, *Eur. J. Biochem.* **72**:453.

Bruening, G., Beachy, R., Scalla, R., and Zaitlin, M., 1976, *In vitro* and *in vivo* translation of the ribonucleic acids of the cowpea strain of tobacco mosaic virus, *Virology* **71**:498.

Butler, P., Finch, J., and Zimmern, D., 1977, Configuration of tobacco mosaic virus RNA during virus assembly, *Nature* **265**:217.

Clark, J. M., Jr. Chang, A. Y., Spiegelman, S., and Reichman, M. E., 1965, The *in vitro* translation of a monocistronic message, *Proc. Natl. Acad. Sci. USA* **54**:1193.

Dasgupta, R. Shih, D. S., C., and Kaesberg, P., 1975, Nucleotide sequence of a viral RNA fragment that binds to eukaryotic ribosomes, *Nature (London)* **256**:624.

Dasgupta, R., Harad, F., and Kaesberg, P., 1976, Blocked 5′ termini in brome mosaic virus RNA, *J. Virol.* **18**:260.

Davies, J. W., and Kaesberg, P., 1974, Translation of virus mRNA: Protein synthesis directed by several virus RNAs in a cell-free extract from wheat germ, *J. Gen. Virol.* **25**:11.

Dawson, J. R. O., Motoyoshi, F., Watts, J. W., and Bancroft, J. B., 1975, Production of RNA and coat protein of a wild-type isolate and a temperature-sensitive mutant of CCMV in cowpea leaves and tobacco protoplasts, *J. Gen. Virol.* **29**:99.

Duda, C. T., Zaitlin, M., and Siegel, A., 1973, *In vitro* synthesis of double-stranded RNA by an enzyme system isolated from tobacco leaves, *Biochim. Biophys. Acta* **319**:62.

Dunn, D., and Hitchborn, J. H., 1965, The use of bentonite in the purification of plant viruses, *Virology* **25**:171.

Efron, D., and Marcus, A., 1973, Translation of TMV-RNA in a cell-free wheat embryo system, *Virology* **53**:343.

El Manna, M., and Bruening, G., 1973, Polyadenylate sequences in the ribonucleic acids of cowpea mosaic virus, *Virology* **56**:198.

Filner, B., and Marcus, A., 1974, Tobacco mosaic virus coat protein synthesis *in vivo:* Analysis of the *N*-terminal acetylation, *Virology* **61**:537.

Fraenkel-Conrat, H., 1956, The role of nucleic acid in the reconstitution of TMV, *J. Am. Chem. Soc.* **78**:882.

Fraenkel-Conrat, H., 1976, RNA polymerase from tobacco necrosis virus infected and uninfected tobacco: Purification of the membrane-associated enzyme, *Virology* **72**:23.

Fritsch, C., Mayo, M. A., and Hirth, L., 1976, *In vitro* translation of tobacco rattle virus RNA, *Ann. Microbiol. (Inst. Pasteur)* **127A**:93.

Fritsch, C., Mayo, M. A., and Hirth, L., 1977, Further studies on the translation of tobacco rattle virus *in vitro* (in press).

Gerlinger, P., Mohier, E., LeMeur, M. A., and Hirth, L., 1977, Monocistronic translation of alfalfa mosaic virus RNAs, *Nucleic Acid Res.* **4**:813.

Gierer, A., and Schramm, G., 1956, Die Infektiosität der Ribonukleinsäure des Tabak-mosaikvirus, *Z. Naturforsch.* **11b**:138 [also *Nature (London)* **177**:702].

Goodwin, P. B., and Higgins, T. J. V., 1974, *In vitro* synthesis of tobacco mosaic virus coat protein, *Proc. Aust. Biochem. Soc.,* **7**:75.

Giege, R., Briand, J. P., Mengual, R., Ebel, J. P., and Hirth, L., 1977, Valylation of the two RNA components of TYMV and specificity of the tRNA aminoacylation reaction, *Proc. Natl. Acad. Sci. USA* **74** (in press).

Gurdon, J. B., Lane, C. D., Woodland, H. R., and Marbaix, G., 1971, Use of frog eggs and oocytes for the study of mRNA and its translation in living cells, *Nature (London)* **233**:177.

Hadidi, A., and Fraenkel-Conrat, H., 1973, Characterization and specificity of soluble RNA polymerase of brome mosaic virus, *Virology* **52**:363.

Haenni, A. L., Prochiantz, A., Bernard, O., and Chapeville, F., 1973, TYMV valyl-RNA as an amino-acid donor in protein biosynthesis, *Nature (London) New Biol.* **241**:166.

Hall, T. C., Shih, D. S., and Kaesberg, P., 1972, Enzyme mediated binding of tyrosine to BMV RNA, *Biochem. J.* **129**:969.

Hariharasubramanian, V., Hadidi, A., Singer, B., and Fraenkel-Conrat, H., 1973, Possible identification of a protein in brome mosaic virus infected barley as a component of viral RNA polymerase, *Virology* **54**:190.

Hashimoto, J., and Okamoto, K., 1975, Partially stripped tobacco mosaic virus-stimulated methionyl-tRNA binding to ribosomes in an *in vitro* wheat embryo system, *Virology* **67**:107.

Higgins, T., Goodwin, P., and Whitfeld, P., 1976, Occurrence of short particles in beans infected with the cowpea strain of TMV. 2. Evidence that the short particles contain the cistron for coat protein, *Virology* **71**:486.

Higgins, T. J. V., Whitfeld, P. R., and Goodwin, P. B., 1974, Small particles containing the coat-protein cistron associated with the cowpea strain of tobacco mosaic virus, *Proc. Aust. Biochem. Soc.* **7**:75.

Horst, J., Fraenkel-Conrat, H., and Mandeles, S., 1971, Terminal heterogeneity at both ends of the satellite tobacco necrosis virus (STNV) RNA, *Biochemistry* **10**:4748.

Hunter, T. R., Hunt, T., Knowland, J., and Zimmern, D., 1976, Messenger RNA for the coat protein of tobacco mosaic virus, *Nature (London)* **260**:759.

Jackson, A. O., Zaitlin, M., Siegel, A., and Francki, R. I. B., 1972, Replication of tobacco mosaic virus. III. Viral RNA metabolism in separated leaf cells, *Virology* **48**:655.

Jacobson, M. F., and Baltimore, D., 1968, Polypeptide cleavages in the formation of poliovirus proteins, *Proc. Natl. Acad. Sci. USA* **61**:77.

Jones, I. M., and Reichmann, M. E., 1973, The proteins synthesized in tobacco leaves infected with tobacco necrosis virus and satellite tobacco necrosis virus, *Virology* **52**:49.

Kado, C. I., and Knight, C. A., 1968, The coat protein gene of tobacco mosaic virus. I. Location of the gene by mixed infection, *J. Mol. Biol.* **36**:15.

Kamen, R., 1970, Characterization of the subunits of Qβ replicase, *Nature (London)* **228**:527.

Kassanis, B., and McCarthy, D., 1967, The quality of virus as affected by the ambient temperature, *J. Gen. Virol.* **1**:425.

Keith, J., 1976, Studies on the chemical structure of the terminal sequences of Rous sarcoma virus RNA and other viral RNAs, Ph.D. thesis, University of California, Berkeley.

Keith, J., and Fraenkel-Conrat, H., 1975, Identification of the 5′ end of Rous sarcoma virus RNA, *Proc. Natl. Acad. Sci. USA* **72**:3347.

Klein, C., Fritsch, C., Briand, J. P., Richards, K. E., Jonard, G., and Hirth, L., 1976, Physical and functional heterogeneity in TYMV RNA: Evidence for the existence of an independent messenger coding for coat protein, *Nucleic Acids Res.* **3**:3043.

Klein, W. H., Nolan, C., Lazar, J. M., and Clark, J. M., Jr., 1972, Translation of satellite tobacco necrosis virus ribonucleic acid. I. Characterization of *in vitro* procaryotic and eucaryotic translation products, *Biochemistry* **11**:2009.

Knowland, J., 1974, Protein synthesis directed by the RNA from a plant virus in a normal animal cell, *Genetics* **78**:383.

Knowland, J., Hunter, T., Hunt, T., and Zimmern, D., 1975, Translation of tobacco mosaic virus RNA and isolation of the messenger for TMV coat protein, *Coll. Inst. Nat. Sante Rech. Med.* **47**:211.

Kohl, R., and Hall, T., 1974, Aminoacylation of RNA from several viruses: amino acid specificity and differential activity of plant, yeast, and bacterial synthetases, *J. Gen. Virol.* **25**:257.

Kondo, M., Gallerani, R., and Weissmann, C., 1970, Subunit structure of Qβ replicase, *Nature (London)* **228**:525.

Lebeurier, G., Nicolaieff, A., and Richards, K. E., 1977, Inside-out model for self-assembly of tobacco mosaic virus, *Proc. Nat. Acad. Sci.* **74**:149.

Leung, D. W., Gilbert, C. W., Smith, R. E., Sasavage, N. L., and Clark, Jr., J. M., 1976, Translation of satellite tobacco necrosis virus ribonucleic acid by an *in vitro* system from wheat germ, *Biochemistry* **15**:4943.

Litvak, S., Tarrago, A., Tarrago-Litvak, L., and Allende, J., 1973, Elongation factor-viral genome interaction dependent on the aminoacylation of TYMV and TMV RNAs, *Nature (London) New Biol.* **241**:88.

Mandeles, S., 1968, Location of unique sequences in tobacco mosaic virus ribonucleic acid, *J. Biol. Chem.* **243**:3671.

May, D. S., and Knight, C. A., 1965, Polar stripping of protein subunits from tobacco mosaic virus, *Virology* **25**:502.

Mayo, M., and Robinson, D., 1975, Revision of estimates of the molecular weights of tobravirus coat proteins, *Intervirology* **5**:313.

Mayo, M. A., Fritsch, C., and Hirth, L., 1976, Translation of tobacco rattle virus RNA *in vitro* using wheat germ extracts, *Virology* **69**:408.

Mohier, E., Hirth, L., LeMeur, M.-A., and Gerlinger, P., 1975, Translation of alfalfa mosaic virus RNAs in mammalian cell-free systems, *Virology* **68**:349.

Mohier, E., Hirth, L., LeMeur, M.-A., and Gerlinger, P., 1976, Analysis of alfalfa mosaic virus 17 S RNA translation products, *Virology* **71**:615.

Morris, T. J., 1974, Two ribonucleoprotein components associated with the cowpea strain of TMV, *Am. Phytopathol. Soc. Proc.* **1**:83.

Nathans, D., Notani, G., Schwartz, J. H., and Zinder, N. D., 1962, Biosynthesis of the coat protein of coliphage f2 by *E. coli* extracts, *Proc. Natl. Acad. Sci. USA* **48**:1424.

Nikolaieff, A., Lebeurier, G., Morel, M.-C., and Hirth, L., 1975, The uncoating of native and reconstituted TMV by dimethylsulphoxide: the polarity of stripping, *J. Gen. Virol.* **26**:295.

Nirenberg, M. W., and Matthaei, J. H., 1961, The dependence of cell-free protein synthesis in *E. coli* upon naturally occurring or synthetic polyribonucleotides, *Proc. Natl. Acad. Sci. USA* **47**:1588.

Öberg, B., and Philipson, L., 1972, Binding of histidine to tobacco mosaic virus RNA, *Biochem. Biophys. Res. Commun.* **48**:927.

Ohno, T., and Okada, Y., 1977, Polarity of stripping of tobacco mosaic virus by alkali and sodium dodecyl sulfate, *Virology* **76**:429.

Paterson, R., 1974, Protein synthesis in tobacco protoplasts infected with tobacco mosaic virus, Ph.D. thesis, University of California, Berkeley.

Paterson, R., and Knight, C. A., 1975, Protein synthesis in tobacco protoplasts infected with tobacco mosaic virus, *Virology* **64**:10.

Pelham, H. R. B., and Jackson, R. J., 1976, An efficient mRNA-dependent translation system from reticulocyte lysates. *Eur. J. Biochem.* **67**:247.

Pelham, R. B., and Stuick, E. J., 1976, Proceedings of the Symposium on Nucleic Acid and Protein Synthesis in Plants, Strasbourg, July 1976.

Perham, R. N., and Wilson, T. M. A., 1976, The polarity of stripping of coat protein subunits from the RNA in tobacco mosaic virus under alkaline conditions, *FEBS Lett.* **62**:11.

Pinck, L., 1975, The 5′-end groups of alfalfa mosaic virus RNAs are m^{7}G^5′ppp^5′Gp, *FEBS Lett.* **59**:24.

Pinck, M., Genevaux, M., and Duranton, H., 1974, Studies on the amino acid acceptor activities of the eggplant mosaic viral RNA and its satellite RNA, *Biochimie* **56**:423.

Pleij, C. W. A., Neeleman, A., van Vloten-Doting, L., and Bosch, L., 1976, Translation of turnip yellow mosaic virus RNA *in vitro:* A closed and an open coat protein cistron, *Proc. Nat. Acad. Sci.* **73**:4437.

Rees, M. W., and Short, M. N., 1965, Variations in the composition of two strains of tobacco mosaic virus in relation to their host, *Virology* **26**:596.

Rees, M. W., and Short, M. N., 1972, The tryptic peptides and terminal sequences of the protein from the cowpea strain of tobacco mosaic virus, *Virology* **50**:772.

Rice, R. H., 1972, Studies on the translation of satellite of tobacco necrosis virus RNA in an *E. coli* cell-free system, Ph.D. thesis, University of California, Berkeley.

Rice, R., and Fraenkel-Conrat, H., 1973, Fidelity of translation of satellite tobacco necrosis virus ribonucleic acid in a cell-free *Escherichia coli* system, *Biochemistry* **12**:181.

Richards, K. E., Morel, M. C., Nicolaieff, A., Lebeurier, G., and Hirth, L., 1975, Location of the cistron of the tobacco mosaic virus coat protein, *Biochimie* **57**:749.

Richards, K., Briand, J. P., Klein, C., and Jonard, G., 1977, Common nucleotides sequences on long and short RNAs of turnip yellow mosaic virus, *FEBS Lett.* **74**:279.

Roberts, B. E., Mathews, M. B., and Bruton, C. J., 1973, Tobacco mosaic virus RNA directs the synthesis of a coat protein peptide in a cell-free system from wheat, *J. Mol. Biol.* **80**:733.

Roberts, B. E., Paterson, B. M., and Sperling, R., 1974, The cell-free synthesis and assembly of viral specific polypeptides into TMV particles, *Virology* **59**:307.

Sakai, F., and Takebe, I., 1972, A non-coat protein synthesized in tobacco mesophyll protoplasts infected by tobacco mosaic virus, *Mol. Gen. Genet.* **118**:93.

Sakai, F., and Takebe, I., 1974, Protein synthesis in tobacco mesophyll protoplasts induced by tobacco mosaic virus infection, *Virology* **62**:426.

Sakai, F., Watts, J. W., Dawson, J. R. O., and Bancroff, J. B., 1977, Synthesis of proteins in tobacco protoplasts infected with cowpea chlorotic mottle virus, *Gen. Virol.* **34**:285.

Salvato, M., 1977, *In vitro* translation of plant viral RNAs, Ph.D. thesis, University of California, Berkeley.

Salvato, M., and Fraënkel-Conrat, H., 1977, Translation of tobacco necrosis virus and its satellite in a cell-free wheat germ system, *Proc. Nat. Acad. Sci.* (in press).

Scalla, R., Boudon, E., and Rigaud, J., 1976, Sodium dodecyl sulfate-polyacrylamide-gel electrophoretic detection of two high molecular weight proteins associated with tobacco mosaic virus infection in tobacco, *Virology* **69**:339.

Schwartz, J. H., 1967, Initiation of protein synthesis under the direction of tobacco mosaic virus RNA in cell-free extracts of *Escherichia coli, J. Mol. Biol.* **30**:309.

Schwinghamer, M. W., and Symons, R. H., 1975, Fractionation of cucumber mosaic virus RNA and its translation in a wheat embryo cell-free system, *Virology* **63**:252.

Shatkin, A. J., Banerjee, A. K., and Both, G. W., 1977, Translation of animal virus mRNAs *in vitro,* in: *Comprehensive Virology,* Vol. 10 (H. Fraenkel-Conrat and Robert R. Wagner, eds.), Plenum Press, New York.

Shih, D. S., and Kaesberg, P., 1973, Translation of brome mosaic viral RNA in a cell-free system derived from wheat embryo. *Proc. Natl. Acad. Sci. USA* **70**:1799.

Shih, D. S., and Kaesberg, P., 1976, Translation of the RNAs of Brome Mosaic Virus: The monocistronic nature of RNA 1 and RNA 2, *J. Mol. Biol.* **103**:77.

Shih, D. S., Kaesberg, P., and Hall, T. C., 1974, Messenger and aminoacylation functions of brome mosaic virus RNA after chemical modification of 3′ terminus, *Nature (London)* **249**:353.

Shih, D. S., Dasgupta, R., and Kaesberg, P., 1976, 7-Methyl-guanosine and efficiency of RNA translation, *J. Virol.* **19**:637.

Siegel, A., Zaitlin, M., and Duda, C. T., 1973, Replication of tobacco mosaic virus. IV. Further characterization of viral-infected RNAs, *Virology* **53**:75.

Siegel, A., Hari, V., Montgomery, I., and Kolacz, K., 1976, A messenger RNA for capsid protein isolated from tobacco mosaic virus infected tissue, *Virology* **73**:363.

Singer, B., 1971, Protein synthesis in virus-infected plants. I. The number and nature of TMV-directed proteins detected on polyacrylamide gels, *Virology* **46**:247.

Singer, B., and Condit, C., 1974, Protein synthesis in virus-infected plants. III. Effects of tobacco mosaic virus mutants on protein synthesis in *Nicotiana tabacum, Virology* **57**:42.

Smith, A., 1973, The initiation of protein synthesis directed by the RNA from encephalomyocarditis virus, *Eur. J. Biochem.* **33**:301.

Steinschneider, A., and Fraenkel-Conrat, H., 1966, Studies of nucleotide sequences in tobacco mosaic virus ribonucleic acid. IV. Use of aniline in stepwise degradation, *Biochemistry* **5**:2735.

Stubbs, J. D., and Kaesberg, P., 1967, Amino acid incorporation in an *E. coli* cell-free system directed by bromegrass mosaic virus ribonucleic acid, *Virology* **33**:385.

Thang, M. N., Dondon, L., and Mohier, E., 1976, Translation of alfalfa mosaic virus RNA. Effect of polyamines, *FEBS Lett.* **61**:85.

Tsugita, A., Fraenkel-Conrat, H., Nirenberg, M. W., and Matthaei, J. H., 1962, *Proc. Natl. Acad. Sci. USA* **48**:846.

van Loon, L. C., and van Kammen, A., 1970, Polyacrylamide disc electrophoresis of the soluble leaf proteins from Nicotiana tabacum var. "Samsun" and "Samsun NN."

11. Changes in protein constitution after infection with tobacco mosaic virus, *Virology* **40**:199.

van Ravenswaay Claasen, J. C., van Leeuwen, A. B. J., Duijts, G. A. H., and Bosch, L., 1967, *In vitro* translation of alfalfa mosaic virus RNA, *J. Mol. Biol.* **23**:535.

Whitfeld, P. R., and Higgins, T. J. V., 1976, Occurrence of short particles in beans infected with the cowpea strain of TMV. I. Purification and characterization of short particles, *Virology* **71**:471.

Wilson, T. M. A., Perham, R. N., Finch, J. T., and Butler, P. J. G., 1976, Polarity of the RNA in the tobacco mosaic virus particle and the direction of protein stripping in sodium dodecyl sulphate, *FEBS Lett.* **64**:285.

Yot, P., Pinck, M., Haenni, A.-L., Duranton, H. M., and Chapeville, F., 1970, Valine-specific tRNA-like structure in turnip yellow mosaic virus RNA, *Proc. Nat. Acad. Sci. USA* **67**:1345.

Zaitlin, M., and Hariharasubramanian, V., 1970, Proteins in tobacco mosaic virus-infected tobacco plants, *Biochem. Biophys. Res. Commun.* **39**:1031.

Zaitlin, M., and Hariharasubramanian, V., 1972, A gel electrophoretic analysis of proteins from plants infected with tobacco mosaic and potato spindle tuber viruses, *Virology* **47**:296.

Zaitlin, M., Beachy, R. N., Bruening, G., Romaine, C. P., and Scalla, R., 1976, Translation of tobacco mosaic virus RNA, Squaw Valley ICN-UCLA.

Ziemiecki, A., and Wood, K. R., 1976, Proteins synthesized by cucumber cotyledons infected with two strains of cucumber mosaic virus, *J. Gen. Virol.* **31**:373.

Zimmern, D., 1975, The 5′ end group of tobacco mosaic virus RNA is m⁷G⁵′ppp⁵′Gp, *Nucleic Acid Res.* **2**:1189.

CHAPTER 5

Protoplasts in the Study of Plant Virus Replication

Itaru Takebe

Institute for Plant Virus Research
Tsukuba Science City, Ibaraki 300-21, Japan

1. INTRODUCTION

In spite of its much longer history, plant virology lags far behind bacterial or animal virology in the understanding of the process of virus replication. One of the reasons for this situation stems from the very nature of plant viruses, that they are not provided with a specialized mechanism for entry through the rigid walls of plant cells. Infection by plant viruses thus relies upon a third agent that produces wounds of one type or another in the plant cell walls. The lack of a penetration function accounts for the extremely small numbers of plant cells which become primarily infected by inoculation, and causes serious difficulty in the studies of virus replication processes.

Another drawback in plant virology has been the lack of plant materials consisting of single cells. It has been difficult until recent years to dissociate plant tissues into single cells, and attempts to utilize suspension-cultured plant cells or unicellular algae for plant virus studies have met with only limited success. Experiments with plant viruses have been done therefore using tissue materials in which the infection stage in individual cells is inevitably randomized because of the cell-to-cell movement of virus. Plant virologists have thus never been provided with an experimental system in which a majority of cells are infected simultaneously without infection being spread to other cells, or in which "one-step virus growth" (Ellis and Delbrück, 1939) can be realized. An understanding of the processes of virus replication relies upon knowledge of the sequence of events during the virus replication cycle, and it is clear that such information is difficult to obtain without a system that permits one-step-type virus replication.

Botanists have known for many years that the cellular entity within cell walls, the protoplast, can be released from the surrounding walls by dissecting plasmolyzed plant tissues. The protoplasts thus isolated are spherical irrespective of the shape of the original cells, and they persist as such if the osmotic pressure of the medium is properly adjusted. It was shown in 1960 that plant protoplasts can be obtained by chemical means, using cell-wall-degrading enzymes (Cocking, 1960). Introduction of the enzymatic method stimulated rapid progress in the large-scale isolation of plant protoplasts (Cocking, 1972) and led also to attempts to use the wall-less single plant cells for plant virus research (Cocking, 1966; Takebe et al., 1968). It was thus found that protoplasts from the leaf tissues of tobacco can be infected by TMV* at very high frequencies without wounding them mechanically (Takebe and Otsuki, 1969). Since then, conditions for a synchronous infection of protoplasts were established with many viruses (Takebe, 1975a,b), and a new avenue opened to the study of the virus replication process in plant cells.

This chapter will begin with a brief account of the method for isolating protoplasts from the leaf mesophyll, and the mesophyll protoplast system will then be characterized in relation to virus infection. The remaining part of the chapter will be devoted to discussion of the current uses of protoplast systems and their implication for the study of plant virus replication. Several review articles have appeared to deal with the significance of protoplasts in plant virus research from various viewpoints (Zaitlin and Beachy, 1974a,b; Takebe, 1975a,b; Sarkar, 1977).

2. PROTOPLASTS FROM LEAF MESOPHYLL

2.1. Isolation

Although protoplasts can be isolated from various plant organs and tissues (Cocking, 1972), those from the leaf mesophyll are used

---

* Abbreviations for virus names: AMV, alfalfa mosaic virus; BBWV, broad bean wilt virus; BMV, brome mosaic virus; CCMV, cowpea chlorotic mottle virus; CGMMV, cucumber green mottle mosaic virus; CMV, cucumber mosaic virus; CPMV, cowpea mosaic virus; PEMV, pea enation mosaic virus; PVX, potato virus X; RDV, rice dwarf virus; RRSV, raspberry ringspot virus; TMV, tobacco mosaic virus; TRV, tobacco rattle virus; TYMV, turnip yellow mosaic virus.

almost exclusively for infection by plant viruses. This is not only because the leaf mesophyll is the tissue where virus propagates most vigorously but also because protoplasts are isolated from this tissue more readily than from any other tissue. Cells in the leaf mesophyll are connected with each other more or less loosely and their walls are relatively thin, so that the tissues are readily amenable to attack by wall-degrading enzymes. Successful isolation of mesophyll protoplasts (Takebe *et al.*, 1968) and their infection by a plant virus (Takebe and Otsuki, 1969) were first accomplished using tobacco, and this species is still used most widely as the source of protoplasts for virus research. More recently, mesophyll protoplasts from cowpea (Hibi *et al.*, 1975; Beier and Bruening, 1975), tomato (Motoyoshi and Oshima, 1975), and Chinese cabbage (Renaudin *et al.*, 1975) were infected with viruses. The method developed in my laboratory to isolate tobacco mesophyll protoplasts will be outlined, because this formed the basis for most of the current procedures for the isolation of mesophyll protoplasts. For technical details, readers are referred to the original literature (Takebe *et al.*, 1968; Otsuki *et al.*, 1974).

In plant leaves, the mesophyll tissues are sandwiched by the upper epidermis and the lower epidermis, which, being overlaid with cuticule, render the leaves impervious to external agents. The first necessary step in the enzymatic isolation of mesophyll protoplasts is thus the removal of the epidermis. Only the lower epidermis needs to be removed, and this is done by manually peeling it with the aid of a forceps. The stripped leaves are cut into small pieces and these are vacuum-infiltrated with and bathed in a solution of crude polygalacturonase (polygalacturonide glycanohydrolase, E.C. 3.2.1.15; "pectinase"). This enzyme dissociates the mesophyll tissues by hydrolyzing the pectic substance which cements neighboring cells. The enzyme solution also contains D-mannitol at 0.7 M to render the solution hypertonic, and low molecular weight potassium dextran sulfate which protects the cells from damage during the tissue dissociation. The leaf pieces bathed in the enzyme solution are shaken in a waterbath of 25°C for successive 3- and 7-min periods, the solution containing released cells being removed after each period to be replaced by fresh enzyme solution. The first 3-min incubation releases predominantly damaged cells from cut edges of leaf pieces, whereas the following 7-min incubation releases cells of spongy parenchyma from the exposed surface of the mesophyll. The leaf pieces are then incubated in fresh enzyme solution for 30–40 min, during which time the palisade parenchyma, which comprises the major portion of the mesophyll, is completely dissociated.

The palisade parenchyma cells thus isolated are washed by low-speed centrifugation and are now suspended in 0.7 M mannitol solution containing cellulase (β-1,4-glucan 4-glucanohydrolase, E.C. 3.2.1.4). Incubation at 37°C with gentle shaking results in the dissolution of cell walls within 30 min, and the elongated palisade cells become spherical protoplasts (Fig. 1). The protoplasts are washed with mannitol solution to remove cellulase and the debris of damaged cells, and are ready for inoculation with virus. Approximately 10^7 protoplasts of palisade parenchyma cells are obtained from 1 g fresh weight of mature tobacco leaves.

Several modifications of the basic procedure as described above have been devised for isolating mesophyll protoplasts. Since manual peeling of the epidermis requires skill and is difficult with some species, the epidermis may be treated with enzymes (Schilde-Rentschler, 1973) or may be injured using abrasives (Beier and Bruening, 1975) to render the mesophyll tissues accessible to the wall-degrading enzymes.

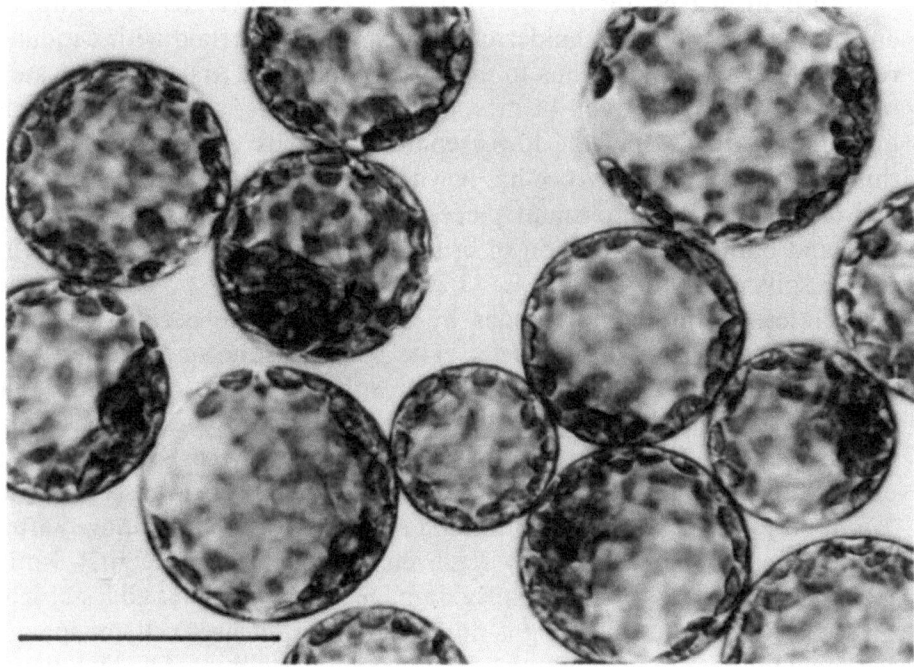

Fig. 1. Protoplasts freshly isolated from the palisade tissue of tobacco leaves. Scale represents 50 μm.

However, these methods are likely to also damage the mesophyll tissues and hence may affect the quantity and quality of protoplasts obtained. A modification called the "one-step procedure" is fairly widely used (Kassanis and White, 1974; Hibi *et al.,* 1975; Beier and Bruening, 1975), in which the stripped leaves are treated with a mixture of polygalacturonase and cellulase instead of being treated consecutively with the two enzymes. Besides being simpler, this procedure has the merit of not requiring the addition of dextran sulfate, the use of which is essential in the original procedure. However, the one-step procedure yields a heterogeneous population of mesophyll protoplasts because it does not permit the separation of palisade from spongy parenchyma cells. Moreover, there are indications that the one-step procedure is more drastic and causes greater trauma to mesophyll cells; the preparations obtained by this method invariably contain substantial numbers of subprotoplasts, smaller spherical bodies lacking part of the cellular content. When inoculated under the same conditions, protoplasts prepared by the one-step procedure give lower levels of infection than protoplasts obtained by the original procedure. A liquid–liquid two-phase separation method was also devised to remove damaged cells from a population of protoplasts (Kanai and Edwards, 1973). This method may be useful for those species whose protoplast preparations contain relatively large numbers of damaged cells.

Yields of mesophyll protoplasts are influenced considerably by the age and the physiological state of source leaves. In general, plants have to be well nourished, and mature leaves should be used soon after they have fully expanded. Younger leaves are readily dissociated by enzymes but the resulting protoplasts are fragile and do not survive subsequent inoculation or culture. Older leaves require longer enzyme treatments and their protoplasts are again unstable. The physiological basis of the stability of protoplasts is poorly understood, so that the optimal conditions of plant growth for protoplast isolation have been worked out empirically. Since these conditions include factors such as temperature, humidity, day length, soil, and method of watering, which usually differ according to where the plants are grown, it is difficult to standardize them, and each laboratory should ascertain its best conditions for plant growth. Once such conditions are established and if leaves are carefully selected, protoplasts can be obtained reproducibly throughout the year. Some efforts were made to better define the growth conditions of source plants (Kubo *et al.,* 1975*b*). Chinese cabbage appears to be less affected by growth conditions than other plants and to supply larger numbers of leaves suitable for protoplast isolation (Renaudin *et al.*, 1975).

Another important factor for the successful isolation of protoplasts is the choice of enzyme preparations. Many commercial pectinases (polygalacturonases) and cellulases are not powerful enough for digesting native cell walls, or they contain impurities which are deleterious to plant cells. Macerozyme R-10 and Cellulase R-10, both manufactured by Kinki Yakult, Nishinomiya, Japan, are satisfactory in these respects and are most widely used.

2.2. Culture

Mesophyll protoplasts do not require a rich medium for the production of virus, because they fix CO_2 through photosynthesis (Nishimura and Akazawa, 1975) and probably also because they have a large pool of precursors. The medium most widely used for culturing virus-infected mesophyll protoplasts has the composition shown in Table 1. Beside mannitol as osmotic stabilizer, it contains several inorganic salts and a plant growth regulator, but has no metabolizable carbohydrate. Protoplasts survive for several days in this medium and actively synthesize RNA and protein (Sakai and Takebe, 1970). However, they do not form walls or initiate cell division, although they are able to do so in richer media (Nagata and Takebe, 1970, 1971). It is not known to what extent nitrogen or phosphorus in the medium of Table 1 contributes to the synthesis of virus. Increasing the concentration of nitrate and phosphate 5 times did not improve the yield of TMV (Kassanis and White, 1974), and a good yield of TMV is reported in protoplasts cultured in plain mannitol solution (Kassanis *et al.*, 1975). These observations suggest that the role of the medium of Table 1 is

TABLE 1

Medium Commonly Used for Culturing Virus-Inoculated Protoplasts

KH_2PO_4	0.2 mM	2,4-Dichlorophenoxyacetic acid	1 μg/ml
KNO_3	1 mM	or 6-benzyladenine	
$MgSO_4$	1 mM	D-Mannitol	0.7 M
$CaCl_2$	10 mM	Cephaloridine	300 μg/ml
KI	1 μM	Rimocidin	10 μg/ml
$CuSO_4$	0.01 μM	pH	5.4

probably to provide a balanced ionic environment rather than to supply nutrients essential for virus synthesis. Cephaloridine added to prevent growth of bacteria may be substituted with carbenicillin (Motoyoshi *et al.*, 1975*b*), aureomycin (Sarkar *et al.*, 1974) or chloramphenicol, and rimocidin to inhibit fungal growth with mycostatin (Motoyoshi *et al.*, 1975*b*).

Mesophyll protoplasts survive longer in the dark than in the light. However, protoplasts inoculated with virus are usually cultured under illumination (2000–3000 lux) because light significantly increases virus yield (Takebe *et al.*, 1968) or is sometimes almost essential for virus replication (Renaudin *et al.*, 1975).

3. INFECTION OF PROTOPLASTS

3.1. Inoculation Procedure

One of the rationales in the attempts to use protoplasts for plant virus studies was the expectation that the wall-less cells would admit virus without being injured physically. This naive idea turned out to be correct when the early studies of Cocking showed that incubation of tomato fruit protoplasts with TMV solution resulted in the uptake of virus (Cocking, 1960) and in infection (Cocking and Pojnar, 1969). However, the efficiency of infection reported in these studies was far from satisfactory, a high concentration of virus (1 mg/ml) and a long incubation time (6 h) being necessary. The use of protoplasts for studying plant virus replication became meaningful, however, when it was found that poly-L-ornithine strikingly stimulated the infection of tobacco mesophyll protoplasts by TMV (Takebe and Otsuki, 1969). An inoculation procedure as described below was subsequently established to effect TMV infection in nearly all protoplasts by brief incubation with a low concentration of virus (Otsuki *et al.*, 1972).

Freshly isolated tobacco mesophyll protoplasts (4 × 10⁶ cells) are pelleted by low-speed centrifugation and allowed to stand as pellet while inoculum TMV is pretreated with poly-L-ornithine. The pretreatment is done by dissolving purified TMV to 2 μg/ml in 10 ml of 0.7 M mannitol solution buffered with potassium citrate at pH 5.2 and containing poly-L-ornithine (molecular weight 130,000) at 2 μg/ml, and by holding the mixture for 10 min at 25°C. The mixture is then added to the protoplasts, which are suspended with 10 ml of 0.7 M mannitol solution immediately before the addition of the virus–poly-L-ornithine mixture. Final concentrations are thus 1 μg/ml TMV, 1 μg/ml poly-L-

TABLE 2

Plant Viruses Inoculated in Protoplasts from Leaf Mesophyll

Virus	Plant	Requirement for poly-L-ornithine[a]	Protoplasts infected[b] (%)	Reference
TMV	Tobacco	E	90	Otsuki *et al.* (1972*a,b*)
	Tomato	E	80	Motoyoshi and Oshima (1975, 1976)
	Petunia	E	47	T. Hibi (personal communication)
	Cowpea	S	57 (7)	Koike *et al.* (1976)
	Chinese cabbage	E	91	Y. Otsuki and I. Takebe (unpublished)
	Barley	E		T. Hibi (personal communication)
CGMMV	Tobacco	E	65	Sugimura and Ushiyama (1975)
CCMV	Tobacco	E	65	Motoyoshi *et al.* (1973*a*)
BMV(V5)	Tobacco	S	77 (45)	Motoyoshi *et al.* (1974*a*)
BMV	Barley	S	30 (variable)	Okuno *et al.*, (1977)
CMV	Tobacco	E	90	Otsuki and Takebe (1973)
	Cowpea	S	95 (95)	Koike *et al.* (1977)
CPMV	Cowpea	S	96 (88)	Hibi *et al.* (1975), Beier and Bruening (1975)
	Tobacco	E	75	Huber *et al.* (1976)
AMV	Tobacco	E	35	Motoyoshi *et al.* (1975)
	Cowpea		6	T. Hibi (personal communication)
PEMV	Tobacco	S	84 (47)	Motoyoshi and Hull (1974)
RRSV	Tobacco	E	99	Barker and Harrison (1977)
BBWV	Broad bean	E	40	Kagi *et al.* (1975)
TRV	Tobacco	E	98	Kubo *et al.* (1975*a*)
PVX	Tobacco	E	70	Otsuki *et al.* (1974)

[a] E (essential), less than 1% of protoplasts are infected in the absence of poly-L-ornithine; S (stimulatory), significant numbers of protoplasts are infected in the absence of poly-L-ornithine (see footnote *b*).

[b] Figures in parentheses indicate percentage of protoplasts infected in the absence of poly-L-ornithine.

ornithine, and 2×10^5/ml protoplasts. After 10 min at 25°C, protoplasts are collected by centrifugation, washed with mannitol solution to remove unadsorbed virus, and then transferred to the culture medium.

The inoculation procedure originally developed for tobacco mesophyll protoplasts and TMV was applicable to other combinations of plant and virus; thus mesophyll protoplasts from seven species have been inoculated with 12 viruses, using essentially the same procedure (Table 2). As new combinations were tried, features peculiar to some viruses or plants have also become apparent with respect to the optimal conditions of inoculation. Some of these features are discussed in the following section.

3.2.   Levels of Infection

In determining the levels of infection of protoplasts, advantage is taken of the fact that protoplasts adhere to glass slides and become permeable to antiserum to virus after fixation with ethanol or acetone. Protoplasts cultured for an appropriate time after inoculation can therefore be stained with fluorescence-labeled antibody to virus without laborious embedding and sectioning (Otsuki and Takebe, 1969). When examined under a fluorescence microscope, infected protoplasts contain fluorescing masses of viral antigen (Fig. 2), so that the percentage of infected protoplasts can be determined readily and exactly. This method can be used with any virus for which specific antiserum of sufficiently high titer can be obtained.

Over 90% of tobacco mesophyll protoplasts are reproductively infected when they are inoculated with TMV by the procedure just described. Similar or even higher levels of infection are reported with

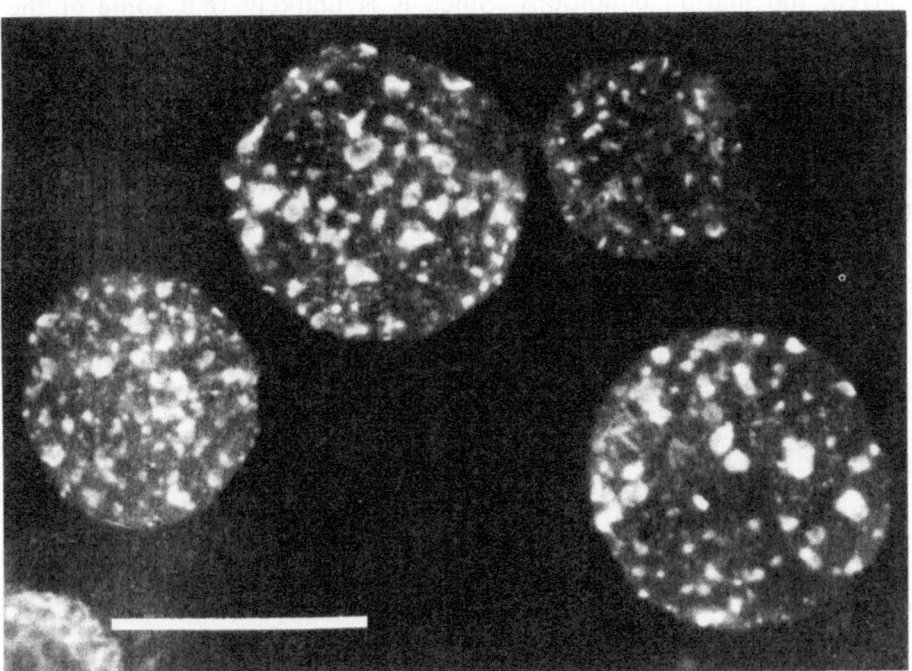

Fig. 2.   Fluorescence micrograph of tobacco protoplasts infected by TMV. Protoplasts were cultured for 24 h after inoculation with TMV and were stained with viral antibody labeled with fluorescein isothiocyanate. The numerous fluorescing masses represent virus aggregates produced in infected protoplasts. Scale represents 50 μm. By courtesy of Dr. Y. Otsuki.

some other combinations of plant and virus (Table 2). These figures show a striking contrast to the extremely low levels of primary infection in intact leaves where less than a thousandth of the leaf cells are initially infected by mechanical inoculation.

Levels of infection of protoplasts are primarily a function of the concentration of inoculum virus. The number of tobacco protoplasts which become infected by TMV is proportional to the logarithm of inoculum concentration, within a certain range (Fig. 3). The same relationship was found also for CMV (Otsuki and Takebe, 1973) and PVX (Otsuki *et al.*, 1974) with tobacco protoplasts and for TYMV with Chinese cabbage protoplasts (Renaudin *et al.*, 1975). The slope of the dosage–infection curve is steeper with multicomponent viruses (Motoyoshi and Hull, 1974). One peculiar aspect of the dosage–infection relationship in protoplasts is that not all protoplasts become infected even when they are inoculated with excessive amounts of virus (Fig. 3). Although the reason for this is not clear, it may suggest that inoculum virus is not evenly distributed among individual protoplasts under the current inoculation conditions. Since it is unlikely that some of the mesophyll cells are inherently "immune" to infection, one may expect that further studies will lead to the inoculation conditions under which literally all protoplasts are infected.

It should be pointed out that the levels of infection of protoplasts are affected also by the specific infectivity of the inoculum virus, a fact to which relatively little attention is paid. Plant virus preparations usually contain rather high proportions of inactive particles, and their specific infectivity is subject to variation according to the method of purification and preservation of the virus. There is an indication that

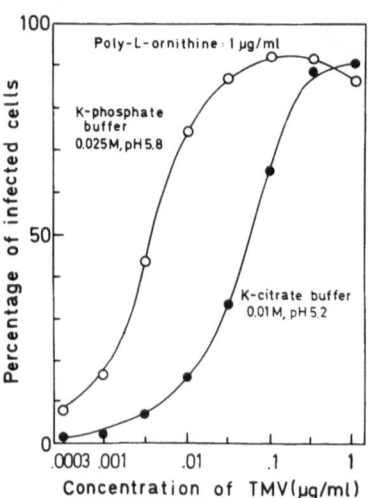

Fig. 3. Levels of infection of tobacco protoplasts as a function of inoculum TMV concentration. Inoculation was performed using citrate buffer (●) and phosphate buffer (○). By courtesy of Dr. Y. Otsuki.

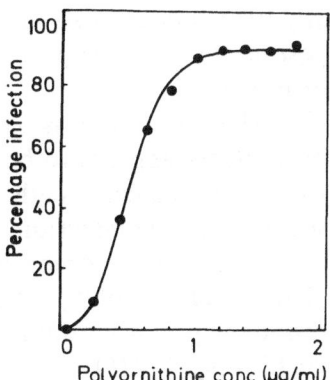

Fig. 4. Effect of poly-L-ornithine on infection of tobacco protoplasts by TMV. Protoplasts were inoculated with TMV at 1 μg/ml.

protoplasts are more exacting than whole leaves with respect to the specific infectivity of virus; CPMV loses infectivity toward cowpea protoplasts apparently much more rapidly than toward cowpea plants (A. van Kammen, personal communication).

Infection of tobacco protoplasts by TMV is greatly stimulated by poly-L-ornithine; few protoplasts become infected when this polycation is not included in the inoculation mixture (Fig. 4). This holds true not only for TMV but also for many other viruses which have been inoculated in protoplasts (Table 2). Poly-L-ornithine is more or less deleterious to protoplasts at concentrations higher than 1 μg/ml. The effect of poly-L-ornithine to stimulate infection is maximal when virus is preincubated for 10–20 min with this polycation before being added to protoplasts (Takebe *et al.*, 1975; Kubo *et al.*, 1975a). Since many plant viruses including TMV have a net negative charge and act as polyanion at the inoculation pH, poly-L-ornithine should form a complex with virus particles during the preincubation, and this complex should play a key role in the infection of protoplasts (Takebe *et al.*, 1975). Enhancement of infection of protoplasts by poly-L-ornithine thus appears to be accounted for primarily by the facilitation of adsorption of virus to the surface of protoplasts. This view is supported by the findings that tobacco mesophyll protoplasts show a net negative charge in cell electrophoresis (T. Nagata, personal communication) and that viruses with higher isoelectric points do not require poly-L-ornithine for infection of tobacco protoplasts (Table 2) (Motoyoshi *et al.*, 1974a; Motoyoshi and Hull, 1974).

Protoplasts from different species apparently differ in their requirement for poly-L-ornithine. Thus, tobacco protoplasts require poly-L-ornithine for infection by CPMV (Huber *et al.*, 1976), whereas cowpea protoplasts do not (Hibi *et al.*, 1975). Significant infection of cowpea protoplasts by TMV (Koike *et al.*, 1976) and by CMV (Koike *et al.*, 1975) occurs also in the absence of poly-L-ornithine (Table 2), suggesting that cowpea protoplasts are less negatively charged than tobacco protoplasts.

The effectiveness of poly-L-ornithine to stimulate infection of protoplasts appears to be related to its molecular size; poly-L-ornithine with a molecular weight of 90,000 was significantly less effective in stimulating the infection of tobacco protoplasts by TMV than the most commonly used preparation with a molecular weight of 130,000 (Takebe *et al.*, 1975). Other polycations such as poly-D-lysine, poly-L-lysine, or poly-L-arginine also stimulate infection of protoplasts (Motoyoshi *et al.*, 1974*b*).

Other factors influencing the levels of infection of protoplasts include pH and the kind of buffer used for inoculation. Lower pH values usually favor the infection by many viruses so that highest levels of infection are obtained at about pH 5, the lower limit of the pH range where protoplasts are stable (Takebe *et al.*, 1975). PVX (Otsuki *et al.*, 1974) and TRV (Kubo *et al.*, 1974) present exceptions to this general trend; infection of tobacco protoplasts by these viruses is relatively insensitive to variation of pH of the inoculation medium. The observed effects of pH on infection of protoplasts should represent a composite of the effects on two different reactions: interaction of virus and poly-L-ornithine and interaction of virus (or virus/poly-L-ornithine complex) and protoplasts.

Citrate has been used in most cases as the inoculation buffer for protoplasts. It was recently found that when phosphate buffer is used in place of citrate the same levels of infection of tobacco protoplasts can be attained with lower TRV concentrations (Kubo *et al.*, 1974). Phosphate shifted the optimum pH for the infection of tobacco protoplasts by TMV to 5.8 as compared with 5.2 using citrate, and at the same time improved the efficiency of infection tenfold (Fig. 3). However, infection of tobacco protoplasts by TMV became much more sensitive to variation of the actual concentration of protoplasts when phosphate rather than citrate was used for inoculation (Y. Otsuki, unpublished). A possibility is suggested that the buffer molecules intervene in the formation of a complex between virus and poly-L-ornithine (Kubo *et al.*, 1976).

3.3. Efficiency of Infection

When tobacco leaves are rubbed with TMV solution, at least 50,000 (Steere, 1955) and usually as many as 1,000,000 (Siegel and

Zaitlin, 1964) TMV particles are needed to give one infection center. With tobacco protoplasts inoculated with 1 μg/ml TMV using citrate buffer, one protoplast is infected for every 80,000 TMV particles added. This figure goes down to 8000 with phosphate buffer, because infection at similar levels can be effected with 0.1 μg/ml virus (Fig. 3). Even smaller numbers of particles are sufficient to cause infection of one protoplast when inoculation is performed with inoculum of nonsaturating concentrations, because the number of infected protoplasts decreases only linearly as the inoculum concentration is reduced exponentially (Fig. 3). These considerations show clearly that the efficiency of TMV infection is strikingly higher in protoplasts than in whole leaves. Similarly, CCMV infects tobacco protoplasts with much higher efficiency than it infects tobacco and other plants (Motoyoshi *et al.*, 1973*a*).

3.4. Number of Virus Particles Involved in Infection

Only a fraction of the inoculum virus adsorbs to protoplasts, and probably not all the adsorbed particles actually initiate infection. Estimation in several laboratories shows that from 600 to 8000 TMV particles adsorb per protoplast at the inoculum concentration of 1 μg/ml (Otsuki *et al.*, 1972*b*; Wyatt and Shaw, 1975; Zhuravlev *et al.*, 1975). Figures within a similar range are reported also for CCMV with tobacco protoplasts (Motoyoshi *et al.*, 1973*b*) and for CPMV with cowpea protoplasts (Hibi *et al.*, 1975). At inoculum concentrations causing infection of 50% of tobacco protoplasts, 30 long and 85 short TRV particles adsorb per protoplast in phosphate buffer, and 250 long and 700 short particles in citrate buffer (Kubo *et al.*, 1976). It is highly probable that the number of virus particles actually involved in infection is much smaller than these figures, since the amounts of adsorbed virus show no bearing on the levels of infection realized (Kubo *et al.*, 1976).

An attempt was made to estimate the number of TMV particles actually involved in infection by determining the number of UV targets in inoculated protoplasts (I. Takebe and A. Ono, unpublished). Protoplasts inoculated with TMV (0.0025 μg/ml) were irradiated with UV immediately after they had been washed to remove excess virus. After 2 days of culture, they were stained with fluorescent antibody to determine the number of infected protoplasts. As shown in Fig. 5, a multitarget inactivation curve was obtained when the number of infected protoplasts was plotted against UV dose, indicating that an

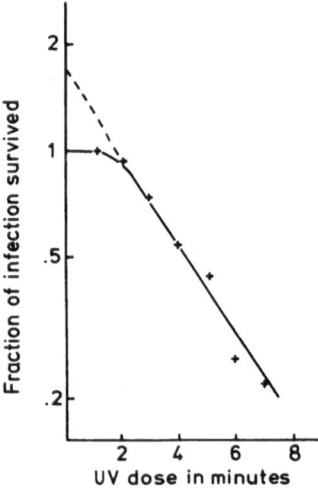

Fig. 5. Effect of UV irradiation of inoculated protoplasts on infection. Tobacco protoplasts inoculated with 0.0025 μg/ml TMV were immediately irradiated with UV. Numbers of infected protoplasts were determined after 44 h of culture by staining the protoplasts with fluorescent antibody. Without irradiation, 50% of the protoplasts were infected.

average of 1.7 TMV particles are involved in the infection of one protoplast at this inoculum concentration. It should be noted that a low concentration of inoculum was used in this experiment which gave rise to infection of 50% of the protoplasts. The results thus show that more than one TMV particle initiates infection in a protoplast even at a nonsaturating concentration of inoculum. Similar experiments with saturating concentrations of inoculum were not possible, because protoplasts were damaged by larger doses of UV required to inactivate virus. It may reasonably be assumed, however, that fairly large numbers of virus particles are involved in the infection of individual protoplasts when a great majority of protoplasts are infected.

3.5. Process of Virus Entry

Electron microscopy of inoculated protoplasts has thus far yielded two opposing views on the way virus particles get into protoplasts. Cocking observed in his early work using tomato fruit protoplasts that TMV particles are attached endwise to the invaginating plasmalemma and are also contained in intracytoplasmic vesicles (Cocking, 1966; Cocking and Pojnar, 1969). He suggested on the basis of these observations that virus enters protoplasts by a process resembling endocytosis in animal cells. Similar observations were made in tobacco mesophyll protoplasts with TMV (Otsuki *et al.*, 1972*b*), CMV (Honda *et al.*, 1974), and PVX (Honda *et al.*, 1975), leading to the hypothesis that the virus–

poly-L-ornithine complex induces endocytic activity in protoplasts (Takebe *et al.*, 1975).

A question was raised, however, by Burgess *et al.* (1973*a,b*) as to the operation of endocytosis in plant protoplasts. They proposed that CCMV particles become attached to areas of the plasmalemma which are damaged by poly-L-ornithine and that they enter protoplasts either directly or as the damage is repaired. Evidence along this line was recently reported also with TRV in tobacco mesophyll protoplasts (Kubo *et al.*, 1976).

3.6. Inoculation with Viral RNA

Tobacco protoplasts become infected when they are incubated with TMV RNA in the presence of poly-L-ornithine or other polycations (Aoki and Takebe, 1969). However, less than 10% of the protoplasts became infected in spite of the high concentration of viral RNA used (1 mg/ml), indicating that 10^9 TMV RNA molecules are needed to infect one protoplast. Most of the added viral RNA should be inactivated by cellular nucleases, although the polycations may provide some protection. Infection of tobacco protoplasts by free viral RNA is reported also with CCMV (Motoyoshi *et al.*, 1973*a*) and with PEMV (Motoyoshi and Hull, 1974). For unknown reasons, the concentration of CCMV RNA needed to infect tobacco protoplasts (Motoyoshi *et al.*, 1973*a*) was much lower than that of TMV RNA.

It was recently reported that an alkaline buffer with high salt concentrations, representing conditions unfavorable to the action of nucleases, strikingly improves the efficiency of infection of protoplasts by TMV RNA (Sarkar *et al.*, 1974). Polycations are not necessary under these conditions and nearly all protoplasts could be infected using TMV RNA concentrations as low as 4–20 μg/ml. If the improvement is in fact due to the inhibition of cellular nucleases, one may expect that these conditions will be useful also for inoculating protoplasts with RNA from other viruses.

4. STUDIES OF PLANT VIRUS REPLICATION USING PROTOPLASTS

Since the first establishment of a protoplast system for TMV, studies of plant virus replication using protoplasts centered around this virus. With other viruses, studies of replication are still in an incipient stage, and little more than the characterization of the growth curve or the estimation of virus production is reported. Before dealing with particular viruses or particular aspects of virus replication, it seems appropriate to recall the fundamental features of the protoplast system in relevance to virus replication.

Virus infection occurs in the majority, in some cases in practically all, of protoplasts by brief incubation with inoculum solution. Since the inoculated protoplasts are washed free of unadsorbed virus and are cultured in the absence of poly-L-ornithine, the chance of secondary infection during culture should be minimal, although some progeny virus may be released into the medium from small numbers of disintegrating protoplasts. We may therefore assume that infection occurs synchronously in protoplasts.

A suspension of protoplasts represents a population of single leaf cells with rather uniform biosynthetic capacity, because they derive from the leaves of similar age and physiological state. A uniform external environment is provided for the protoplasts, since they are bathed in liquid medium and are completely separated from each other. Synchronous infection should therefore give rise to a synchronous replication of virus in protoplasts, so that all the protoplasts are roughly at the same stage of virus replication at any time after inoculation. With protoplasts, we are looking at the course of virus replication in one single protoplast being amplified by a factor which is equal to the number of infected protoplasts.

4.1. Tobacco Mosaic Virus

4.1.1. Growth Curve

The time course of tobacco mosaic virus replication in protoplasts can be followed by determining the amounts of intracellular virus by infectivity assay. A typical example of the TMV growth curve in tobacco protoplasts is shown in Fig. 6. A small amount of infectivity present at time zero represents inoculum virus adsorbed to protoplasts, and the subsequent drop in its amount may be interpreted to reflect uncoating. Production of progeny virus is evident at 6 h postinfection and proceeds exponentially in the early periods of the replication cycle. Replication in the later periods is more or less linear. A growth curve essentially similar to that of Fig. 6 was obtained by counting the number of TMV particles in ultrathin sections of tobacco protoplasts (Hibi and Yora, 1972).

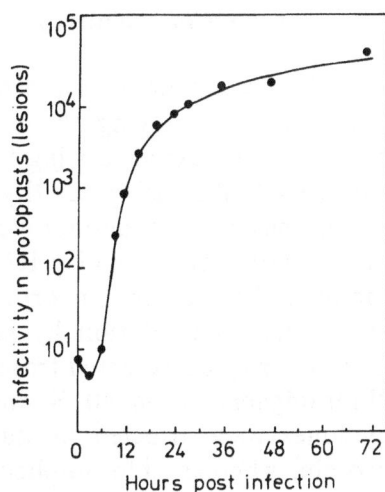

Fig. 6. Time course of TMV replication in synchronously infected tobacco protoplasts.

4.1.2. Yield of Virus

With protoplasts, it is possible to estimate the virus yield per cell, because the number of infected protoplasts can be exactly determined. This is usually done by comparing the infectivity extractable from protoplasts with that of standard virus preparation of a known concentration (Otsuki *et al.*, 1972*a*), assuming that the virus produced in protoplasts has the same specific infectivity as that of the standard virus. This assumption was shown to be correct with TMV, since the virus yield estimated by infectivity assay showed reasonable agreement with the values obtained by measuring the amount of viral RNA in polyacrylamide gels (Aoki and Takebe, 1975) or the amount of virus collected by precipitation with polyethyleneglycol (Y. Otsuki, unpublished). It is clear that an overestimation for virus yield in protoplasts will result if a virus preparation of lower specific infectivity is used as a standard. Values ranging from 1×10^6 to 9×10^6 virus particles or from 6×10^{-5} to 50×10^{-5} µg virus per cell are reported with TMV in tobacco protoplasts (Takebe and Otsuki, 1969; Hibi and Yora, 1972; Kassanis and White, 1974). With leaves, it is difficult to estimate virus yield per cell, because the number of infected cells is usually unknown. Indirect estimations show that $0.5–2.5 \times 10^6$ TMV particles are produced in a tobacco leaf cell (Harrison, 1955; Rappaport and Wildman, 1957; Weintraub and Ragetli, 1964). Virus yield in protoplasts is thus at least comparable to that in the cells within leaves.

4.1.3. Effects of Inhibitors

Protoplasts obviously provide better defined conditions than leaf materials for studying the effects of inhibitors on virus replication, because complexities arising from uneven distribution of chemicals are avoided. Studies using healthy tobacco protoplasts (Sakai and Takebe, 1970) showed that actinomycin D at 10 μg/ml inhibited [^{14}C]uracil incorporation into cellular RNA by 71%. Cycloheximide at 0.1 μg/ml inhibited [^{14}C]leucine incorporation into total protoplast protein by 80%, whereas inhibition by chloramphenicol at 200 μg/ml was only 28%. As may be expected from the specific action of cycloheximide and chloramphenicol on 80 S and 70 S ribosome systems, respectively, cycloheximide affected primarily the incorporation into cytoplasmic protein, whereas chloramphenicol affected incorporation into chloroplast protein (Sakai and Takebe, 1970).

The effects of these inhibitors on TMV replication in tobacco protoplasts were studied by Takebe and Otsuki (1969). The inhibitors were added to protoplasts immediately after inoculation and were present throughout their culture. In confirmation of the earlier finding using leaf material (Sänger and Knight, 1963), actinomycin D did not affect TMV replication in protoplasts. In contrast, 2-thiouracil significantly inhibited virus replication as measured by infectivity assay. It is unlikely that 2-thiouracil inhibits viral RNA synthesis, since it has little effect on [^{14}C]uracil incorporation into cellular RNA (Sakai and Takebe, 1970). It is possible that the analogue of uracil is incorporated into viral RNA, resulting in the formation of noninfectious particles. Cycloheximide completely inhibited TMV replication in protoplasts, while chloramphenicol had no effect at all, indicating that the 80 S cytoplasmic ribosomes and not the 70 S chloroplast ribosomes are responsible for the translation of viral RNA.

A recent study showed that TMV replication in tobacco protoplasts is inhibited by gliotoxin, formycin B, and blasticidin S (I. Takebe and K. Shimizu, unpublished). Mechanisms of action of these inhibitors on virus replication are poorly understood. Comparative studies using healthy and infected protoplasts will show whether they specifically affect virus replication or indirectly inhibit virus synthesis through their effects on the metabolism of host cells. On the other hand, inhibitors with known mechanisms of action may be effectively used with protoplasts to provide valuable information about virus replication, because protoplasts permit programmed addition or withdrawal of such inhibitors at various stages of the replication cycle.

4.1.4. Replication of Viral RNA

Replication of TMV RNA in synchronously infected tobacco protoplasts was followed by Aoki and Takebe (1975). Inoculated protoplasts were cultured in the presence of actinomycin D and [^{32}P]phosphate, and RNA extracted at intervals after inoculation was analyzed by electrophoresis in polyacrylamide gels. By virtue of the absence of cell walls, protoplasts could be solubilized with sodium dodecylsulfate (SDS), permitting phenol extraction of RNA without mechanically breaking the cells. More than 70% of the RNA synthesized after infection was accounted for by virus-related RNAs, because the synthesis of cellular RNA was effectively blocked by actinomycin D.

The inoculated protoplasts synthesized three species of TMV-related RNA which were not made in uninoculated protoplasts (Fig. 7). The RNA produced in largest amount was identified as single-stranded TMV RNA. The other two species were present in much smaller amounts and could be separated from the single-stranded TMV RNA by means of cellulose chromatography. One of them was soluble in 1 M NaCl, was resistant to RNase, and yielded RNA with the size of viral RNA upon denaturation with dimethylsulfoxide. Its molecular weight, estimated using segments of double-stranded RDV RNA, as well as its base composition was close to the value expected for double-stranded RNA consisting of TMV RNA and the RNA complementary to it.

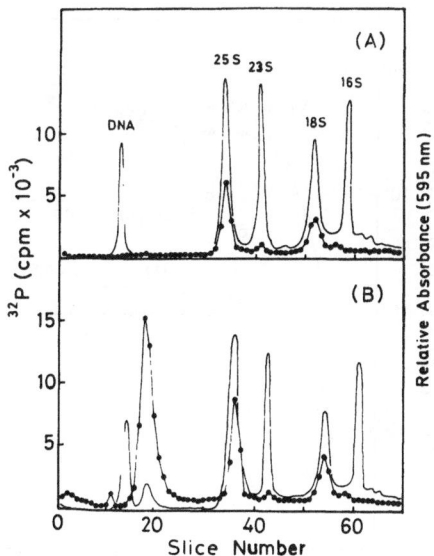

Fig. 7. Polyacrylamide gel electrophoresis of ^{32}P-labeled RNA from uninfected (A) and TMV-infected (B) tobacco protoplasts. RNA was extracted from protoplasts after 20 h of culture in the presence of actinomycin D. Absorbance at 595 nm of gels stained with methylene blue (——) and ^{32}P radioactivity (—●—). From Aoki and Takebe (1975) by permission.

This RNA was thus analogous in structure to the replicative form (RF) of bacteriophage RNA. The third species was insoluble in 1 M NaCl, yielded RF by RNase treatment, and was heterogeneous with respect to size, the modal value for its molecular weight being 6.7×10^6. The structure of replicative intermediate (RI) was therefore assigned to this RNA. The double-stranded forms of TMV RNA are reported to occur also in infected tobacco leaves (Jackson *et al.*, 1971, 1972; Kielland-Brandt and Nilsson-Tillgren, 1973).

The time course of synthesis of the TMV-related RNAs was also studied using synchronously infected tobacco protoplasts, and was correlated to the production of progeny virus particles (Fig. 8) (Aoki and Takebe, 1975). Synthesis of the single-stranded viral RNA was detectable at 4 h postinfection, but it could have started earlier, because a substantial amount of newly synthesized molecules was already present at this time. The synthesis of viral RNA was exponential until 8 h postinfection but turned linear at about 10 h postinfection and remained so thereafter. More than half of the final yield of viral RNA was therefore synthesized at a linear rate.

When the course of viral RNA synthesis was compared with that of virus particle production, it was evident that RNA replication outstrips assembly of virus particles in the initial phase of virus replication. About 10^5 viral RNA molecules were thus synthesized in a protoplast by 8 h postinfection, whereas the amount of progeny virus was lit-

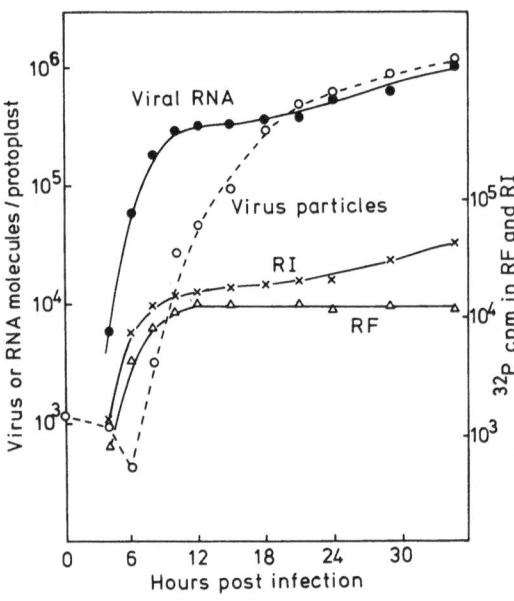

Fig. 8. Time course of synthesis of TMV-related RNAs in synchronously infected tobacco protoplasts. The number of single-stranded viral RNA molecules was calculated from radioactivity in the viral RNA band in polyacrylamide gels, assuming that its specific radioactivity is constant throughout the replication cycle. The number of virus particles was calculated from the results of infectivity assay of protoplast homogenates.

tle more than 10^3 particles, as estimated from the infectivity in the protoplast extract. This was also substantiated by comparing the total vs. assembled viral RNA by infectivity. Protoplasts harvested 9 h postinfection were homogenized to inactivate unassembled viral RNA, and RNA extracted before and after the homogenization was compared for infectivity. It was thus found that only 4% of the total viral RNA survived homogenization, showing that most of the viral RNA made by this time exists in a free or only partially coated form. Similar experiments with protoplasts harvested 24 h postinfection showed that 88% of the total viral RNA is not accessible to cellular nucleases, thus confirming the close agreement in Fig. 8 between the number of viral RNA molecules and that of virus particles in the later periods of virus replication.

The results obtained with synchronously infected protoplasts show that the replication cycle of TMV in individual tobacco leaf cells may be divided into three successive phases. In the initial phase (0–10 h postinfection), exponential synthesis of viral RNA is followed by exponential production of virus particles, with a time lag of 4–5 h. Only a small fraction of the viral RNA is assembled into complete virus particles in this phase. In the transient phase (10–20 h postinfection), the synthesis of viral RNA proceeds at a linear rate, while the assembly of virus particles still goes on more or less exponentially. Most of the viral RNA is incorporated into complete virus particles toward the end of this phase. In the final phase (20 h postinfection and later), assembly of virus particles proceeds linearly, keeping pace with the synthesis of viral RNA.

The identification of the RF and RI of TMV RNA in infected protoplasts suggested their role as intermediates in the synthesis of TMV RNA. The time course of synthesis of these forms was also largely compatible with this idea (Fig. 8). At 4 h postinfection, the earliest time the newly made viral RNA was detected, as much as 40% of the total radioactivity in TMV-related RNAs was accounted for by RF and RI, and this ratio decreased continuously as more viral RNA was synthesized. Pulse-chase type experiments were also performed to establish the intermediate role for these RNAs. However, the results were not sufficiently clear-cut, most probably because the large precursor pools in the mature tobacco cells interfered with the stoichiometric flow of radioactivity between precursors and products (Aoki and Takebe, 1975).

It has been known for some years that a TMV-related RNA of low molecular weight (3.5×10^5) occurs in infected tobacco leaves (Jackson *et al.*, 1972; Siegel *et al.*, 1973) and in the polysomes isolated from such leaves (Beachy and Zaitlin, 1975). More recently, a molecular weight of 2.5×10^5 was assigned, and it was shown that this RNA represents the 3′-terminal 750 nucleotides of TMV RNA containing the coat protein cistron. The RNA isolated from infected leaves directed the synthesis of TMV coat protein in the wheat germ cell-free system, showing that it can act as the coat protein messenger (Hunter *et al.*, 1976; Siegel *et al.*, 1976). In contrast to the findings with leaf materials, no positive evidence was obtained for the presence of such RNA in infected protoplasts (Aoki and Takebe, 1975). This discrepancy may be due to the initial incorrect assignment of molecular weight or to the long labeling period used with protoplasts which may have obscured the presence of a short-lived RNA. In any case, the 2.5×10^5 dalton RNA must be found in infected protoplasts if it actually serves as the *in vivo* messenger for TMV coat protein, and its production must be correlated with the synthesis of coat protein.

4.1.5. Synthesis of Virus-Specified Proteins

Sakai and Takebe (1972, 1974) studied the synthesis of TMV-specified proteins using tobacco protoplasts. Even with protoplasts in which almost all the cells are infected, protein synthesis induced by infection comprised only a very small fraction of total protein synthesis, because host protein synthesis is not significantly affected by infection. Actinomycin D was of limited use to suppress host protein synthesis in short-term experiments since the average half-life of tobacco messenger RNAs was as long as 4 h (Sakai and Takebe, 1970). It was found, however, that UV irradiation of protoplasts immediately after inoculation is useful to reduce host protein synthesis without seriously interfering with TMV replication (Sakai and Tabebe, 1974). The apparent insensitivity of virus replication to UV probably indicates that virus is not yet uncoated at the time of irradiation and that fairly large numbers of virus particles participate in the infection of individual protoplasts.

After irradiation with UV, protoplasts were cultured in the presence of [^{14}C]leucine and actinomycin D, and the total extractable protein was analyzed by electrophoresis in SDS polyacrylamide gels. About 50% of the protein synthesis was due to infection under these conditions. The radioactivity profile of the protein from the inoculated protoplasts revealed the presence of three proteins which were absent in uninoculated protoplasts (Fig. 9). The fastest-moving protein was identified as TMV coat protein since it comigrated with the authentic

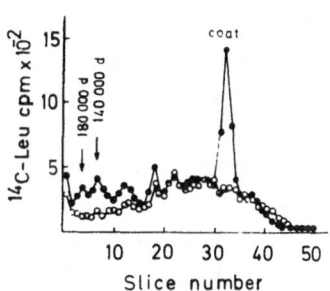

Fig. 9. Electrophoresis profiles of [^{14}C]leucine-labeled proteins from TMV-infected (●) and uninfected (○) tobacco protoplasts in SDS polyacrylamide gels. Protoplasts were labeled for 12 h. From Sakai and Takebe (1974) by permission.

sample and since it was not labeled with radioactive methionine or histidine, amino acids which are absent in the coat protein. The other two proteins had high molecular weights (140,000 and 180,000), were produced in much smaller amounts than coat protein, and were labeled also with methionine and histidine. Various denaturation treatments failed to alter the mobility of these proteins, indicating that they do not consist of subunits. In contrast to coat protein, the high molecular weight proteins were found predominantly in the particulate fraction of protoplast homogenates sedimenting between 1000 and 20,000g. These proteins apparently correspond to the 155,000- and 195,000-dalton proteins which are reported to occur in TMV-infected tobacco leaves (Zaitlin and Hariharasubramanian, 1972).

It is highly probable that at least one of the high molecular weight proteins synthesized in infected protoplasts is specified by the viral genome, although direct evidence for this is still lacking. The possibility that both are the translation products of TMV RNA is suggested by the report that TMV RNA directs the synthesis of proteins with molecular weights of 140,000 and 165,000 in *Xenopus* oocytes and in reticulocyte lysate (Knowland, 1974; Hunter *et al.*, 1976). If this is the case, there must be overlapping sequences in the two proteins, because TMV RNA is not large enough to accommodate their cistrons separately. An alternative possibility is that only one of the large proteins made in infected protoplasts is specified by the viral genome, while the other is a host protein whose synthesis is stimulated by infection. In any case, there are indications that TMV RNA replicase is close in size to these proteins; an enzyme catalyzing the synthesis of the minus strand of TMV RNA upon addition of its plus strand was solubilized from a particulate fraction of infected tobacco leaves, and this activity cosedimented with human γ-globulin, suggesting an approximate molecular weight of 160,000 (Zaitlin *et al.*, 1973). (See Chapter 4 for further discussion of this question.)

The time course of the synthesis of the coat and the 140,000-dalton proteins was followed in the synchronously infected and UV-irradiated protoplasts, and was correlated with viral RNA replication and progeny particle production (Fig. 10) (Sakai and Takebe, 1974). The course of the latter two processes was similar to that in nonirradiated protoplasts (Fig. 8), except that there was an overall delay of several hours. Most significantly, a conspicuous difference was revealed between the coat and the 140,000-dalton protein not only in regard to amounts produced (Fig. 9) but also in their course of synthesis (Fig. 10). The course of synthesis of the 140,000-dalton protein paralleled that of viral RNA replication, whereas that of coat protein closely resembled the course of assembly of virus particles. Synthesis of the 140,000-dalton protein thus reached the maximal rate about 4 h earlier than coat protein synthesis, but the rate declined in the later periods, whereas coat protein continued to be produced at a near maximal rate throughout the later periods of virus replication. These results clearly indicate that the frequency of translation of individual cistrons in the viral genome is regulated separately. The mode of *in vivo* translation of TMV RNA is thus incompatible with the monocistronic model of translation in animal picornaviruses, in which viral RNA is translated into a large, single polypeptide which is subsequently cleaved into products of individual cistrons (reviewed by Sugiyama *et al.*, 1972). The results in Fig. 10 also show that the rate of assembly of TMV particles is limited by the synthesis of coat protein.

Synthesis of TMV-related proteins in infected tobacco protoplasts was also studied by Paterson (1974) and Paterson and Knight (1975). They did not use UV to suppress host protein synthesis, but rather used autoradiography in combination with electrophoresis at several gel concentrations to resolve virus-related proteins from host proteins. In spite of the somewhat different experimental conditions, the results obtained by Paterson and Knight (1975) were quite similar to those

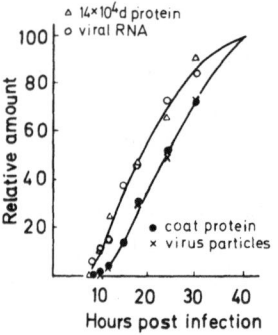

Fig. 10. Time course of production of TMV-specified proteins, TMV RNA, and TMV particles in synchronously infected tobacco protoplasts. Data are expressed as the percentage of the maximum value attained at 40 h postinfection.

obtained by Sakai and Takebe (1974). The amounts of the high molecular weight proteins were reported, however, to decrease after they had reached a maximal level at 24 h postinfection. At about the same time, coat protein synthesis also leveled off temporarily, but no explanation is given for this rather strange observation.

4.1.6. Virus Replication Cycle

Studies with protoplasts are providing for the first time some basic information on the process of TMV replication in individual infected cells. While the information so far obtained is certainly limited, such information may be used in combination with that obtained with other systems to tentatively construct the sequence of events during the replication cycle of TMV in protoplasts. An assumption is made in the following considerations that the 140,000-dalton protein synthesized in protoplasts represents the replicase of TMV RNA.

More than one inoculum virus particle usually enters each protoplast to initiate infection. The infecting particles are rapidly uncoated to expose the replicase cistron which occupies the two-thirds of TMV RNA near the 5′ end. Where and how the virus rods are uncoated in protoplasts remain completely unknown. The replicase cistron of the parental RNA is now translated using 80 S ribosomes; the methylated, blocked 5′-terminal group (Zimmern, 1975; Keith and Fraenkel-Conrat, 1975) may play an active role in this translation. It is not known whether the translation occurs on free or membrane-bound polysomes, but the product of translation is associated with some cellular structures lighter than the nucleus or the chloroplasts. The possibility may be considered that two types of replicase are produced from the overlapping cistrons in TMV RNA (Hunter *et al.*, 1976).

The first replicase molecules made on the parental RNA use the same RNA as the template and produce progeny plus strands via double-stranded intermediate forms. The progeny strands are then translated to produce more replicase, and at the same time serve as the template for new progeny strands. Both replicase and viral RNA thus increase exponentially during the initial phase of the replication cycle. Most of the viral RNA synthesized in this phase is not immediately incorporated into virus rods but remains for some time as free or partially assembled molecules, because production of coat protein does not immediately catch up with the exponential rate of synthesis of viral RNA. This is perhaps not surprising because as many as 2130 coat protein subunits are required to fully encapsidate every TMV RNA molecule.

The initially exponential increase of viral RNA becomes linear at about 10 h postinfection, when the synthesis of RF and RI also levels off. It thus appears that no new minus strand is synthesized in the later periods (see also Kielland-Brandt and Nilsson-Tillgren, 1973). The reason for this is obscure, but it may simply be due to the accumulation of coat protein which may bind to an increasing proportion of viral RNA to limit the availability of the template. Also unknown is the exact mechanism by which coat protein is now synthesized at a much higher rate than replicase. One possibility may be that coat protein is translated from a separate monocistronic messenger RNA which may be generated by specific processing of the full-length TMV RNA or by transcription of a part of viral RNA (Hunter et al., 1976), although this has not yet been demonstrated to occur in protoplasts. The vigorous production of coat protein results in the encapsidation of almost all the viral RNA molecules at about 20 h postinfection.

Once most of the existing viral RNA is encapsidated, the rate of replicase synthesis declines. The mechanism ensuring translation of the coat protein cistron at high frequency should operate also in the final phase of the virus replication cycle, where coat protein continues to be made at a near maximal rate. Any new viral RNA made in this phase is rapidly assembled into virus rods.

The picture of the TMV replication cycle described above shows many missing links which should be found by future studies. The two high molecular weight proteins should obviously be better characterized and their interrelation elucidated. The question of whether viral RNA is synthesized in the nucleus (Smith and Schlegel, 1965) or on a membraneous structure in the cytoplasm (Ralph et al., 1971) has not yet been settled. The plus strand of viral RNA should serve as the template for the minus strand and also as the messenger for viral proteins, but we do not know how the dual functions are coordinated. It is not known whether translation of the replicase cistron is repressed by TMV coat protein as is the case in RNA bacteriophages (reviewed by Sugiyama et al., 1972, and Kozak and Nathans, 1972), and our knowledge on TMV-specific polysomes is conflicting (Kiho, 1972; Beachy and Zaitlin, 1975). Assuming that coat protein is translated from its monocistronic messenger, we do not know how the short piece of TMV RNA is generated. We may expect that some of these questions will be approached using protoplasts and will be correlated with the virus replication cycle.

4.1.7. Interaction between Strains and Mutants

On the basis of experiments using leaf systems, it has been hypothesized that inoculated TMV particles exclude each other during infection so that only one TMV particle can participate in the infection of a leaf cell (Siegel and Zaitlin, 1964). Experiments with protoplasts are yielding evidence which is clearly inconsistent with this hypothesis. For example, infection of protoplasts by TMV shows a multitarget-type response to inactivation by UV (Fig. 5), suggesting that more than one inoculum particle enters each protoplast to initiate replication.

Clearer evidence against the operation of exclusion in protoplasts came from the work of Otsuki and Takebe (1976c), who showed that tobacco protoplasts can be doubly infected not only by TMV and an unrelated virus (Otsuki and Takebe, 1976a) but also by two strains of TMV. The common and the tomato strains used in this study are closely related to each other (Hennig and Wittmann, 1972), yet differ to such an extent that antisera specific to each of them could be obtained by cross-absorption. Protoplasts inoculated with a mixture of the two strains were cultured for 24 h; one portion was stained with fluorescent antibody specific to the common strain, and another portion was stained with fluorescent antibody specific to the tomato strain. Scoring under a fluorescence microscope showed that 90% of the protoplasts contained the common strain and 85% contained the tomato strain. It was thus clear that 80% of the protoplasts were doubly infected and produced particles of both strains.

Parallel replication of the common and tomato strains in the same protoplasts was demonstrated also by analyzing the antigenic constitution of individual progeny particles produced in the mixedly inoculated protoplasts (Otsuki and Takebe, 1976b). Progeny virus rods purified from such protoplasts were treated separately with specific γ-globulins against the common and tomato strains, respectively. The reaction of individual virus rods with globulin molecules was examined under an electron microscope using a technique adapted from that of leaf-dip serology (Ball, 1971). It was found that 77% of the virus rods produced in the mixedly inoculated protoplasts combined with globulin specific to the common strain, and 86% combined with globulin specific to the tomato strain, showing that 63% of the rods contain coat protein of both strains. The mixedly coated particles would not have been produced unless the two strains replicate within the same cell and are assembled at the same site.

While there is no doubt that the common and tomato strains of

TMV can replicate within one cell, this does not mean that the two strains replicate independently. In fact, a phenomenon resembling the cross-protection in plants could be seen with protoplasts (Otsuki and Takebe, 1976c). For example, smaller numbers of protoplasts became infected by the common strain when the mixed inocula contained excessive amounts of the tomato strain. The competition is likely to occur at the stage of virus replication rather than at the stage of adsorption or penetration, because UV-inactivated particles of the tomato strain did not show the competition. Furthermore, protoplasts became refractory to infection by the common strain when they were infected 8 h or more previously with the tomato strain. The "protection" is apparently based on the relatedness of the viruses, because previous infection by CMV did not protect protoplasts against challenge inoculation with the common strain of TMV. One may expect that a detailed study of this phenomenon will provide an insight into the mechanism of cross-protection at the plant level, which has remained obscure for so long.

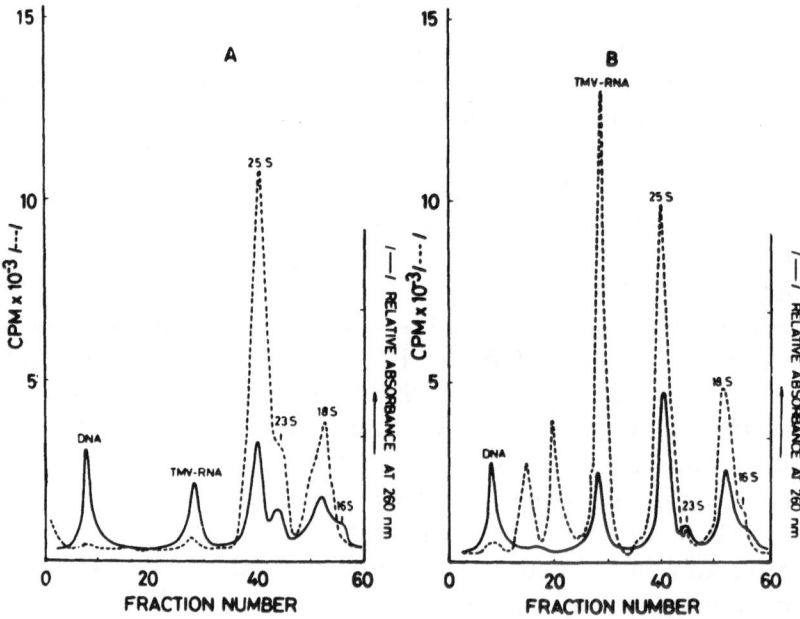

Fig. 11.   Polyacrylamide gel electrophoresis of ³²P-labeled RNA extracted from the attached half of a tobacco leaf inoculated 8 days previously (A) and from the protoplasts isolated from the other half of the same leaf (B). [³²P]Phosphate was fed to the attached half leaf and to the isolated protoplasts for a period of 6 h. From Föglein *et al.* (1975) by permission.

The high levels of double infection of protoplasts by two closely related strains of TMV suggest the feasibility of studying genetic complementation between defective mutants of TMV. A recent study showed indeed that a temperature-sensitive mutant of TMV can replicate at a nonpermissive temperature when inoculated to protoplasts together with wild-type TMV (I. Takebe and K. Shimidzu, unpublished). The nitrous acid-induced TMV mutant Ni 118 produces little virus at 34°C, because its coat protein is denatured at this temperature and consequently cannot be assembled into virus rods (Jockusch, 1968). When protoplasts were inoculated with a mixture of Ni 118 and *vulgare* (wild type) and held at 34°C, substantial amounts of Ni 118 were produced as assayed on a differential host, in contrast to the negligible amounts produced in the protoplasts inoculated with Ni 118 alone. This shows that double infection by Ni 118 and *vulgare* occurred in some protoplasts and that the Ni 118 RNA produced in such protoplasts was coated with *vulgare* protein. The amounts of Ni 118 produced at 34°C in the mixedly inoculated protoplasts were not so large, however, as might be expected from the high frequencies of double infection by the common and tomato strains of TMV. It remains to be seen whether this is because Ni 118 and *vulgare* interfere more strongly with each other than the common and tomato strains.

4.1.8. Control of Virus Replication in Leaf Tissues

Comparative studies using protoplasts and leaf materials provide information on some aspects of virus replication at a tissue level. Föglein *et al.* (1975) isolated protoplasts from one-half of a tobacco leaf which was inoculated with TMV 8–10 days previously and in which virus had accumulated to high levels. Replication of viral RNA in such protoplasts was studied by measuring the incorporation of [^{32}P]phosphate into viral RNA and was compared with that in the opposite half leaf which remainded attached to the plant. Electrophoresis of RNA extracted from these materials showed that a burst of TMV RNA synthesis occurred in the isolated protoplasts, whereas little viral RNA was synthesized in the leaf half left attached to the plant (Fig. 11). The striking contrast cannot be ascribed to possible difference between the two systems in the uptake of radioactive phosphate, because the cellular RNA species were labeled to the same extent in both systems. Similar results were also obtained with protoplasts isolated from systemically infected leaves or from the "dark green islands" (Atkinson and Matthews, 1970) of such leaves. These findings seem to indicate that a control prevails in the leaf tissues to set a limit to virus replication in leaf cells or to prevent infection of cells in particular areas. Leaf cells are apparently released from such control when the tissues are dissociated.

TMV replication in protoplasts from the necrotic-responding tobacco varieties represents another example of the difference between protoplasts and leaf materials with respect to virus replication. Cells in the leaves of such varieties produce only limited amounts of virus, because they undergo necrosis while actively synthesizing virus. Otsuki *et al.* (1972a) compared TMV replication in protoplasts and in leaf disks of the necrotic-responding tobacco varieties. Virus replication in the leaf disks leveled off as necrotic local lesions appeared. Surprisingly, however, protoplasts from the same varieties did not necrose at all and continued to synthesize virus, so that as much virus was finally produced as in protoplasts from systemic varieties. It thus appears that the necrotic response to TMV infection occurs only at the tissue level and not in isolated protoplasts.

The two examples described here illustrate a way in which protoplasts may be useful for disclosing aspects of virus replication in intact plants which have so far been overlooked or only poorly understood. For example, if the necrotic reaction is determined genetically, conditions must exist under which the reaction comes to expression also in protoplasts. Once such conditions are found, an effective approach will be possible to attack the biochemical basis of the necrotic response, one of the long-standing questions in plant virology.

4.1.9. Resistance

Genes conferring resistance to TMV infection have been introduced into tomato plants (Pelham, 1966). Tomato lines homozygous for one of these genes, $Tm-2^a$, are symptomless and produce little virus upon infection with a tomato strain of TMV. In contrast, protoplasts isolated from such lines were found to be as readily infected by the same strain of TMV and to produce as much virus as the protoplasts from susceptible parent lines (Motoyoshi and Oshima, 1975). This finding clearly shows that the resistance conferred by $Tm-2^a$ is not due to the inherent inability of mesophyll cells to support virus replication. $Tm-2^a$ possibly controls virus replication in individual leaf cells through a mechanism which functions only in the intact plant or, alternatively, it may control cell-to-cell movement of virus within leaf tissues. The interesting observation made with protoplasts should trigger more detailed studies with leaf materials on the mechanism of resistance controlled by $Tm-2^a$.

It is likely that other classes of resistance genes also exist which directly interfere with virus infection or replication. Indeed, Motoyoshi and Oshima (1977) showed more recently that protoplasts from tomato lines homozygous for another resistance gene, Tm, are immune to infection by a common and a tomato strain of TMV. Resistance genes of this class should be extremely valuable for providing insights into the virus replication cycle, because it should be possible with protoplasts to pinpoint the stage at which these genes block virus infection or replication.

The studies by Motoyoshi and Oshima (1975, 1977) show that protoplasts offer a powerful tool to characterize various resistance genes. Comparative studies of resistance genes in different classes should be invaluable for understanding the mechanisms by which virus replication is controlled by the genetic makeup of host cells.

4.1.10. Uncoating

Only one report has so far dealt with the uncoating of TMV in protoplasts (Wyatt and Shaw, 1975). Protoplasts were inoculated with TMV whose RNA was labeled with [^{32}P]phosphate and the protein with [^{35}S]sulfate. Virus particles were reextracted from the inoculated protoplasts after various periods of infection and were analyzed by centrifugation in sucrose gradients. About 5% of the ^{35}S and 3% of the ^{32}P radioactivity retained by the protoplasts were found at the top of the gradient after 30 min of infection or later, with simultaneous broadening of the virus zone toward the lighter region. It thus appeared that a small fraction of the adsorbed virus underwent dissociation within 30 min. If this represents uncoating of those particles which actually initiate infection, the time is consistent with the replication cycle in protoplasts, since a substantial amount of viral RNA was made by 4 h postinfection (Fig. 8). However, much uncertainty is associated with interpretation of these results, because as many as 8×10^3 virus particles are retained per protoplast and most of them probably do not participate in infection. As mentioned earlier, it is now possible to effect high levels of infection of protoplasts using a virus concentration of 0.01 μg/ml (Fig. 3), which is 100 times lower than that used by Wyatt and Shaw (1975). A clearer picture of the uncoating of infecting TMV particles may emerge under such conditions where a much larger fraction of the adsorbed particles should take part in infection.

4.2. Cowpea Chlorotic Mottle Virus

4.2.1. Virus Replication

Cowpea chlorotic mottle virus produces mild symptoms on inoculated tobacco leaves but does not invade tobacco plants systemically. Motoyoshi *et al.* (1973*a*) showed that tobacco protoplasts are readily infected by this virus and produce 10^7 progeny particles per protoplast within 48 h. Tobacco protoplasts thus provide a good synchronous system for this multicomponent virus whose replication cycle in infected cells has been largely unknown (Lane, 1974). It is interesting to note that significant numbers (about 7%) of the protoplasts become infected also when they are inoculated with free CCMV RNA at relatively low concentration (1 μg/ml) (Motoyoshi *et al.*, 1973*a*). The high efficiency of infection by free viral RNA might enable studies of the function of individual RNA species of CCMV using protoplasts.

4.2.2. Replication of Viral RNAs

Studies by Bancroft *et al.* (1975) using CCMV-infected tobacco protoplasts provided some information pertaining to the *in vivo* replication of CCMV RNA. As labeled with [^{32}P]phosphate and analyzed by electrophoresis in gels, synthesis of viral RNA was detectable at 7 h postinfection. Four species of CCMV RNA were synthesized, apparently at unequal rates; RNA 3 was made first and most rapidly so that this species predominated throughout the replication cycle. Assuming the equimolar incorporation of RNAs 3 and 4 into the middle component of CCMV, it was estimated that less than half of the RNA 3 synthesized is encapsidated. The relative proportion of RNA species changed markedly at an elevated temperature (35°C); the amount of RNA 1 was strongly reduced, while that of RNA 2 increased. RNase-resistant forms were found for RNAs 1, 2, and 3, but not for RNA 4, suggesting that the three larger species are made on their own minus strands whereas the smallest species is made on the minus strand of RNA 3.

4.2.3. Synthesis of Virus-Specified Proteins

Proteins synthesized in tobacco protoplasts upon infection by CCMV were analyzed by Sakai *et al.* (1977) using the techniques developed for studying TMV-specific proteins (Sakai and Takebe, 1974), except that protoplasts were irradiated with UV before rather than after inoculation. Three species of protein with molecular weights of 20,000, 36,000, and 100,000 were synthesized by tobacco protoplasts upon infection by CCMV. The smallest protein comigrated with the authentic CCMV coat protein in SDS gels and was found predominantly in the soluble fraction of the protoplast homogenates. Its synthesis was detectable at 12 h postinfection and proceeded at a linear rate for at least 60 h (Fig. 12). The other two proteins were produced in much smaller amounts than coat protein, and were found associated with some subcellular structures. The 36,000-dalton protein is identical in size to one of the *in vitro* translation products of CCMV RNA 3 (Davies and Kaesberg, 1974) and is presumably the replicase subunit, because it is synthesized only in the early period of virus replication cycle (Fig. 12). Pulse-chase-type experiments showed that this protein is not the precursor of coat protein. Although the nature of the largest protein is not known, it is probably a translation product of RNA 1 or 2, both of which are sufficiently large to code for this high molecular weight protein.

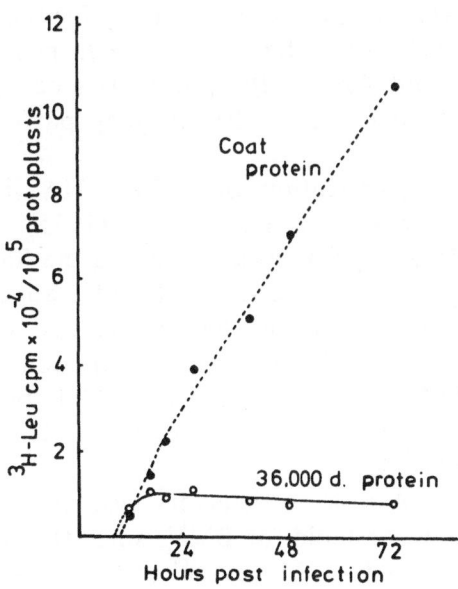

Fig. 12. Time course of synthesis of CCMV-specified proteins in synchronously infected tobacco protoplasts. By courtesy of Dr. F. Sakai.

4.2.4. Replication of a Temperature-Sensitive Mutant

J. R. O. Dawson *et al.* (1975) studied the replication of a tempera-ture-sensitive mutant of CCMV in tobacco protoplasts. The mutant replicated normally at 25°C but produced neither virus nor free coat protein at 35°C. Virus produced in protoplasts at 25°C was degraded *in situ* when the protoplasts were subsequently transferred to the nonper-missive temperature. Little RNA 1 was made at 35°C, while other RNAs were synthesized normally. Since the same trend was seen also with wild-type CCMV at 35°C (see above), it was concluded that the mutant has no fault in the replication of viral RNA. The absence of coat protein at the nonpermissive temperature was interpreted to indi-cate a mutation in the coat protein cistron as the result of which the cistron is not translated or its translation product is rapidly degraded at 35°C.

4.3. Brome Mosaic Virus

The commonly used strain of brome mosaic virus infects neither tobacco plants nor tobacco protoplasts (Motoyoshi *et al.*, 1973a). However, a variant V5 of BMV, which can be separated from the com-mon strain by electrophoresis, was found to infect both tobacco plants and protoplasts (Motoyoshi *et al.*, 1974a). Poly-L-ornithine was not essential but was stimulatory for the infection of tobacco protoplasts by BMV V5, reflecting the near neutral isoelectric point of this virus. About 40% of the protoplasts became infected using 50 μg/ml BMV V5, and 3.5×10^6 progeny particles were produced in an infected protoplast.

Replication of BMV RNA in tobacco protoplasts was briefly reported by Bancroft *et al.* (1975). As was the case also with CCMV, RNA 3 predominated among the four BMV RNA species synthesized. However, more RNAs 1 and 2 appeared to be synthesized early in the replication cycle than in the case of CCMV. In addition to the four BMV RNA species, an anomalous RNA with a molecular weight of 0.56×10^6 was found at 24 h postinfection but not later. RNase-resistant forms were found for RNAs 1, 2, and 3, but again not for RNA 4.

A more satisfactory system of synchronous infection seems to be now available for BMV, since the relatively low efficiency of infection reported by Motoyoshi *et al.* (1974a) was improved to such an extent that 70–90% of tobacco protoplasts can be infected using 2.5 μg/ml

BMV V5 (F. Sakai, personal communication). BMV has the advantage that its RNA species (Shih *et al.*, 1972; Dasgupta *et al.*, 1975) and their *in vitro* translation products (Shih and Kaesberg, 1973, 1976) are best characterized among multicomponent viruses. BMV replicase has also been isolated and partially purified (Hadidi and Fraenkel-Conrat, 1973; Hariharasubramanian *et al.*, 1973). Extensive studies on BMV RNA replication and translation using protoplasts will be valuable, and may disclose the replication cycle of bromoviruses. Protoplasts may also be used to approach the intriguing question of why V5 but not its parent isolate of BMV can infect tobacco.

An alternative system of synchronous infection for BMV was recently introduced by Okuno *et al.* (1977), who were able to infect barley leaf protoplasts with this virus. This system has the advantage of using the natural host and should permit studies using any BMV strain. However, barley protoplasts sometimes accumulate an unidentified substance during culture which emits fluorescence similar in color to that of fluorescein isothiocyanate (T. Hibi, personal communication). This creates some difficulty in determining the levels of infection by means of the fluorescent antibody technique.

4.4. Cucumber Mosaic Virus

A synchronous system of infection by CMV was established using tobacco protoplasts (Otsuki and Takebe, 1973), and replication of viral RNA in this system was followed by Takanami *et al.* (1977). Viral RNA synthesis was detectable by [^{3}H]uracil incorporation at 6 h postinfection and was most active at 12 h. All of the four species of CMV RNA were synthesized, but RNA 3 was produced in much larger amounts than other species throughout the replication cycle. Synthesis of RNA 3 in excess of other species thus appears to be a common feature of bromo- and cucumoviruses. RF was found not only for RNAs 1, 2, and 3 but also for RNA 4. When a CMV strain with the 5th RNA component was used, RNA 5 was produced in large amounts and its RF and RI were detected.

Cytological studies of CMV-infected tobacco protoplasts showed that this virus is assembled not only in the cytoplasm but also in the nucleus (Otsuki and Takebe, 1973; Honda *et al.*, 1974). It would be of interest to see whether or not the synthesis of viral RNA or protein also occurs in the nucleus.

CMV was also inoculated to cowpea protoplasts (Koike *et al.*, 1975). No necrotic death of cowpea protoplasts could be observed after infection by CMV, whereas the same virus incites necrotic local lesions on cowpea leaves.

4.5. Cowpea Mosaic Virus

A protoplast system was made available for CPMV using primary leaves of cowpea (Hibi *et al.*, 1975; Beier and Bruening, 1975). Leaves suitable as the source of protoplasts can be obtained as early as 10 days after germination, but the conditions of seedling growth must be strictly controlled. Cowpea protoplasts have the advantage that poly-L-ornithine is not required for their infection by some viruses, including CPMV (Hibi *et al.*, 1975; Rottier, 1976) and CMV (Koike *et al.*, 1975). Infection by CPMV can be brought about in nearly all the protoplasts, and more than 10^6 virus particles per protoplast are produced within 2 days. This system should thus enable extensive studies of replication for this two-component virus. Preliminary attempts were made to study the function of individual components of CPMV using protoplasts (Rottier, 1976). The middle component could be purified to such an extent that it does not cause infection of cowpea protoplasts when inoculated singly but causes infection in 70% of protoplasts when inoculated together with the bottom component.

Although tobacco plants are not a good host for CPMV, tobacco protoplasts were found to be readily infected by this virus (Huber *et al.*, 1977). CPMV replication in tobacco protoplasts had a lag period about 10 h longer than that of CPMV in cowpea protoplasts or that of TMV in tobacco protoplasts. The rate of virus replication was also slower than in the homologous systems. However, the CPMV concentration in tobacco protoplasts finally reached a level similar to that in cowpea protoplasts. The "cytopathic structure" produced in CPMV-infected cowpea cells (De Zoeten *et al.*, 1974) and protoplasts (Hibi *et al.*, 1975) appeared also in tobacco protoplasts, indicating that it is characteristic of virus and not of host. The availability of protoplast systems from two different plants may help to disclose host-specific aspects in CPMV replication.

4.6. Tobacco Rattle Virus

Very high levels of infection (up to 98% of protoplasts infected) have been obtained by inoculating tobacco protoplasts with TRV at 1 μg/ml (Kubo *et al.*, 1975a). About 2×10^5 long and 6×10^5 short

Fig. 13. Accumulation of products of TRV replication in synchronously infected tobacco protoplasts. ●, Infectious nucleoprotein; ○, infectious RNA; ▲, virus antigen assayed using antibody-sensitized latex. In samples taken 1 h after inoculation, no infectious RNA or virus antigen was detected, and only 0.03 unit of infectious nucleoprotein was found. However, 1.0 was added to each of these values for convenience of plotting. Redrawn from Harrison *et al.* (1976) by permission.

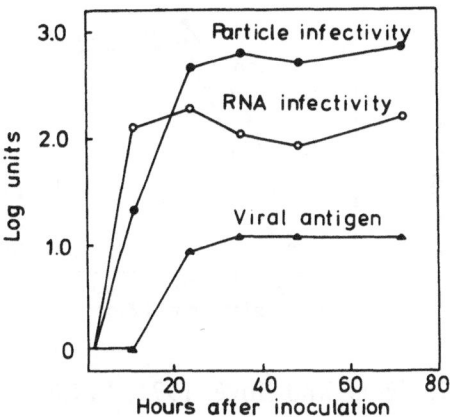

particles per protoplast were produced within 40 h. Inoculation with long particles alone resulted in the production of infectious RNA but neither viral antigen nor virus particles were formed. Infection could be effected also by inoculating protoplasts first with long particles and several hours later with short particles, or *vice versa* (Harrison *et al.*, 1976).

The replication cycle of TRV in tobacco protoplasts was recently studied in some detail (Harrison *et al.*, 1976). Synthesis of long RNA species was detectable by infectivity at 7 h postinfection and increased until 12 h, at which time it reached a constant level, whereas nucleoprotein particles were produced by 9 h and continued to increase until about 40 h (Fig. 13). The course of viral antigen synthesis was similar to that of nucleoprotein production, suggesting that the latter process is limited by the rate of coat protein synthesis (Fig. 13). Infectious RNA made by 9 h thus appeared to be incorporated into nucleoprotein particles about 4–5 h later. Determination of the amounts of long and short particles showed that they are not assembled in parallel (Fig. 14). Long particles predominated until 16 h, but were gradually outnumbered by short particles, ending up with the ratio of 1:4 for long and short particles at 40 h postinfection. Nearly all the long particles were associated with mitochondria throughout the replication cycle, whereas the short ones were predominantly free in the cytoplasm except for the first few hours.

4.7. Turnip Yellow Mosaic Virus

TYMV is unique in that replication of its RNA takes place in close association with chloroplasts (Ushiyama and Matthews, 1970;

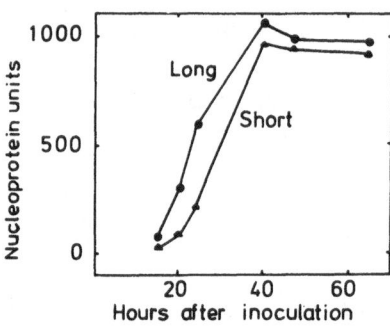

Fig. 14. Accumulation of long-particle (●) and short-particle (▲) nucleoprotein in tobacco protoplasts synchronously infected by TRV. Redrawn from Harrison et al. (1976) by permission.

Lafléche and Bové, 1971; Lafléche et al., 1972). Recently, Chinese cabbage protoplasts proved to be an excellent system for a synchronous replication of TYMV (Renaudin et al., 1975). More than 90% of protoplasts became infected by inoculation with 1 μg/ml TYMV and produced 1–2 × 10⁶ virus particles per protoplast within 48 h. In the infected Chinese cabbage protoplasts, all of the chloroplasts aggregated into one large mass, enabling the investigator to distinguish between infected and uninfected protoplasts without recourse to the fluorescent antibody technique. No appreciable amount of TYMV was produced in Chinese cabbage protoplasts when they were cultured in the dark. Either carbon dioxide or oxygen was also required for TYMV replication in protoplasts (Renaudin et al., 1976), indicating that energy for virus replication is supplied by photosynthesis. However, chloramphenicol did not affect TYMV replication in Chinese cabbage protoplasts, showing that the protein-synthesizing system of chloroplasts is not involved in TYMV replication.

TYMV failed to infect tobacco protoplasts, while TMV was found to replicate well in Chinese cabbage protoplasts (Y. Otsuki and I. Takebe, unpublished). It would be of interest to see whether this virus is unable quite to initiate infection in tobacco protoplasts, or whether it can carry out some early steps of replication without going further. One might speculate, for example, that TYMV may be uncoated in tobacco protoplasts, but that their chloroplasts are incompatible with TYMV with respect to viral RNA replication.

4.8. Potato Virus X

PVX is the only flexuous plant virus thus far successfully inoculated to protoplasts. Satisfactory levels of infection (up to 70% of protoplasts infected) were attained by inoculating tobacco protoplasts with 5 μg/ml PVX (Otsuki *et al.*, 1974). This virus accumulated in tobacco protoplasts in such large amounts that virus aggregates occupied a substantial fraction of the cytoplasmic volume. One peculiar feature of PVX replication in protoplasts is that it is affected by actinomycin D. When present throughout the replication cycle, the drug markedly suppressed PVX replication during the first 24 h, although nearly as much virus was produced after 48 h in the presence as in the absence of actinomycin D. The number of infected protoplasts, as determined by the fluorescent antibody technique, also decreased significantly when actinomycin D was added within 6 h postinfection.

PVX induces the formation of characteristic inclusion bodies in infected cells (Shalla and Shepard, 1972). Electron microscopy of synchronously infected tobacco protoplasts showed that active virus replication always preceded genesis of the inclusion body, indicating that this structure is not involved in PVX replication (Shalla and Petersen, 1973; Honda *et al.*, 1975). Protoplasts should be similarly useful for studying the function of inclusion bodies induced by other viruses.

5. CONCLUDING REMARKS

Studies of plant virus replication in protoplasts can take the following advantages of the protoplast system which are not shared by the conventional leaf materials: (1) synchrony of infection, (2) high proportion of infected cells, (3) high efficiency of infection, (4) pipettability, (5) precise control of experimental conditions, and (6) facile isolation of virus-related structures and molecules. A few examples of the use of protoplasts for the study of virus replication have been discussed in this chapter. It is clear that such studies are still in very early stages of development and much is left to be done in the future. Protoplasts may also be used in ways that have not been tried so far. For example, De Zoeten *et al.* (1976) located the site of PEMV RNA replication in the nucleus by electron microscopic autoradiography combined with the fractionation of subcellular structures. Such experiments should be far easier with protoplasts and should greatly contribute to the understanding of the process of virus replication *in vivo*. Protoplasts should also be useful for characterizing virus-specific polysomes and for correlating their formation to the virus replication cycle.

It should be pointed out that progress in the general techniques of plant virology is needed for some of the more advanced uses of protoplasts. Protoplasts are undoubtedly the best available material with which to identify the function of individual components of divided viral genomes. It is increasingly clear, however, that such studies require more rigorous purification of genome components than can be achieved by the current methods (Kubo *et al.*, 1975*a*; Rottier, 1976), because a trace of contamination by other components is picked up by protoplasts due to their high efficiency of infection. Also, experiments on the fate of infecting virus particles in protoplasts will be meaningful only when an inoculum virus of sufficiently high specific infectivity becomes available.

We may safely assume that the process of virus replication is basically the same in isolated protoplasts and in the cells in leaves. The fact should be kept in mind, however, that protoplasts are maintained in an artificial environment which differs in many respects from the natural milieu of leaf cells. It is possible that the difference in environment influences the physiology and the metabolism of leaf cells and hence modifies virus replication to some extent. In this respect, Lazar *et al.* (1973) reported that a hypertonic condition triggers *de novo* synthesis of RNase in tobacco leaf cells, and Mäder *et al.* (1976) found that the peroxidase level rises in tobacco protoplasts cultured *in vitro*. Although some information is available for RNA and protein synthesis (Sakai and Takebe, 1970) and for photosynthesis (Kanai and Edwards, 1973; Nishimura and Akazawa, 1975), relatively little is known about the metabolism of isolated plant protoplasts. We should be alert to the possibility that some features of virus replication in protoplasts may be due to the peculiar environment in which they are placed.

Comparative studies of virus replication in leaves and in isolated protoplasts suggest that some mechanisms may operate in the intact leaf to control virus replication. Thus protoplasts isolated from fully infected tobacco leaves resume vigorous viral RNA synthesis (Föglein *et al.*, 1975) and protoplasts carrying the *N* gene escape necrotic collapse during active virus replication (Otsuki *et al.*, 1972*a*). These findings suggest that care should be taken to apply the knowledge obtained with protoplasts to account for the events in intact leaves. It is worthwhile to note in this respect that systems approaching synchrony of infection have been developed using intact plants (Nilsson-Tillgren *et al.*, 1969; W. O. Dawson *et al.*, 1975). While these systems lack many of the advantages inherent in protoplasts, they are clearly valuable because information from such systems should supplement the knowledge obtained with protoplasts, a system of strictly cellular level.

ACKNOWLEDGMENTS

I am grateful to Drs. B. D. Harrison, T. Hibi, A. van Kammen, S. Kubo, Y. Otsuki, and F. Sakai for supplying prepublication materials. Assistance by Mrs. K. Shimidzu in compiling and typewriting the reference list is gratefully acknowledged.

6. REFERENCES

Aoki, S., and Takebe, I., 1969, Infection of tobacco mesophyll protoplasts by tobacco mosaic virus ribonucleic acid, *Virology* **39**:439.

Aoki, S., and Takebe, I., 1975, Replication of tobacco mosaic virus RNA in tobacco mesophyll protoplasts inoculated *in vitro*, *Virology* **65**:343.

Atkinson, P. H., and Matthews, R. E. F., 1970, On the origin of dark green tissue in tobacco leaves infected with tobacco mosaic virus, *Virology* **40**:344.

Ball, E. M., 1971, Leaf-dip serology, in: *Methods in Virology*, Vol. V (K. Maramorosch and H. Koprowski, eds.), pp. 445–450, Academic Press, New York.

Bancroft, J. B., Motoyoshi, F., Watts, J. W., and Dawson, J. R. O., 1975, Cowpea chlorotic mottle and brome mosaic viruses in tobacco protoplasts, in: *Modification of the Information Content of Plant Cells* (R. Markham, D. R. Davis, D. A. Hopwood, and R. W. Horne, eds.), pp. 133–160, North-Holland, Amsterdam.

Barker, H., and Harrison, B. D., 1977, Infection of tobacco mesophyll protoplasts with raspberry ringspot virus alone and together with tobacco rattle virus, *J. Gen. Virol.* **35**:125.

Beachy, R. N., and Zaitlin, M., 1975, Replication of tobacco mosaic virus. VI. Replicative intermediate and TMV-RNA-related RNAs associated with polyribosomes, *Virology* **63**:84.

Beier, H., and Bruening, G., 1975, The use of an abrasive in the isolation of cowpea leaf protoplasts which support the multiplication of cowpea mosaic virus, *Virology* **64**:272.

Burgess, J., Motoyoshi, F., and Fleming, E. N., 1973a, Effect of poly-L-ornithine on isolated tobacco mesophyll protoplasts: Evidence against stimulated pinocytosis, *Planta* **111**:199.

Burgess, J., Motoyoshi, F., and Fleming, E. N., 1973b, The mechanism of infection of plant protoplasts by viruses, *Planta* **112**:323.

Cocking, E. C., 1960, A method for the isolation of plant protoplasts and vacuoles, *Nature (London)* **187**:927.

Cocking, E. C., 1966, An electron microscopic study of the initial stages of infection of isolated tomato fruit protoplasts by tobacco mosaic virus, *Planta* **68**:206.

Cocking, E. C., 1972, Plant cell protoplasts—Isolation and development, *Annu. Rev. Plant Physiol.* **23**:29.

Cocking, E. C., and Pojnar, E., 1969, An electron microscopic study of the infection of isolated tomato fruit protoplasts by tobacco mosaic virus, *J. Gen. Virol.* **4**:305.

Dasgupta, R., Shih, D. S., Saris, C., and Kaesberg, P., 1975, Nucleotide sequence of a viral RNA fragment that binds to eukaryotic ribosomes, *Nature (London)* **256**:624.

Davies, J. W., and Kaesberg, P., 1974, Translation of virus mRNA: Protein synthesis directed by several RNAs in a cell-free extract from wheat germ, *J. Gen. Virol.* **25**:11.

Dawson, J. R. O., Motoyoshi, F., Watts, J. W., and Bancroft, J. B., 1975, Production of RNA and coat protein of a wild-type isolate and a temperature-sensitive mutant of cowpea chlorotic mottle virus in cowpea leaves and tobacco protoplasts, *J. Gen. Virol.* **29**:99.

Dawson, W. O., Schlegel, D. E., and Lung, M. C. Y., 1975, Synthesis of tobacco mosaic virus in intact tobacco leaves systemically inoculated by differential temperature treatment, *Virology* **65**:565.

De Zoeten, G. A., Assink, A. M., and van Kammen, A., 1974, Association of cowpea mosaic virus-induced double-stranded RNA with a cytopathological structure in infected cells, *Virology* **59**:341.

De Zoeten, G. A., Powell, C. A., Gaard, G., and German, T. L., 1976, *In situ* localization of pea enation mosaic virus double-stranded ribonucleic acid, *Virology* **70**:459.

Ellis, E. L., and Delbrück, M., 1939, The growth of bacteriophage, *J. Gen. Physiol.* **22**:365.

Föglein, F. J., Kalpagam, C., Bates, D. C., Premecz, G., Nyitrai, A., and Farkas, G. L., 1975, Viral RNA synthesis is renewed in protoplasts isolated from TMV-infected Xanthi tobacco leaves in an advanced stage of virus infection, *Virology* **67**:74.

Hadidi, A., and Fraenkel-Conrat, H., 1973, Characterization and specificity of soluble RNA polymerase of brome mosaic virus, *Virology* **52**:363.

Hariharasubramanian, V., Hadidi, A., Singer, B., and Fraenkel-Conrat, H., 1973, Possible identification of a protein in brome mosaic virus infected barley as a component of viral RNA polymerase, *Virology* **54**:190.

Harrison, B. D., 1955, Studies on the multiplication of plant virus in inoculated leaves, Ph. D. thesis, University of London.

Harrison, B. D., Kubo, S., Robinson, D. J., and Hutcheson, A. M., 1976, The multiplication cycle of tobacco rattle virus in tobacco mesophyll protoplasts, *J. Gen. Virol.* **33**:237.

Hennig, B., and Wittmann, H. G., 1972, Tobacco mosaic virus: Mutants and strains, in: *Principles and Techniques in Plant Virology* (C. I. Kado and H. O. Agrawal, eds.), pp. 546–594, Van Nostrand Reinhold, New York.

Hibi, T., and Yora, K., 1972, Electron microscopy of tobacco mosaic virus infection in tobacco mesophyll protoplasts, *Ann. Phytopathol. Soc. Jap.* **38**:350.

Hibi, T., Rezelman G., and van Kammen, A., 1975, Infection of cowpea mesophyll protoplasts with cowpea mosaic virus, *Virology* **64**:308.

Honda, Y., Matsui, C., Otsuki, Y., and Takebe, I., 1974, Ultrastructure of tobacco mesophyll protoplasts inoculated with cucumber mosaic virus, *Phytopathology* **64**:30.

Honda, Y., Kajita, S., Matsui, C., Otsuki, Y., and Takebe, I., 1975, An ultrastructural study of the infection of tobacco mesophyll protoplasts by potato virus X, *Phytopathol. Z.* **84**:66.

Huber, R., Rezelman, G., Hibi, T., and van Kammen, A., 1977, Cowpea mosaic virus infection of protoplasts from Samsun tobacco leaves, *J. Gen. Virol.* **34**:315.

Hunter, T. R., Hunt, T., Knowland, J., and Zimmern, D., 1976, Messenger RNA for the coat protein of tobacco mosaic virus, *Nature* (*London*) **260**:759.

Jackson, A. O., Mitchell, D. M., and Siegel, A., 1971, Replication of tobacco mosaic virus. I. Isolation and characterization of double-stranded forms of ribonucleic acid, *Virology* **45**:182.

Jackson, A. O., Zaitlin, M., Siegel, A., and Francki, R. I. B., 1972, Replication of tobacco mosaic virus. III. Viral RNA metabolism in separated leaf cells, *Virology* **48**:655.

Jockusch, H., 1968, Two mutants of tobacco mosaic virus temperature-sensitive in two different functions, *Virology* **35**:94.

Kagi, T., Ozaki, T., and Inoue, T., 1975, Preparation of mesophyll protoplasts of broad bean and their infection by BBWV, *Ann. Phytopathol. Soc. Jap.* **41**:107 (Abstr.).

Kanai, R., and Edwards, G. E., 1973, Purification of enzymatically isolated mesophyll protoplasts from C_3, C_4, and crassulacean acid metabolism plants using an aqueous dextran-polyethylene glycol two phase system, *Plant Physiol.* **52**:484.

Kassanis, B., and White, R. F., 1974, A simplified method of obtaining tobacco protoplasts for infection with tobacco mosaic virus, *J. Gen. Virol.* **24**:447.

Kassanis, B., White, R. F., and Woods, R. D., 1975, Inhibition of multiplication of tobacco mosaic virus in protoplasts by antibiotics and its prevention by divalent metals, *J. Gen. Virol.* **28**:185.

Keith, J., and Fraenkel-Conrat, H., 1975, Tobacco mosaic virus RNA carries 5′-terminal triphosphorylated guanosine blocked by 5′-linked 7-methylguanosine, *FEBS Lett.* **57**:31.

Kielland-Brandt, M. C., and Nilsson-Tillgren, T., 1973, Studies on the biosynthesis of TMV. V. Determination of TMV RNA and its complementary RNA at different times after infection, *Mol. Gen. Genet.* **121**:229.

Kiho, Y., 1972, Polycistronic translation of plant viral ribonucleic acid, *Jap. J. Microbiol.* **16**:259.

Knowland, J., 1974, Protein synthesis directed by the RNA from a plant virus in a normal animal cell, *Genetics* **78**:383.

Koike, M., Hibi, T., and Yora, K., 1976, Infection of cowpea protoplasts by tobacco mosaic virus, *Ann. Phytopathol. Soc. Jap.* **42**:105 (Abstr.).

Koike, M., Hibi, T., and Yora, K., 1977, Infection of cowpea mesophyll protoplasts with cucumber mosaic virus, *Virology* (in press).

Kozak, M., and Nathans, D., 1972, Translation of the genome of a ribonucleic acid bacteriophage, *Bacteriol. Rev.* **36**:109.

Kubo, S., Harrison, B. D., and Robinson, D. J., 1974, Effects of phosphate on the infection of tobacco protoplasts by tobacco rattle virus, *Intervirology* **3**:382.

Kubo, S., Harrison, B. D., Robinson, D. J., and Mayo, M. A., 1975*a*, Tobacco rattle virus in tobacco mesophyll protoplasts: Infection and virus multiplication, *J. Gen. Virol.* **27**:293.

Kubo, S., Harrison, B. D., and Robinson, D. J., 1975*b*, Defined conditions for growth of tobacco plants as sources of protoplasts for virus infection, *J. Gen. Virol.* **28**:255.

Kubo, S., Robinson, D. J., Harrison, B. D., and Hutcheson, A. M., 1976, Uptake of tobacco rattle virus by tobacco protoplasts and the effect of phosphate on infection, *J. Gen. Virol.* **30**:287.

Lafléche, D., and Bové, J. M., 1971, Virus de la mosaique jaune du navet: Site cellulaire de la replication du RNA viral, *Physiol. Veg.* **9**:487.

Lafléche, D., Bové, C., Dupont, G., Mouchés, C., Astier, T., Carnier, M., and Bové, J. M., 1972, Site of viral RNA replication in the cells of higher plants: TYMV RNA synthesis on the chloroplast outer membrane system, in: *RNA Viruses/Ribosomes* (*Proceedings of Eighth FEBS Meeting*), Vol. 27, pp. 43–71, North-Holland, Amsterdam.

Lane, L. C., 1974, The bromoviruses, in: *Advances in Virus Research,* Vol. 19 (M. A.

Lauffer, F. B. Bang, K. Maramorosch, and K. M. Smith, eds.), pp. 151–220, Academic Press, New York.

Lazar, G., Borbély, G., Udvardy, J., Premecz, G., and Farkas, G. L., 1973, Osmotic shock triggers an increase in ribonuclease level in protoplasts isolated from tobacco leaves, *Plant Sci. Lett.* **1**:53.

Mäder, M., Meyer, Y., and Bopp, M., 1976, Zellwandregeneration und Peroxidase-Isoenzym-Synthese isolierter Protoplasten von *Nicotiana tabacum* L., *Planta* **129**:33.

Motoyoshi, F., and Hull, R., 1974, The infection of tobacco protoplasts with pea enation mosaic virus, *J. Gen. Virol.* **24**:89.

Motoyoshi, F., and Oshima, N., 1975, Infection with tobacco mosaic virus of leaf mesophyll protoplasts from susceptible and resistant lines of tomato, *J. Gen. Virol.* **29**:81.

Motoyoshi, F., and Oshima, N., 1976, The use of tris-HCl buffer for inoculation of tomato protoplasts with tobacco mosaic virus, *J. Gen. Virol.* **32**:311.

Motoyoshi, F., and Oshima, N., 1977, Expression of genetically controlled resistance to tobacco mosaic virus infection in isolated tomato leaf mesophyll protoplasts, *J. Gen. Virol.* **34**:499.

Motoyoshi, F., Bancroft, J. B., Watts, J. W., and Burgess, J., 1973*a*, The infection of tobacco protoplasts with cowpea chlorotic mottle virus and its RNA, *J. Gen. Virol.* **20**:177.

Motoyoshi, F., Bancroft, J. B., and Watts, J. W., 1973*b*, A direct estimate of the number of cowpea chlorotic mottle virus particles absorbed by tobacco protoplasts that become infected, *J. Gen. Virol.* **21**:159.

Motoyoshi, F., Bancroft, J. B., and Watts, J. W., 1974*a*, The infection of tobacco protoplasts with a variant of brome mosaic virus, *J. Gen. Virol.* **25**:31.

Motoyoshi, F., Watts, J. W., and Bancroft, J. B., 1974*b*, Factors influencing the infection of tobacco protoplasts by cowpea chlorotic mottle virus, *J. Gen. Virol.* **25**:245.

Motoyoshi, F., Hull, R., and Flack, I. H., 1975, Infection of tobacco mesophyll protoplasts by alfalfa mosaic virus, *J. Gen. Virol.* **27**:263.

Nagata, T., and Takebe, I., 1970, Cell wall regeneration and cell division in isolated tobacco mesophyll protoplasts, *Planta* **92**:301.

Nagata, T., and Takebe, I., 1971, Plating of isolated tobacco mesophyll protoplasts on agar medium, *Planta* **99**:12.

Nilsson-Tillgren, T., Kolehmainen-Sevéus, L., and von Wettstein, D., 1969, Studies on the biosynthesis of TMV. I. A system approaching a synchronized virus synthesis in a tobacco leaf, *Mol. Gen. Genet.* **104**:124.

Nishimura, M., and Akazawa, T., 1975, Photosynthetic activities of spinach leaf protoplasts, *Plant Physiol.* **55**:712.

Okuno, T., Furusawa, I., and Hiruki, C., 1977, Infection of barley protoplasts with brome mosaic virus, *Phytopathology* **67**:610.

Otsuki, Y., and Takebe, I., 1969, Fluorescent antibody staining of tobacco mosaic virus antigen in tobacco mesophyll protoplasts, *Virology* **38**:497.

Otsuki, Y., and Takebe, I., 1973, Infection of tobacco mesophyll protoplasts by cucumber mosaic virus, *Virology* **52**:433.

Otsuki, Y., and Takebe, I., 1976*a*, Double infection of isolated tobacco mesophyll protoplasts by unrelated plant viruses, *J. Gen. Virol.* **30**:309.

Otsuki, Y., and Takebe, I., 1976*b*, Interaction of tobacco mosaic virus strains in doubly infected tobacco protoplasts, *Ann. Microbiol.* **127A**:21 (Abstr.).

Otsuki, Y., and Takebe, I., 1976*c*, Double infection of isolated tobacco leaf protoplasts by two strains of tobacco mosaic virus, in: *Biochemistry and Cytology of Plant-Parasite Interaction* (K. Tomiyama, J. M. Daly, I. Uritani, H. Oku, and S. Ouchi, eds.), pp. 213–222, Kodansha, Tokyo.

Otsuki, Y., Shimomura, T., and Takebe, I., 1972a, Tobacco mosaic virus multiplication and expression of the N gene in necrotic responding tobacco varieties, *Virology* **50**:45.

Otsuki, Y., Takebe, I., Honda, Y., and Matsui, C., 1972b, Ultrastructure of infection of tobacco mesophyll protoplasts by tobacco mosaic virus, *Virology* **49**:188.

Otsuki, Y., Takebe, I., Honda, Y., Kajita, S., and Matsui, C., 1974, Infection of tobacco mesophyll protoplasts by potato virus X, *J. Gen. Virol.* **22**:375.

Paterson, R., 1974, Protein synthesis in tobacco protoplasts infected with tobacco mosaic virus, Ph.D. thesis, University of California, Berkeley.

Paterson, R., and Knight, C. A., 1975, Protein synthesis in tobacco protoplasts infected with tobacco mosaic virus, *Virology* **64**:10.

Pelham, J., 1966, Resistance in tomato to tobacco mosaic virus, *Euphytica* **15**:258.

Ralph, R. K., Bullivant, S., and Wojcik, S. J., 1971, Cytoplasmic membranes, a possible site of tobacco mosaic virus RNA replication, *Virology* **43**:713.

Rappaport, I., and Wildman, S. G., 1957, A kinetic study of local lesion growth on *Nicotiana glutinosa* resulting from tobacco mosaic virus infection, *Virology* **4**:265.

Renaudin, J., Bové, J. M., Otsuki, Y., and Takebe, I., 1975, Infection of Brassica leaf protoplasts by turnip yellow mosaic virus, *Mol. Gen. Genet.* **141**:59.

Renaudin, J., Gandar, J., and Bové, J. M., 1976, Replication of TYMV in Chinese cabbage protoplasts, *Ann. Microbiol.* **127A**:61.

Rottier, P. J. M., 1976, Inoculation of *Vigna* protoplasts with separate components of CPMV, *Ann. Microbiol.* **127A**:113 (Abstr.).

Sakai, F., and Takebe, I., 1970, RNA and protein synthesis in protoplasts isolated from tobacco leaves, *Biochim. Biophys. Acta* **224**:531.

Sakai, F., and Takebe, I., 1972, A non-coat protein synthesized in tobacco mesophyll protoplasts infected by tobacco mosaic virus, *Mol. Gen. Genet.* **118**:93.

Sakai, F., and Takebe, I., 1974, Protein synthesis in tobacco mesophyll protoplasts induced by tobacco mosaic virus infection, *Virology* **62**:426.

Sakai, F., Watts, J. W., Dawson, J. R. O., and Bancroft, J. B., 1977, Synthesis of proteins in tobacco protoplasts infected with cowpea chlorotic mottle virus, *J. Gen. Virol.* **34**:285.

Sänger, H. L., and Knight, C. A., 1963, Action of actinomycin D on RNA synthesis in healthy and virus infected tobacco leaves, *Biochem. Biophys. Res. Commun.* **13**:455.

Sarkar, S., 1977, Use of protoplasts for plant virus studies, in: *Methods in Virology,* Vol. VI (K. Maramorosch and H. Koprowski, eds.), pp. 435–456, Academic Press, New York.

Sarkar, S., Upadhya, M. D., and Melchers, G., 1974, A highly efficient method of inoculation of tobacco mesophyll protoplasts with ribonucleic acid of tobacco mosaic virus, *Mol. Gen. Genet.* **135**:1.

Schilde-Rentschler, L., 1973, A simpler method for the preparation of plant protoplasts, *Z. Naturforsch.* **27b**:208.

Shalla, T. A., and Petersen, L. J., 1973, Infection of isolated plant protoplasts with potato virus X, *Phytopathology* **63**:1125.

Shalla, T. A., and Shepard, J. F., 1972, The structure and antigenic analysis of amorphous inclusion bodies induced by potato virus X, *Virology* **49**:654.

Shih, D. S., and Kaesberg, P., 1973, Translation of brome mosaic viral ribonucleic acid in a cell-free system derived from wheat embryo, *Proc. Natl. Acad. Sci. USA* **70**:1799.

Shih, D. S., and Kaesberg, P., 1976, Translation of the RNAs of brome mosaic virus: the monocistronic nature of RNA 1 and RNA 2, *J. Mol. Biol.* **103**:77.

Shih, D. S., Lane, L. C., and Kaesberg, P., 1972, Origin of the small component of brome mosaic virus RNA, *J. Mol. Biol.* **64**:353.

Siegel, A., and Zaitlin, M., 1964, Infection process in plant virus diseases, *Annu. Rev. Phytopathol.* **2**:179.

Siegel, A., Zaitlin, M., and Duda, C. T., 1973, Replication of tobacco mosaic virus. IV. Further characterization of viral related RNAs, *Virology* **53**:75.

Siegel, A., Hari, V., Montgomery, I., and Kolacz, K., 1976, A messenger RNA for capsid protein isolated from tobacco mosaic virus-infected tissue, *Virology* **73**:363.

Smith, S. H., and Schlegel, D. E., 1965, The incorporation of ribonucleic acid precursors in healthy and virus-infected plant cells, *Virology* **26**:180.

Steere, R. L., 1955, Concepts and problems concerning the assay of plant viruses *Phytopathology* **45**:196.

Sugimura, Y., and Ushiyama, R., 1975, Cucumber green mottle mosaic virus infection and its bearing on cytological alterations in tobacco mesophyll protoplasts, *J. Gen. Virol.* **29**:93.

Sugiyama, T., Korant, B. D., and Lonberg-Holm, K. K., 1972, RNA virus gene expression and its control, *Annu. Rev. Microbiol.* **26**:467.

Takanami, Y., Kubo, S., and Imaizumi, S., 1977, Synthesis of single- and double-stranded cucumber mosaic virus RNAs in tobacco mesophyll protoplasts, *Virology* (in press).

Takebe, I., 1975a, The use of protoplasts in plant virology, *Annu. Rev. Phytopathol.* **13**:105.

Takebe, I., 1975b, Protoplasts from leaf mesophyll and their infection by plant viruses, *Rev. Plant Protection Res.* **8**:136.

Takebe, I., and Otsuki, Y., 1969, Infection of tobacco mesophyll protoplasts by tobacco mosaic virus, *Proc. Natl. Acad. Sci. USA* **64**:843.

Takebe, I., Otsuki, Y., and Aoki, S., 1968, Isolation of tobacco mesophyll cells in intact and active state, *Plant Cell Physiol.* **9**:115.

Takebe, I., Otsuki, Y., Honda, Y., and Matsui, C., 1975, Penetration of plant viruses into isolated tobacco leaf protoplasts, in: *Proceedings of the First Intersectional Congress of the International Association of Microbiological Societies,* Vol. 3 (T. Hasegawa, ed.), pp. 55-64. Science Council of Japan, Tokyo.

Ushiyama, R., and Matthews, R. E. F., 1970, The significance of chloroplast abnormalities associated with infection by turnip yellow mosaic virus, *Virology* **42**:293.

Weintraub, M., and Ragetli, H. W. J., 1964, Studies on the metabolism of leaves with localized virus infections. Particulate fractions and substrates in TMV-infected *Nicotiana glutinosa, Can. J. Bot.* **42**:533.

Wyatt, S. D., and Shaw, J. G., 1975, Retention and dissociation of tobacco mosaic virus by tobacco protoplasts, *Virology* **63**:459.

Zaitlin, M., and Beachy, R. N., 1974a, The use of protoplasts and separated cells in plant virus research, *Adv. Virus Res.* **19**:1.

Zaitlin, M., and Beachy, R. N., 1974b, Protoplasts and separated cells: Some new vistas for plant virology, in: *Tissue Culture and Plant Science 1974* (H. E. Street, and P. J. King, eds.), pp. 265-285, Academic Press, New York.

Zaitlin, M., and Hariharasubramanian, V., 1972, A gel electrophoretic analysis of proteins from plants infected with tobacco mosaic and potato spindle tuber viruses, *Virology* **47**:296.

Zaitlin, M., Duda, C. T., and Petti, M. A., 1973, Replication of tobacco mosaic virus. V. Properties of the bound and solubilized replicase, *Virology* **53**:300.

Zhuravlev, Y. N., Pisetskaya, N. F., Shumilova, L. A., Musorok, T. I., and Reifman, V. G., 1975, Attachment of labeled TMV to tobacco mesophyll protoplasts, *Virology* **64**:43.

Zimmern, D., 1975, The 5′ end group of tobacco mosaic virus RNA is $m^7G^{5'}ppp^{5'}Gp$, *Nucleic Acids Res.* **2**:1189.

CHAPTER 6

Viroids

T. O. Diener and A. Hadidi

Plant Virology Laboratory, Plant Protection Institute
Agricultural Research Service
U.S. Department of Agriculture
Beltsville, Maryland 20705

1. INTRODUCTION

Viroids have been recognized recently as the smallest agents of infectious disease. Viroids differ from viruses by the absence of a dormant phase (virions) and by genomes that are much smaller than those of known viruses (Diener, 1971b). The term "viroid" has been introduced to describe infectious nucleic acids which have properties similar to those of the causal agent of potato spindle tuber disease (Diener, 1971b). Presently known viroids consist solely of a low molecular weight RNA of about 75,000–130,000. Introduction of this RNA into susceptible hosts leads to autonomous replication of the RNA, and, in some hosts, to disease.

Previously, the term "viroid" has been defined as "any prophylactic vaccine" (*Stedman's Medical Dictionary*, 1942) or "any biological specific used in immunization" (*Dorland's Illustrated Medical Dictionary*, 1944). In 1946, the term was redefined by Altenburg to denote hypothetical, ultramicroscopic organisms that are useful symbionts, occur universally within cells of larger organisms, and are capable, by mutation, of giving rise to viruses. These two earlier meanings of "viroid" were judged to be obsolete at the time it was defined for a third time (Diener, 1971b, 1973b).

The first viroid was discovered in efforts to purify and characterize the agent of the potato spindle tuber disease, a disease which, for many years, had been assumed to be of viral etiology (Diener and Raymer, 1971). Diener and Raymer (1967) reported that the infectious agent of the disease is a free RNA and that conventional virus particles are, apparently, not present in infected tissue. Later, sedimentation and gel electrophoretic analyses conclusively demonstrated that the infectious RNA has a very low molecular weight (Diener, 1971b) and that the agent therefore basically differs from conventional viruses.

Four other plant diseases have now been linked with the presence of viroids: citrus exocortis (Semancik and Weathers, 1972b; Sänger, 1972), chrysanthemum stunt (Diener and Lawson, 1973; Hollings and Stone, 1973), chrysanthemum chlorotic mottle (Romaine and Horst, 1975), and cucumber pale fruit (Van Dorst and Peters, 1974; Sänger *et al.*, 1976). In all of these cases, low molecular weight RNA has been isolated from diseased plants, purified by polyacrylamide gel electrophoresis, and shown to be infectious (these represent the minimal criteria necessary to establish the presence of a viroid).

One additional example of a potential viroid disease has been described. Randles (1975) suspects that cadang-cadang (a disease of coconut palms of enormous economic importance in the Philippines) is caused by a viroid. In this case, a low molecular weight RNA of the appropriate size present only in diseased tissue has been isolated. The infectivity of this new RNA species has not yet been demonstrated.

The recognition of viroids as a newly identified class of pathogens raises several questions that have potentially important implications for microbiology, molecular biology, plant pathology, animal pathology, and medicine.

2. BIOLOGICAL PROPERTIES

2.1. Propagation Hosts and Environmental Factors

2.1.1. Potato Spindle Tuber Viroid (PSTV)

PSTV is conveniently propagated in tomato (*Lycopersicon esculentum* Mill. cv. Rutgers) (Raymer and O'Brien, 1962). To obtain early symptom expression, plants are inoculated at the cotyledonary stage and maintained in a greenhouse at 30–35°C. During winter months and in locations with low light intensity, supplementary lighting is essential.

Vigorously growing plants develop symptoms earlier than slowly growing plants; thus application of fertilizer may be advantageous. Under
optimal conditions and with a high-titer inoculum, first symptoms
regularly appear 10–14 days after inoculation (Fig. 1). Leaf epinasty
and stunting of plants are typical symptoms of PSTV in tomato; leaf
and stem necrosis also develop in infected plants. Leaves are harvested
4–8 weeks after inoculation and are stored frozen until used.

PSTV may also be propagated in Sheyenne tomato (Singh and
Bagnall, 1968) or in *Scopolia sinensis* Hemsl. (Singh *et al.,* 1974)
plants.

2.1.2. Citrus Exocortis Viroid (CEV)

CEV is propagated in "Etrog" citron (*Citrus medica* L.)
(Semancik and Weathers, 1968) or in *Gynura aurantiaca* (Bl.) DC.
(Semancik and Weathers, 1972*a*). Symptoms in both hosts consist of
necrosis of midveins and epinasty of young developing leaves and severe
stunting. Bark scaling is a definite symptom of CEV in trifoliate
orange, *Poncirus trifoliata* (L.) Raft (Olson and Shull, 1956).

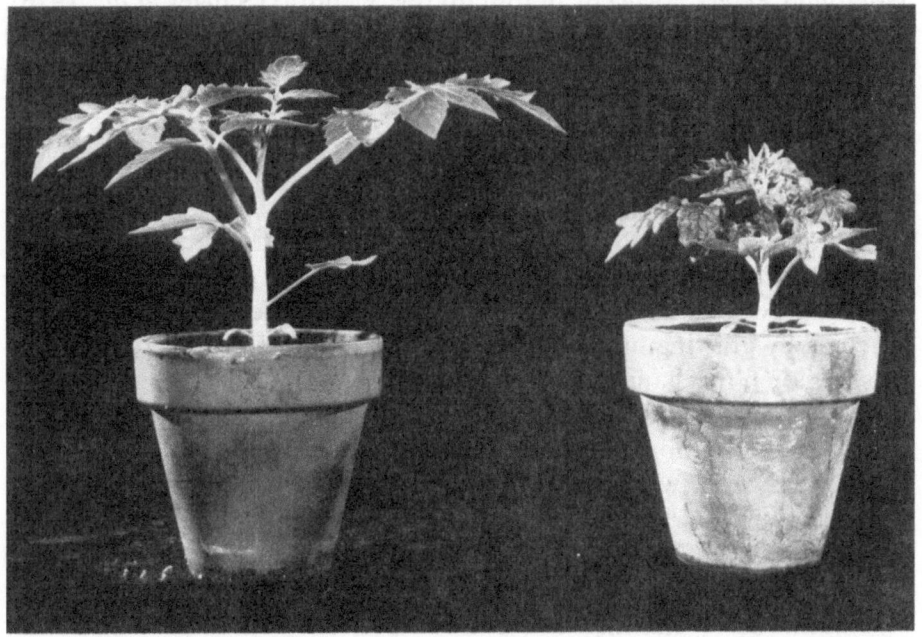

Fig. 1.   Rutgers tomato plants. Right: Plant with symptoms of PSTV, 20 days postinoculation. Left: Uninoculated control plant of same age.

2.1.3. Chrysanthemum Stunt Viroid (CSV)

CSV may be propagated in either *Senecio cruentus* DC. (Brierley, 1953) (florists' cineraria) or *Chrysanthemum morifolium* Ramat. cv. Mistletoe. Cineraria leaves are harvested just as they begin to show leaf curl and distortion; highest infectivity titers occur at any time during fall and winter months (Diener and Lawson, 1973).

2.1.4. Chrysanthemum Chlorotic Mottle Viroid (ChCMV)

ChCMV is propagated in *Chrysanthemum morifolium* cv. Deep Ridge. Systemically infected leaves with symptoms varying from extensive mottling to complete chlorosis are harvested 3–5 weeks after inoculation (Romaine and Horst, 1975).

2.1.5. Cucumber Pale Fruit Viroid (CPFV)

CPFV may be propagated in cucumber (*Cucumis sativus* L.) (Van Dorst and Peters, 1974) or in tomato (cv. Rentita) (Sänger *et al.,* 1976). This viroid-incited disease is characterized by pale fruits, crumbled flowers, and rugosity and chlorosis on the leaves of cucumber (Van Dorst and Peters, 1974).

2.2. Inoculation Procedures

All viroids described so far are mechanically transmissible, either readily or with some difficulty. Although other means of transmission (such as by grafting or by dodder bridges) are possible, all recent work was based on mechanical transmission.

With PSTV, CSV, and ChCMV, standard inoculation procedures used with conventional viruses and viral RNAs are suitable.

In our work with PSTV, tomato plants are dusted with 600-mesh carborundum and are inoculated by lightly rubbing cotyledons and terminal portions of the plants with cotton-tipped applicators dipped into viroid suspension in 0.02 M phosphate buffer, pH 7.

With CEV, slashing of stems or petioles with a razor blade or knife dipped into inoculum is more efficient than inoculation by rubbing of carborundum-dusted leaves (Garnsey and Whidden, 1970). Often, a combination of razor slashing and rubbing has been used with

CEV (Semancik and Weathers, 1968) and with CPFV (Van Dorst and Peters, 1974).

2.3. Bioassay of Viroids

Estimation of viroid concentration is essential in efforts to purify and characterize the infectious molecules. In crude extracts and partially purified preparations, such estimates can only be obtained by measuring biological activity of viroids, i.e., symptom formation in susceptible plants. As with conventional plant viruses, infectivity assays rely on the percentage of inoculated plants becoming systemically infected or, in cases where a hypersensitive host is available, on the number of local lesions produced as a consequence of infection. Although local lesion assays are inherently more accurate than systemic assays, the latter type of assay has been used more often than the former in viroid work, either because local lesion hosts are not available or because assays based on local lesions posed difficulties.

2.3.1. Systemic Bioassay of Viroids

The use of systemic infections for the determination of the relative concentration of a biologically active entity is complicated by many factors (see Brakke, 1970), particularly if relatively small differences in titer are to be determined. Fortunately, much work with viroids does not require an accurate knowledge of relative viroid titer. Often, certain procedures result in large effects and approach all-or-nothing type responses.

For the assay of PSTV in tomato, an empirical "infectivity index" was developed which takes into consideration the dilution end point, the percentage of plants infected at each dilution, and the time required for symptom expression (Raymer and Diener, 1969). These three factors are used in the index as a means of estimating relative viroid concentration.

As soon as the first plant in an experiment begins to develop symptoms, readings are initiated and are continued at 2-day intervals until no further increase in the number of plants with symptoms has occurred for two or three consecutive readings. The experiment is then terminated. The type of data obtained by this method is illustrated in Table 1, together with the method used to compute an "infectivity index" based on such data.

TABLE 1

PSTV Symptom Expression in Rutgers Tomato Plants as a Function of Dilution and Time[a]: Calculation of an Infectivity Index

Dilution	Infectivity Days after inoculation								Sum[c]	Multiplier[d]	Product[e]
	10	12	14	16	18	20	22	24			
10^{-1}	1/3[b]	3/3	3/3	3/3	3/3	3/3	3/3	3/3	22	1	22
10^{-2}				3/3	3/3	3/3	3/3	3/3	15	2	30
10^{-3}					3/3	3/3	3/3	3/3	12	3	36
10^{-4}						1/3	2/3	2/3	5	4	20
10^{-5}							2/3	2/3	4	5	20
10^{-6}							2/3	2/3	4	6	24
10^{-7}							1/3	1/3	2	7	14
10^{-8}								0/3	0	8	0
								Total = Infectivity index:			166

[a] Data were obtained with a viroid concentrate obtained by extraction of infected leaf tissue with 0.5 M K_2HPO_4, chloroform, and n-butanol, followed by phenol treatment and ethanol precipitation.
[b] Number of plants with symptoms/number of plants inoculated.
[c] Sum of all plants showing symptoms at all dates for each dilution.
[d] Negative log of the dilution.
[e] Sum × multiplier for each dilution.

Evidently, the more concentrated the viroid preparation, the earlier symptoms appear. The index is computed by adding together the number of plants at each dilution over the entire recording period, multiplying this figure by the negative log of the dilution, and adding together these products for all the dilutions tested. This index permits discrimination between treatments that might achieve the same dilution end points but differ both in the earliness with which symptoms are expressed and in the number of plants infected. Undoubtedly, with this method, the difference in viroid titer is underestimated, since a tenfold difference in dilution is represented by a difference of only 1 in the multiplier. On the other hand, the infectivity index gives relatively little weight to individual plants that express symptoms later, after having been inoculated with a highly diluted viroid preparation. Thus much of the variability inherent in an assay of this type is "dampened out."

With careful and consistent inoculation techniques, however, spurious results are rare, and in these cases a more realistic index may be computed by using the actual dilution factor as multiplier (Diener, 1971b) instead of its negative logarithm.

Semancik and Weathers (1972c) expressed relative infectivity titers of CEV preparations by determining the total number of "infected plant days" on three to five *Gynura* plants inoculated with one concentration of inoculum only. The authors considered this procedure satisfactory, because the dilution–response curve was found to be reasonably linear within a certain range of "relative infectivity units" (Semancik and Weathers, 1972c).

2.3.2. Local Lesion Assay of Viroids

So far, local lesion hosts have been discovered only for CSV and PSTV. With CSV, local starch lesions are detected on inoculated leaves of *Senecio cruentus* (florists' cineraria) 12–18 days after inoculation, provided that the plants are grown with light intensities not higher than 2000 ft-c and at 18–26°C (Lawson, 1968). Increased starch lesion formation is favored by an 18-h light period with 500 ft-c fluorescent illumination and a constant temperature of 21°C. Variation in lesion counts among cineraria plants and between leaves on a single plant, however, precludes their use for detecting small differences in CSV concentration (Lawson, 1968).

With PSTV, Singh (1971) reported that *Scopolia sinensis,* a solanaceous plant species, produces necrotic local lesions 7–10 days after inoculation with the severe strain and 10–15 days after inoculation with the mild strain. Singh later stressed that local lesion development is critically dependent on environmental conditions (Singh, 1973). Local lesions developed best on leaves of plants at 22–23°C; plants maintained at 28–31°C developed mostly systemic symptoms without conspicuous local lesions. A low light intensity of 400 ft-c favored local lesion development.

2.4. Host Range*

PSTV is able to systemically infect plants of several families (Table 2), especially species of the Solanaceae (O'Brien and Raymer, 1964; Singh and O'Brien, 1970; Diener *et al.,* 1972; Singh, 1973; Hadidi and Fraenkel-Conrat, 1974). Singh (1973) has also reported that PSTV infects *Pyrracanthum villisum* Lam., *P. sysimbrifilium* Lam., *Solanum*

---

* Common names of host species, when available, were obtained from *Standardized Plant Names* (1942) and/or *Manual of Cultivated Plants* (1969).

TABLE 2

Host Range of Potato Spindle Tuber Viroid (PSTV)

Family and species	Family and species
Amaranthaceae	Solanaceae (*Continued*)
Gomphrena globosa L., common globe amaranth	*Nicotiana alata* Link & Otto, winged tobacco
Boraginaceae	*Nicotiana bigelovii* (Torr.) Wats., Indian tobacco
Myosotis sylvatica Hoffm., woodland forget-me-not	*Nicotiana bonariensis* Lehm.
Campanulaceae	*Nicotiana chinensis* Fisch. ex Lehm.
Campanula medium L., Canterbury bells	*Nicotiana clevelandii* Gray
Caryophyllaceae	*Nicotiana glauca* Grah., tree tobacco
Cerastium tomentosum L., snow-in-summer cerastium	*Nicotiana glutinosa* L.
	Nicotiana goodspeedii Wheeler
Dianthus barbatus L., sweet william carnation	*Nicotiana clevelandii* × *Nicotiana glutinosa* Christie
Compositae	*Nicotiana knightiana* Goodspeed
Gynura aurantiaca (Bl.) DC., Java velvet plant; velvet plant	*Nicotiana langsdorffii* Weinm.
	Nicotiana longiflora Cav.
Convolvulaceae	*Nicotiana megalosiphon* Heurck. & Meull.
Convolvulus tricolor L., dwarf glorybind	*Nicotiana nudicaulis* Wats.
Dipsaceae	*Nicotiana paniculata* L.
Scabiosa japonica Miq., Japanese scabious	*Nicotiana plumbaginifolia* Viv.
Sapindaceae	*Nicotiana quadrivalvis* Pursh
Cardiospermum halicacabum L.	*Nicotiana raimondii* Macbride
Scrophulariaceae	*Nicotiana repanda* Willd. ex Lehm.
Penstemon richardsonii Dougl., Richardson penstemon	*Nicotiana rotundifolia* Lindl.
Solanaceae	*Nicotiana rustica* L., Aztec tobacco or Indian tobacco
Atropa bella-donna L., belladona	*Nicotiana* X *sanderae* Hort. ex W. Wats.
Browallia demissa L. = *B. Americana* L.	*Nicotiana solanifolia* Walp.
Browallia grandiflora Grah., bigflower browallia	*Nicotiana sylvestris* Speg. & Comes
	Nicotiana tabacum L., common tobacco
Browallia viscosa H.B.K., stricky browallia	*Nicotiana texana* Hort. Par ex Maxim.
Capsicum frutescens L. = *C. microcarpum* DC., bush red pepper	*Nicotiana viscosa* Lehm.
	Nierembergia coerulea Sealy, cupflower
Capsicum nigrum Willd.	*Petunia axillaris* (Lam.) B.S.P. = *P. nyctaginiflora* Juss., whitemoon petunia
Cyphomandra betacea (Cav.) Sendtn., tree tomato	*Petunia hybrida* Vilm., common petunia
Datura metel L., Hindu Datura	*Petunia inflata* Fries, inflated petunia
Datura stramonium L., jimsonweed	*Petunia violacea* Lindl., violet petunia
Lycopersicon esculentum Mill., common tomato	*Physalis alkekengi* L., strawberry groundcherry
Lycopersicon pimpinellifolium (L.) Mill, currant tomato	*Physalis angulata* L., cut leaf groundcherry
Nicandra physalodes (L.) Pers., apple of Peru	*Physalis floridana* Rydberg = *P. pubescens* L., downy groundcherry
	Physalis franchetii Mast. = *P. alkekengi* L. var. *franchetii* (Mast.) Mak.

TABLE 2

(Continued)

Family and species	Family and species
Solanaceae (*Continued*)	Solanaceae (*Continued*)
Physalis heterophylla Nees., clammy groundcherry	*Solanum gracile* Otto ex W. Baxt.
Physalis ixocarpa Brot. ex Hornem.	*Solanum guineense* L., Guinea nightshade
Physalis minima L.	*Solanum hendersonii* Hort. ex W. F. Wight, Jerusalem cherry
Physalis parviflora Hort. ex Zuccagni	*Solanum hibiscifolium* Rusby
Physalis peruviana L. = *P. edulis* Sims, Peruvian groundcherry; cape gooseberry	*Solanum humile* Bernh. ex Willd.
Physalis philadelphica Lam.	*Solanum judaicum* Bess.
Physalis pruinosa L., hairy groundcherry	*Solanum kitaibelii* Schult.
Physalis somnifera L.	*Solanum laciniatum* Ait.
Physalis viscosa L.	*Solanum luteum* Mill., yellow nightshade
Salpiglossis sinuata Ruiz & Pav. = *S. variabilis* Hort., scalloped salpiglossis	*Solanum maritimum* Meyen ex Nees
Salpiglossis spinescens Clos. (mixed hybrids)	*Solanum melongena* L., garden eggplant
Saracha jaltomata Schlecht.	*Solanum memphiticum* J. F. Gmel.
Saracha umbellata DC.	*Solanum miniatum* Bernh. ex Willd.
Schizanthus pinnatus Ruiz & Pav., wingleaf butterfly flower	*Solanum nigrum* L., black nightshade
Schizanthus retusus Hook., orange-rose butterfly flower	*Solanum nitidibaccatum* Bitt.
Scopolia sinensis Hemsl.	*Solanum nodiflorum* Jacq.
Scopolia spp.	*Solanum ochroleucum* Bast.
Solanum aethiopicum L., Ethiopian nightshade	*Solanum olgae* Pojark.
Solanum alatum Moench, shrub nightshade	*Solanum ottonis* Hyl.
Solanum americanum Mill.	*Solanum papita* Rydb.
Solanum atriplicifolium Gill. ex Nees	*Solanum paranense* Dusen
Solanum auriculatum Ait. = *S. mauritianum* Scop., violet nightshade	*Solanum persicum* Willd. ex Roem. & Schult.
Solanum aviculare G. Forst., Australian nightshade	*Solanum pseudo-capsicum* L., Jerusalem cherry
Solanum bonariense L.	*Solanum pyracanthum* Jacq.
Solanum capsicastrum Link, ex. Schau., false Jerusalem cherry	*Solanum rantonnettii* Carr. ex Lescuy., Paraguay nightshade
Solanum carolinense L., Carolina horsenettle	*Solanum saponaceum* Dun.
Solanum cervantesii Lag.	*Solanum sinaicum* Boiss.
Solanum chlorocarpum Schur	*Solanum sisymbrifolium* Lam.
Solanum ciliatum Lam.	*Solanum sodomeum* L., apple-of Sodom nightshade
Solanum cornutum Lam., horned nightshade	*Solanum surattense* Burm. f.
Solanum decipiens Opiz	*Solanum tomentosum* L.
Solanum depilatum Kitag.	*Solanum tuberosum* L., potato
Solanum diflorum Vellozo	*Solanum tripartitum* Dun.
Solanum dulcamara L., bitter nightshade	*Solanum umbellatum* Mill.
	Solanum verbascifolium L., Mullein nightshade
	Valerianaceae
	Valeriana officinalis L., common valerian

humistratum Rshw., and *S. macroglobularum* Rshaw. These plant species, however, are not listed in literature dealing with plant classification and naming, i.e., *Index Kewensis* and J. C. Willis's *Dictionary of Flowering Plants and Ferns.* Consequently, these hosts are not listed in Table 1. In most species, however, no obvious symptoms develop. The viroid is easily transmitted by inoculation of sap (O'Brien and Raymer, 1964) and by contaminated grafting and cutting tools. Seed transmission of PSTV in solanaceous plants has been reported (Hunter *et al.,* 1969; Singh, 1970). At present, two strains of PSTV, mild and severe, are known which cross-protect one against the other in tomato (Fernow, 1967). In potato fields, the mild strain of PSTV prevails over the severe one (Singh *et al.,* 1970), and the mild and severe strains have been reported to cause up to 24% and 64%, respectively, reduction in potato yield (Singh *et al.,* 1971).

The reported host range of CEV (Table 3) (Olson and Shull, 1956; Childs *et al.,* 1958; Weathers *et al.,* 1967; Garnsey and Whidden, 1970) is narrower than that of PSTV. However, the two viroids elicit similar

TABLE 3
Host Range of Citrus Exocortis Viroid (CEV)

Family and species	Family and species
Compositae	Solanaceae (*Continued*)
Gynura aurantiaca (Bl.) DC., Java velvet plant	*Petunia hybrida* Vilm., petunia
	Petunia violacea Lindl., violet petunia
Gynura sarmentosa (Bl.) DC. = *G. procumbens* (Lour.) Merr.	*Physalis floridana* Rydberg.
	Physalis ixocarpa Brot. ex Hornem., tomatillo groundcherry
Rutaceae	*Physalis peruviana* L., Peruvian groundcherry; cape gooseberry
Citrus aurantifolia (Christm.) = *C. limonica,* Swingle, lime	*Scopolia carniolica* Jacq., European scopolia
Citrus aurantium L., sour orange	*Scopolia lurida* Dun.
Citrus jambhiri Lush., rough lemon	*Scopolia physaloides* Dun.
Citrus limon Burm. f., Eureka lemon	*Scopolia sinensis* Hemsl.
Citrus medica L., Etrog citron	*Scopolia stramonifolia* (Wall.) Semenova
Citrus paradisi, Macf., grapefruit	*Scopolia tangutica* Maxim.
Citrus reticulata Blanco., Mandarin orange	*Solanum aculeatissimum* Jacq., soda-apple nightshade
Citrus sinensis (L.) Osbeck., sweet orange	*Solanum dulcamara* L., bitter nightshade
Citrus sinensis X *Poncirus trifoliata,* rusk orange	*Solanum hispidum* Pers.
Poncirus trifoliata (L) Raft., trifoliate orange	*Solanum integrifolium* Poir., Ethiopian eggplant
Solanaceae	*Solanum marginatum* L. f.
Lycopersicon esculentum Mill., common tomato	*Solanum quitoense* Lam.
	Solanum topiro Humb. & Bonpl. ex Dunal
Petunia axillaris (Lam.) B.S.P., Whitemoon petunia	*Solanum tuberosum* L., potato

TABLE 4

Host Range of Chrysanthemum Stunt Viroid (CSV)

Family and species
Compositae
Chrysanthemum carinatum Schousb., annual chrysanthemum, tricolor chrysanthemum
Chrysanthemum coccineum Willd., florists' pyrethrum, common pyrethrum
Chrysanthemum parathenium (L.) Bernh., feverfew chrysanthemum
Senecio cruentus (L'Her.) DC., common cineraria, florists' cineraria
Sonchus asper (L.) Hill, prickley sowthistle
Verbesina encelioides (Cav.) Benth. & Hook., golden crownbeard
Zinnia elegans Jacq., common zinnia, youth-and-old-age

responses in tomato, potato, *Scopolia* spp., *Gynura aurantiaca,* and *Petunia hybrida* (Semancik and Weathers, 1972a; Singh and Clark, 1973). These results led to the conclusion that PSTV and CEV were closely related, if not identical, strains of a single pathogenic agent (Singh and Clark, 1973; Semancik *et al.,* 1973a). Recent results indicate, however, that the two RNAs do not have the same primary sequence (see below). CEV is transmitted mechanically by grafting and pruning tools. Treatment of CEV-contaminated tools with RNase greatly reduces the infectivity of CEV (Garnsey and Whidden, 1974), which suggests that RNase could be useful as a practical sterilizing agent for CEV.

CSV is confined to plants in the composite family. Attempts to infect herbaceous plant species outside the family Compositae have failed (Hollings and Stone, 1973). Plant species susceptible to infection by CSV are shown in Table 4. Stunt disease spreads rapidly by foliage contact and by handling plants. The viroid is not transmitted through chrysanthemum seeds (Hollings and Stone, 1973).

At present, no systematic study of the host range of ChCMV has been reported. *Chrysanthemum morifolium* (Ramat.) Hemsl. is the only known host. ChCMV is extremely unstable in crude extract; however, grinding of infected tissue in alkaline buffer (pH 7.5–9) significantly increases the stability and infectivity of the agent (Romaine and Horst, 1975). CSV and ChCMV do not seem to be related because CSV infection does not protect against subsequent infection by ChCMV (Romaine and Horst, 1975). A latent infectious agent that protects against ChCMV infection was found in cultivars of *Chrysanthemum morifolium* (Horst, 1975). At present, the identity of the latent agent has not been determined; however, it is possible that the agent is a strain of ChCMV.

CPFV is mechanically transmissible and is able to infect a large number of cucurbitaceous species (Van Dorst and Peters, 1974) as well as tomato (Sänger *et al.,* 1976). With cadang-cadang disease of coconut, no successful transmission, mechanically or otherwise, to any plant species, including coconut palm, has been reported (Randles, 1975).

2.5. Cytopathic Effects

Comparison of sections prepared from uninfected and PSTV-infected tomato leaves and petioles revealed a marked hypertrophy of nuclei in the infected tissue. Also, protoplasmic streaming was found to be consistently more active in cells from infected than in those from healthy tissue (Diener, 1971c).

Electron microscopic examination of thin sections of CEV-infected *Gynura* leaves revealed the appearance of paramural bodies or boundary formations at the cell-plasma membrane interface (Semancik and Vanderwoude, 1976). The components of these formations may fuse to form vesicles or membrane proliferations while usually remaining near the cell surface.

2.6. Subcellular Location *in Situ*

Bioassays of subcellular fractions from PSTV-infected tissue disclosed that appreciable infectivity is present only in the original tissue debris and in the fraction containing nuclei. Chloroplasts, mitochondria, ribosomes, and the soluble fraction contain no more than traces of infectivity. Furthermore, when chromatin was isolated from infected tissue, most infectivity was associated with it and could be extracted as free RNA with phosphate buffer (Diener, 1971a). These and other experiments suggest that, *in situ,* PSTV is associated with the nuclei, and particularly with the chromatin, of infected cells. The significant amount of infectivity regularly present in the tissue debris most probably is a consequence of incomplete extraction of nuclei by the method chosen (Kuehl, 1964), but the possibility that some PSTV is associated with cell membranes cannot be ruled out at present.

The association of PSTV with chromatin may explain its heterogeneous sedimentation properties in crude extracts (see below). In addition to free PSTV, PSTV associated with chromatin fragments of varying size may be present, and the latter entities may constitute the faster-sedimenting portions of infectious material.

Experiments with CEV (Sänger, 1972) disclosed that the infectious RNA is similarly located in the nuclei of infected cells and that it exists in close association with the chromatin. Purified fractions of chloroplasts, ribosomes, and mitochondria prepared from CEV-infected *Gynura* plants were devoid of infectivity (Sänger, 1972). Recently, Semancik *et al.* (1976) have reported that CEV in *Gynura* is associated not only with nuclei-rich preparations but also with a plasma membrane-like component of the endomembrane system. Evidence of the association of CEV with plasma membrane components was obtained by analyzing 1000–80,000*g* fractions from CEV-infected *Gynura* on equilibrium sucrose density gradients, followed by assaying of each collected density gradient fraction for infectivity and for activity of enzyme markers of cell components. Although CEV infectivity was associated with the plasma membrane-like component, the activity of DNA-directed RNA polymerase associated with that component was unusually high. It is known that the activity of that enzyme in higher plants is specifically associated with cellular nuclei and chloroplasts. Contamination of the plasma membrane-like component with nuclear membranes and/or chloroplast fragments could readily explain the association of infectivity with the plasma component.

3. EVIDENCE FOR EXISTENCE OF VIROIDS

3.1. Sedimentation Properties and Nuclease Sensitivity

Early work had shown that in crude extracts from potato or tomato leaves affected with the potato spindle tuber disease, most of the infectious material sediments at very low rates (approximately 10 S), making it unlikely that the extracted infectious agent is a conventional virus particle. As the agent was found to be insensitive to treatment with various organic solvents, lipid-containing virus particles of low density also appeared to be ruled out. Treatment of crude extracts with phenol affected neither the infectivity nor the sedimentation properties of the agent. In view of these findings, it was proposed that the agent is a free nucleic acid. Incubation of crude extracts with nucleases revealed that the agent is sensitive to ribonuclease, but not to deoxyribonuclease (Diener and Raymer, 1967). The observation that the agent could readily be concentrated by ethanol precipitation and resuspension in a small volume of buffer is compatible with the concept that the extractable agent is a free nucleic acid. Incubation of extracts with ribonuclease in media of high ionic strength disclosed that the agent partially survives this treatment. This property, as well as the elution pattern from columns of methylated serum albumin, suggested that the extractable agent may be a double-stranded RNA (Diener and Raymer, 1967, 1969).

Singh and Bagnall (1968) extracted infectious nucleic acid from PSTV-infected tissue and compared some of its properties with those of PSTV in crude extracts. They found that, compared with the agent in a crude extract, the RNA had a greater infectivity dilution end point and higher thermal inactivation point, and was more sensitive to ribonuclease. Also, when infectivity of a crude extract was removed by heating or by incubation with ribonuclease, it could be restored by treatment with phenol (Singh and Bagnall, 1968). From comparative centrifugation studies, the authors concluded that no free infectious RNA was present in crude extracts, but did not specify what the RNA was bound to.

Results similar to those of Diener and Raymer (1967) were reported by Semancik and Weathers (1968), who worked with citrus exocortis disease. They found that most infectivity present in clarified extracts prepared from infected tissue remained in the supernatant solution after high-speed centrifugation; the authors came to the conclusion that the infectious entity possesses a sedimentation coefficient of about 10–15 S. Because of these results and because no typical virus particles could be observed in electron micrographs of infectious aliquots, the authors suggested that "the virus might represent an infectious nucleic acid form perhaps analogous to either the unstable form of tobacco rattle virus, the nonassembling mutants of tobacco mosaic virus, or a protein-free, double-stranded RNA molecule."

A third plant pathogen, the agent of chrysanthemum stunt disease, was shown by Lawson (1968) to have properties in crude extracts somewhat similar to those of PSTV and CEV. CSV, in partially purified form, sediments in sucrose gradients with rates of about 5–7.5 S, whereas in crude extracts it sediments more heterogeneously and faster-sedimenting infectious material is always present (Diener and Lawson, 1973). CSV displays properties characteristic of nucleic acids in crude extracts, such as insensitivity to treatment with organic solvents and sensitivity to treatment with RNase but not to treatment with DNase or to precipitation with ethanol (Diener and Lawson, 1973; Hollings and Stone, 1973).

Romaine and Horst (1975) reported that the predominant infectious species of ChCMV sediments between 6 and 14 S, but with minor species sedimenting between 18 and 23 S and 35 and 40 S. ChCMV has a high sensitivity to RNase in crude extracts as well as in a more purified state and is resistant to treatment with DNase, chloroform, *n*-butanol, phenol, and sodium dodecylsulfate (SDS). Sänger *et al.* (1976) reported recently that the sedimentation coefficient of CPFV is 6.5 S and that of PSTV or CEV is 6.7 S.

Coconut palms with cadang-cadang contain two apparently disease-specific RNA species—one of them with a sedimentation coefficient of 7.5 S (Randles, 1975). RNase treatment of crude sap from diseased palm causes the loss of the two disease-specific RNA species from subsequent nucleic acid preparations.

3.2. Absence of Virions

Although there is little doubt that the slowly sedimenting infectious entities in preparations from PSTV-, CEV-, CSV-, ChCMV, and CPFV-infected tissues are free RNA molecules, the question arises as to whether these infectious entities exist as such *in situ* or whether they are released from conventional virus particles during extraction.

A systematic study of this question with PSTV led to results that are incompatible with the concept that conventional viral nucleoprotein particles exist in PSTV-infected tissue (Diener, 1971a). Diener demonstrated that the sedimentation properties of the faster-sedimenting infectious material which is present in crude extracts (and which could presumably consist of virions) are not significantly altered by treatment of crude extracts with phenol or with phenol in the presence of SDS. These results make it unlikely that the RNA is bound to protein or that it is present in the form of complete or partially degraded virions. This conclusion was strengthened by the observation that highly purified RNA preparations from PSTV-infected tissue also contain infectious material that sediments at faster rates than would be expected of free RNA (Diener, 1971a). If the faster-sedimenting infectious material were composed of viral nucleoprotein particles, these particles would have most unusual properties. On the one hand, their protein coat would have to be loose enough to allow access to ribonuclease (since all infectivity is sensitive to treatment with ribonuclease); yet, on the other hand, these structures would have to be resistant to treatment with phenol and SDS. As there are apparently no known nucleoproteins with these properties, Diener (1971a) concluded that the faster-sedimenting infectious material is not composed of viral nucleoprotein particles.

This conclusion was further strengthened by the observation that, *in situ,* PSTV is sensitive to treatment with ribonuclease. Vacuum infiltration of ribonuclease solutions into PSTV-infected leaves resulted in complete or nearly complete loss of infectivity under conditions where the infectivity of conventional virus particles was not affected (Diener, 1971c).

Zaitlin and Hariharasubramanian (1972) analyzed proteins isolated from PSTV-infected leaves and compared them with proteins isolated from uninfected leaves. They found no evidence for the production in infected leaves of proteins that could be construed as coat proteins under conditions where coat protein of a defective strain of tobacco mosaic virus could readily be demonstrated (see Chapter 3).

No evidence of conventional virus particles has been obtained in preparations of CEV (Semancik and Weathers, 1968), CSV (Diener and Lawson, 1973; Hollings and Stone, 1973), ChCMV (Romaine and Horst, 1975), cadang-cadang (Randles, 1975), or CPFV (Sänger *et al.,* 1976).

3.3. Molecular Weight Estimates of Native Viroids

The low sedimentation rate of PSTV is consistent with a viral genome of conventional size ($\geq 10^6$ daltons) only if the RNA is double-stranded or multistranded. Early experiments indeed indicated that the RNA might be double-stranded (Diener and Raymer, 1969), but later results showed that its chromatographic properties are not compatible with this hypothesis (Diener, 1971c).

Evidently, determination of the molecular weights of viroids is of great importance in elucidating their structure. This determination is difficult, because the agents occur in infected tissue in very small amounts and are therefore difficult to separate from host RNA and to purify in amounts sufficient for conventional biophysical analyses.

A concept elaborated by Loening (1967) made it feasible to determine the molecular weight of PSTV, using infectivity as the sole parameter. Combined sedimentation and gel electrophoretic analyses conclusively showed that the infectious RNA has a very low molecular weight (Diener, 1971b). A value of 5×10^4 was compatible with the experimental results (Diener, 1971b). This conclusion was confirmed by the ability of PSTV to penetrate into polyacrylamide gels of high concentration (small pore size), from which high molecular weight RNA molecules are excluded (Diener and Smith, 1971). Singh and Clark (1971) reported some results that appear also to indicate that

PSTV is an RNA of low molecular weight. They concluded from a determination of the electrophoretic mobility of PSTV in a 7.5% polyacrylamide gel that "peak infectivity corresponded to a particle size of 4–5 Svedberg units."

On the basis of its electrophoretic mobility in 5% polyacrylamide gels, Semancik and Weathers (1972b) came to the conclusion that CEV is a low molecular weight RNA. They estimated that the RNA has a molecular weight of 1.25×10^5. Sänger (1972), on the other hand, estimated that CEV has a molecular weight of $5–6 \times 10^4$. Diener and Lawson (1973) showed by a combination of isokinetic density gradient centrifugation and electrophoresis in 20% polyacrylamide gels that CSV is a low molecular weight RNA similar to, but distinct from, PSTV.

Although these determinations conclusively demonstrate that presently known viroids are low molecular weight RNAs, the molecular weight values arrived at must be regarded with caution for two reasons. First, all determinations are based on the electrophoretic mobility in polyacrylamide gels of native RNA molecules relative to RNA standards of known molecular weight. The electrophoretic mobilities of RNA, however, are a function not only of their molecular weights (or, more correctly, of their molecular volumes) but also of their particular secondary and tertiary structures (Boedtker, 1971). Thus, if viroids should appreciably differ in structure from RNA standards used, the reported molecular weight values could be substantially in error. Second, results with PSTV suggest that the RNA may occur in several states of aggregation (Diener, 1971b). Some of the values reported, therefore, may be based on aggregates, and not on the monomeric form of the RNA.

When native PSTV was analyzed in 3%, 5%, or 7.5% polyacrylamide gels, paucidisperse distribution of the RNA was observed, with apparent molecular weight values of about 5×10^4 and 1×10^5 (Diener, 1971b). Because of the 1:2 ratio of the apparent molecular weights and because of the fact that all of the PSTV entered 20% polyacrylamide gels and migrated with an apparent molecular weight of 5×10^4 (Diener and Smith, 1971), the hypothesis was advanced that native PSTV occurs in several states of aggregation, and that electrophoresis in gels of high concentration (small pore size) leads to disaggregation to the monomeric form of the RNA (Diener, 1971b; Diener and Smith, 1971).

In the case of CEV, Semancik et al. (1973b) reported that under nondenaturing conditions, at gel concentrations of less than 8–10%, the RNA migrates with an apparent molecular weight of about 1×10^5, whereas at gel concentrations greater than 8–10% it migrates with an apparent molecular weight of about 5×10^4. The authors accepted the 1×10^5 value as correct and concluded that the migration of native CEV in high-percentage gels is aberrant, "presumably resulting from its unusual structural properties."

Evidently, the discrepancy in the reported apparent molecular weights of native PSTV (5×10^4) and native CEV ($1–1.25 \times 10^5$) is not a consequence of different experimental results, but of different interpretation of essentially identical results. If, as postulated, the greater electrophoretic mobility of CEV in gels of high concentration, as compared with that in gels of low concentration, were due to its aberrant mobility in the former gels, it is difficult to understand why this process should not gradually become more pronounced as the gel concentration is increased. This clearly is not the case. At a gel concentration of 8–10%, an abrupt change in migration rate occurs and no intermediate values are observed (Semancik *et al.*, 1973*b*).

This sudden change in apparent molecular weight can readily be explained by the assumption that above a critical gel concentration (below a critical pore size) disaggregation of a dimer to a monomer occurs. This explanation appears plausible in view of the reported 1:2 ratio of the respective molecular weight values. Furthermore, Sänger (1972) reported an apparent molecular weight of $5–6 \times 10^4$ for native CEV, irrespective of whether the RNA was analyzed in gels of 5%, 10%, 15%, or 20% concentration.

Equilibrium sedimentation analysis of viroids resulted in molecular weight estimates of 1.27×10^5 for PSTV, 1.19×10^5 for CEV, and 1.10×10^5 for CPFV (Sänger *et al.*, 1976).

Chromatography of PSTV from *Scopolia sinensis* Hemsl. on Bio-Gel P200 revealed the presence of three infectious species of low molecular weight RNA (Singh *et al.*, 1974). The smallest infectious form was reported to be in the size range of tRNA, as estimated by its position in the gel filtration profile.

3.4. Identification of Viroids as Physical Entities

Although the above experiments clearly demonstrated that viroids are low molecular weight RNAs, further characterization of the molecules was not possible without isolation of the RNAs as physically recognizable entities. As a first step toward purification of PSTV, the RNA was extracted and purified from relatively large quantities of infected tomato leaves (Diener, 1972*a*). Identically extracted and purified preparations from healthy plants served as controls. Figure 2A shows the UV absorption profile of an RNA preparation from healthy leaves after electrophoresis in a 20% polyacrylamide gel. In addition to 5 S RNA, at least three additional UV-absorbing components are discernible in the gel (I, III, and IV). Evidently, these components are minor low molecular weight constituents of cellular RNA.

Figure 2B shows the UV absorption and infectivity distribution profiles of an identically obtained RNA preparation from PSTV-infected leaves after electrophoresis in a 20% polyacrylamide gel. In addition to 5 S RNA, four UV-absorbing components are discernible. The positions in the gel of three of these (I, III, and IV) coincide with those of components found in the preparation from healthy leaves. In addition, another prominent component is discernible (II). Bioassay of individual gel slices demonstrated that infectivity coincides with this component (Fig. 2B). This coincidence, the high level of infectivity, and the fact that component II could not be detected in preparations from healthy leaves constitute strong evidence that component II is PSTV.

These results therefore confirmed by physical means earlier conclusions that were based entirely on infectivity assays (Diener, 1971*b*; Diener and Smith, 1971). Isolation of PSTV as a ribonuclease-sensitive, UV-absorbing component demonstrates that the infectious agent is, indeed, an RNA, and since this RNA is able to penetrate into 20% polyacrylamide gels and to move through such gels as a monodisperse, UV-absorbing band, the low molecular weight of the RNA is confirmed.

4. PURIFICATION

These observations made it possible to isolate and purify PSTV in amounts sufficient for biophysical and biochemical analyses. To purify PSTV, preparations from which DNA, ribosomal RNAs, tRNA, and polysaccharides had previously been removed (Diener, 1971*b*) were subjected to electrophoresis for 16 h in 20% polyacrylamide gels. Under these conditions, PSTV migrates close to the bottom of the gel and is more completely separated from component III (Fig. 2B). The gel portion containing PSTV was excised from each gel. PSTV-containing portions from many gels were combined, and the RNA was eluted by homogenization of the gel slices in buffer. PSTV was then separated from the gel particles (and reconcentrated) by centrifugation, followed

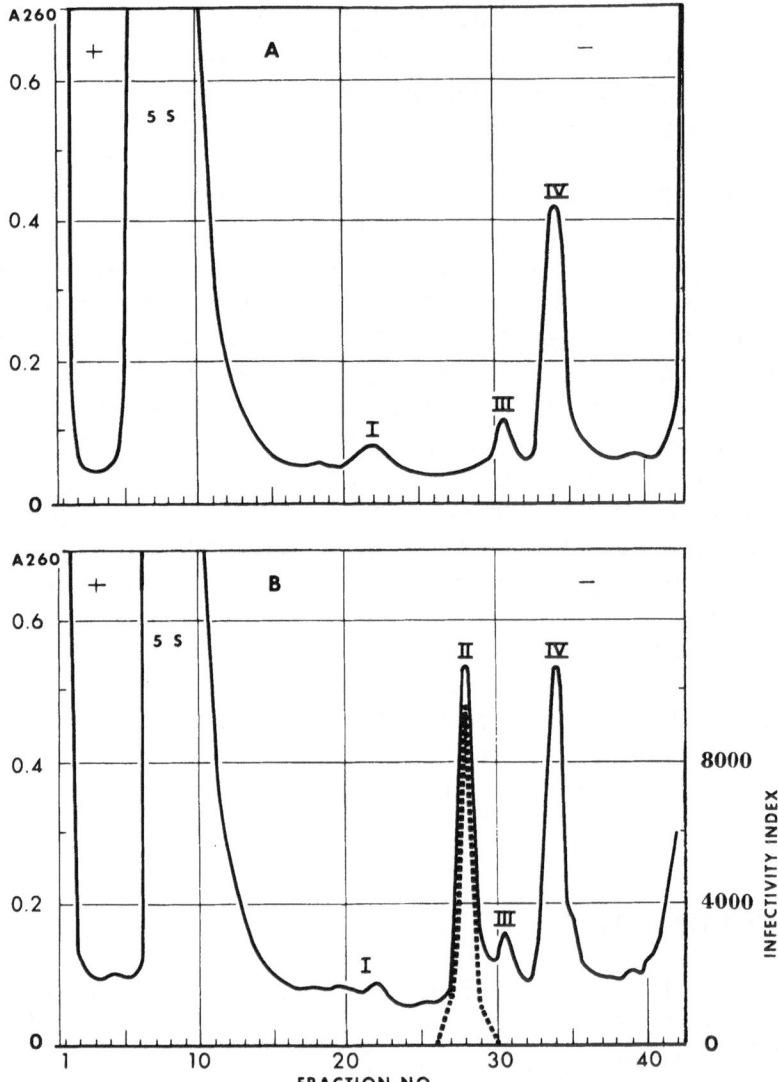

Fig. 2. A: UV absorption profile of RNA preparation from healthy tomato leaves after electrophoresis in a 20% polyacrylamide gel for 7.5 h at 4°C (5 mA per tube, constant current). B: UV absorption (——) and infectivity distribution (-----) of RNA preparation from PSTV-infected tomato leaves after electrophoresis in a 20% polyacrylamide gel (same conditions as in A). 5 S, 5 S ribosomal RNA; I, III, IV, unidentified minor components of cellular RNA; II, PSTV; A_{260}, absorbance at 260 nm. Electrophoretic movement from right to left. From Diener (1972a).

by hydroxylapatite chromatography of the supernatant solution. An impurity that elutes from the gels together with PSTV was removed by a procedure that involves shaking of the preparation with methoxyethanol (Diener, 1973c).

Analysis of the final preparations by polyacrylamide gel electrophoresis revealed that only one UV-absorbing component is consistently discernible in the gels. Comparison of this component with PSTV in less highly purified preparations (Diener, 1972b) disclosed that both have identical electrophoretic mobilities. Furthermore, infectivity distribution in the gels coincides with the UV-absorbing component. These observations indicate that the UV-absorbing component is PSTV and that the preparations are essentially free of contaminating nucleic acids (Diener and Smith, 1973).

With CEV also, a UV-absorbing component present in preparations from infected leaves, but not in preparations from healthy ones, could be detected in polyacrylamide gels (Semancik and Weathers, 1972b; Semancik et al., 1973a). Deviations from coincidence of the absorbance peak with infectivity distribution in the gels were noticed, but these deviations were ascribed to technical difficulties involved in scanning and cutting the same gel (Semancik and Weathers, 1972b).

Readers who are interested in detailed methods of viroid purification are referred to a recent review article on that subject (Diener et al., 1977).

5. PHYSICAL AND CHEMICAL PROPERTIES

Although purification of PSTV and CEV is now feasible, the separation procedure is laborious and yields only microgram quantities of purified viroid. With supplies so far available, the following physical and chemical properties of viroids have been studied.

5.1. Molecular Weight

With the availability of purified PSTV, a redetermination of its molecular weight based not on its biological activity but on its absorption of UV light became possible. For this purpose, a method described by Boedtker (1971) appeared particularly promising, as it is supposed to permit the determination of the molecular weight of an RNA independent of its conformation.

With this method, RNAs are treated with formaldehyde at 63°C, a treatment which, according to Boedtker (1971) completely denatures the RNAs, i.e., destroys their secondary and tertiary structures. Consequently, the electrophoretic migration of formylated RNAs in polyacrylamide gels is a function of their molecular weights, but not of their particular conformations.

To apply this method to PSTV, it was necessary to compare its rate of migration in gels with those of formylated RNAs of known molecular weights. Of all marker RNAs available, the electrophoretic mobility of formylated tobacco ringspot satellite virus (SAT) RNA (Schneider, 1971) was closest to that of formylated PSTV. Hence this RNA was most useful as a molecular weight marker, particularly in gels with small pore size, from which high molecular weight RNAs are excluded.

Since the molecular weight of SAT RNA had so far been estimated only from its sedimentation coefficient by use of an empirical formula (Schneider, 1971), it was important to determine its molecular weight by gel electrophoresis of the RNA after treatment with formaldehyde.

Accordingly, formylated SAT RNA was analyzed by electrophoresis, in the presence of formaldehyde, using formylated tRNA, 5 S RNA, and other rRNAs, and carnation mottle virus (CarMV) RNA (Waterworth and Kaper, 1972) as molecular weight markers (Diener and Smith, 1973).

A linear relationship was found between the electrophoretic mobility of each RNA (expressed as the ratio of its movement in the gel to that of a visible marker, bromophenol blue dye) and the logarithm of its molecular weight. The results indicate that the molecular weight of SAT RNA lies between 7.7×10^4 and 8.4×10^4.

Formylated PSTV was next analyzed by electrophoresis together with formylated SAT RNA, 5 S RNA, and tRNA as markers. Figure 3 shows the results of one analysis. The electrophoretic mobility of formylated PSTV is slightly greater than that of formylated SAT RNA. This result and those of additional experiments indicate that the molecular weights of PSTV and SAT RNA are similar and that, therefore, the molecular weight of PSTV is within the range of 7.5×10^4 to 8.5×10^4 (Diener and Smith, 1973).

The pronounced discrepancy between this value and that obtained with native PSTV (5×10^4) is most likely due to the compact structure of the RNA (see below) and illustrates the substantial error inherent in efforts to estimate molecular weights of viroids by gel electrophoresis of native molecules.

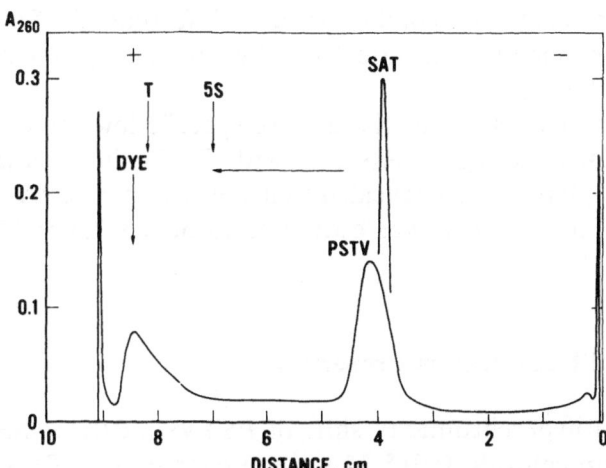

Fig. 3. UV absorption profile of formylated PSTV after electrophoresis (in the presence of formaldehyde) in a 5% polyacrylamide gel. The position of formylated SAT RNA (SAT), as determined in separate gels, is indicated by the top of the UV-absorbing peak (shown at same scale as that of PSTV). The positions of other formylated marker RNAs are shown by arrows. Abbreviations: T, tRNA; 5 S, 5 S ribosomal RNA; SAT, tobacco ringspot satellite virus RNA. Electrophoretic movement from right to left. From Diener and Smith (1973).

A molecular weight estimate for PSTV in urea of 8.9×10^4 was obtained by electron microscopy (Sogo *et al.*, 1973) (see below). This value is in excellent agreement with the values obtained from analysis of heat-denatured, formylated PSTV in polyacrylamide gels (Diener and Smith, 1973). McClements and Kaesberg (1977) determined the size of formylated and nonformylated PSTV by electron microscopy. The molecular weight for the linear molecule of PSTV was estimated to be 1.1×10^5 and that of a newly described circular molecule 1.37×10^5 (see below). Equilibrium sedimentation analyses of denatured, circular molecules of PSTV, CEV, and CPFV led to molecular weight estimates of 1.27×10^5, 1.19×10^5, and 1.10×10^5, respectively (Sänger *et al.*, 1976).

Semancik *et al.* (1973a) estimated the molecular weight of CEV and PSTV in 5% gels under nondenaturing conditions and reported that both viroids have an identical size, 1.25×10^5. Dickson *et al.* (1975) analyzed PSTV and CEV, under identical conditions in polyacrylamide gels, using denaturing and nondenaturing conditions at different gel concentrations. PSTV moved faster than CEV when the electrophoretic analyses were done under nondenaturing conditions—5%, 10%, or 15%

gel—or under denaturing conditions of 98% formamide–5% gel. PSTV and CEV components of identical mobility were only observed in 98% formamide–10% gel.

A comparative study of the disease-specific low molecular weight RNA of cadang-cadang (ccRNA-1) with PSTV in denaturing form-amide polyacrylamide gels revealed that the size of ccRNA-1 is smaller than that of PSTV, and it was estimated to be 6.3–7.3×10^4 (Randles *et al.*, 1976).

5.2. Thermal Denaturation Properties

The total hyperchromicity shift of PSTV in $0.01 \times$ SSC (SSC is 0.15 M sodium chloride–0.015 M sodium citrate, pH 7.0) is about 24% and the T_m about 50°C (Diener, 1972*a*). The thermal denaturation curve (Fig. 4) indicates that PSTV is not a regularly base-paired struc-ture, such as double-stranded RNA, since in this case denaturation would be expected to occur over a narrower temperature range and at higher temperatures (Miura *et al.*, 1966). PSTV could, however, be an

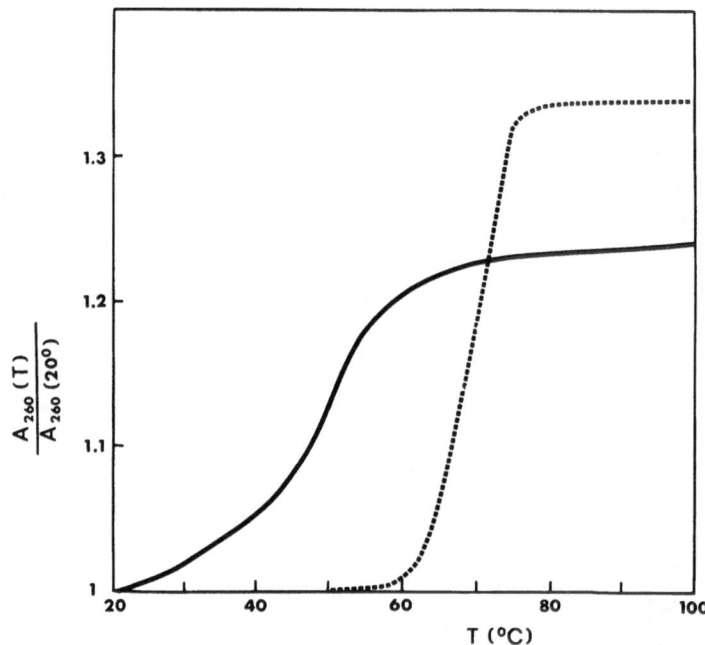

Fig. 4. Thermal denaturation curves of PSTV (——) and of double-stranded rice dwarf virus RNA (-----) in $0.01 \times$ SSC.

irregularly base-paired, single-stranded RNA molecule, similar to transfer RNA, in which single-stranded regions alternate with base-paired regions.

Determination of the thermal denaturation properties of PSTV dissolved in buffer of higher ionic strength (0.1 × SSC) confirmed these conclusions since, again, denaturation occurred over a wide temperature range. Under these conditions, T_m was about 54°C (Diener, unpublished observations).

Semancik *et al.* (1975) reported that CEV in 0.1 × SSC showed a T_m of 52°C, with a hyperchromic shift of about 22%. Sänger *et al.* (1976) reported a T_m of about 51°C for CPFV and a hyperchromic shift of 22% in 0.01 M sodium cacodylate, pH 6.8, 1 mM EDTA. The smallest RNA (8.4 × 10⁴) associated with cadang-cadang disease of coconut was reported to exhibit a thermal denaturation curve with an approximate 10% hyperchromic shift and a T_m of about 58°C in 0.1 × SSC (Randles, 1975). The thermal denaturation curve of CEV, CPFV, or of the smallest RNA of cadang-cadang disease suggests some basepairing which is atypical of either a double-stranded or a single-stranded RNA but which, again, most closely resembles that of PSTV.

5.3. Radiation Sensitivity

In view of the low molecular weight of PSTV, it was of interest to determine its sensitivity to irradiation with UV light. Although one might expect that a small molecule, such as PSTV, would be considerably more resistant to UV irradiation than a conventionally sized viral RNA or DNA, the effect of size on UV sensitivity of nucleic acids is not well understood (Adams, 1970).

Exposure of purified PSTV or of tobacco ringspot virus or its satellite to UV radiation of 254 nm showed that the inactivation dose for PSTV and satellite virus is 70–90 times as large as that for tobacco ringspot virus (Diener *et al.*, 1974) (Fig. 5). Although other explanations are possible (Diener *et al.*, 1974), this marked difference in sensitivity to UV radiation most likely is a consequence of the smaller size (smaller target volume) of PSTV and satellite RNA, as compared with tobacco ringspot virus RNA.

Semancik *et al.* (1973*b*) exposed preparations of CEV and tobacco mosaic virus to ionizing radiation and determined from comparative rates of biological inactivation a molecular weight of 1.1×10^5 for the target size of CEV.

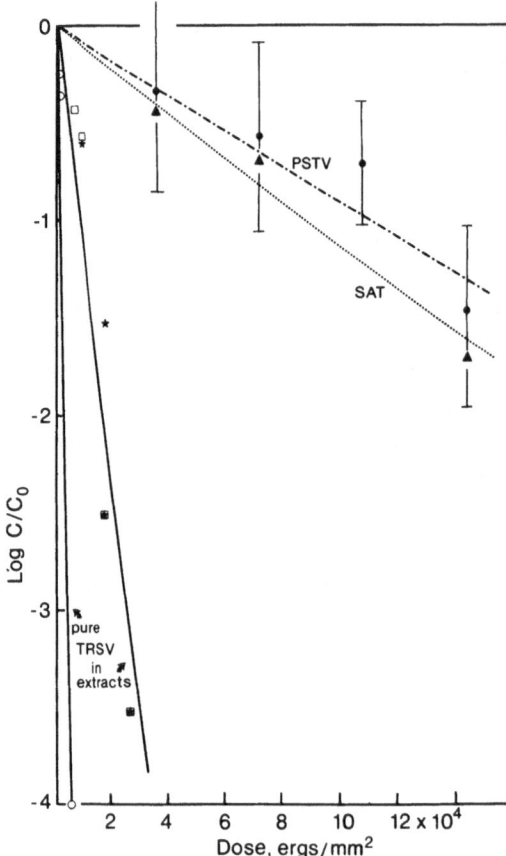

Fig. 5. Inactivation of PSTV, SAT, and TRSV by ultraviolet light of 254 nm. Logarithm of survival ratios (C/C_0) plotted as a function of incident dose. ●, Purified PSTV; vertical bars, 95% fiducial limits for ratios to controls; ▲, purified SAT; ○, purified TRSV. From Diener *et al.* (1974).

5.4. Electron Microscopy of Viroids

Sogo *et al.* (1973) processed purified preparations of PSTV for electron microscopy by the protein monolayer spreading technique of Kleinschmidt and Zahn (1959). When PSTV preparations in 4 M sodium acetate were spread onto a hypophase of distilled water, very short structures, mostly in compact aggregates but occasionally as separate particles, were revealed. These structures could not be detected in nucleic acid-free controls and they were absent from preparations treated with ribonuclease.

Because of the association of PSTV molecules in aggregates, it was difficult to draw conclusions as to their length and structure. Consequently, methods which promised to dissociate the aggregates and to make possible the visualization of individual PSTV molecules were investigated. Indeed, large numbers of individual short strands of relatively uniform length were visible when PSTV preparations in 8 M urea were spread. No such strands were discernible in control samples or after treatment with ribonuclease. The average length of molecules was found to be about 50 nm.

Since the mass per unit length is unknown, the lengths of PSTV molecules were compared with those of nucleic acids of known molecular weight, which were added to PSTV preparations and were thus treated identically.

Figure 6 shows an electron micrograph of a mixture of a double-stranded DNA, namely, coliphage T_7 DNA and PSTV. Measurements indicated that T_7 DNA is about 280 times longer than PSTV. It is also apparent that the width of PSTV is similar to that of T_7 DNA. Assuming that the molecular weight of T_7 DNA is 25×10^5 (Lang, 1970) and that PSTV in urea is formed by two more or less base-paired strands (as either a hairpin or a double helix), then one obtains a molecular weight estimate for PSTV of 8.9×10^4.

Electron microscopy of mixtures of PSTV and formaldehyde-denatured viral RNA [carnation mottle virus RNA (Kaper and Waterworth, 1973), which has a molecular weight of about 1.35×10^6] revealed that PSTV is thicker than this single-stranded RNA and that the viral RNA is about 17 times longer than denatured PSTV (Sogo *et al.*, 1973). This comparison leads to a molecular weight estimate of 7.9×10^4 for PSTV.

The molecular weight estimates obtained by electron microscopy are, therefore, in excellent agreement with the values obtained from analysis of heat-denatured, formylated PSTV in polyacrylamide gels.

Recently, McClements and Kaesberg (1977) examined nondenatured and denatured PSTV by electron microscopy, utilizing the spreading technique of Inman and Schnös (1970). The mean length of the main distribution of nondenatured PSTV was found to be 0.05 ± 0.1 μm and is identical to that reported by Sogo *et al.* (1973) for native PSTV. Under denaturing conditions, using formamide, PSTV preparations contained, in addition to the native particles, two single-stranded RNA components of differing sizes, one linear with a mean length of 0.09 ± 0.1 μm and one circular with a mean length (circumference) of 0.11 ± 0.01 μm. Pretreatment of PSTV with formaldehyde by the method of Boedtker (1971), followed by formamide treatment, revealed that PSTV contained mainly the linear and circular molecules and the linear component was about 4 times more common than the circular. From length measurements of formylated and non-formylated PSTV, the estimated molecular weight for the linear molecule is 1.1×10^5 and for the circular is 1.37×10^5. Both components exist in collapsed, highly base-paired structures under

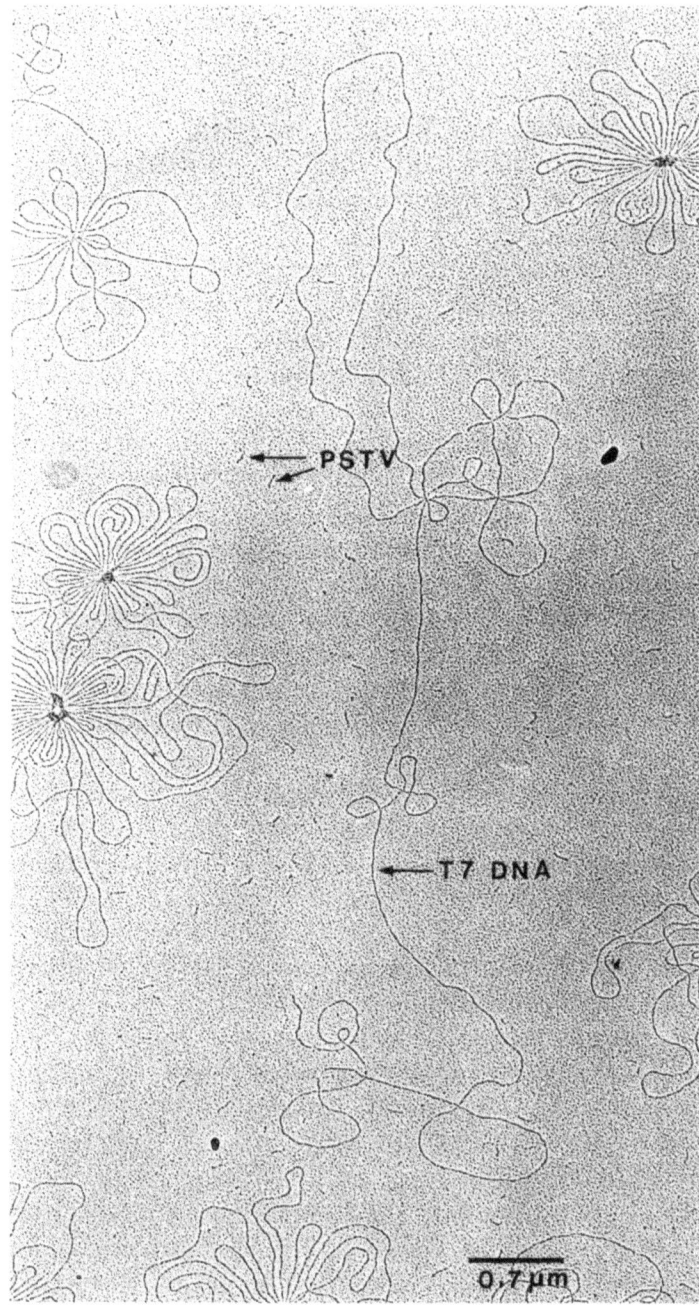

Fig. 6.   Electron micrograph of PSTV mixed with a double-stranded DNA, coliphage
T₇ DNA. Native T₇ DNA (0.8 μg/ml) was mixed with PSTV (0.4 μg/ml) previously
heated for 10 min at 63°C in the presence of 8 M urea, followed by quenching in ice
water. Note that double-stranded T₇ DNA and PSTV have similar widths. Courtesy of
T. Koller and J. M. Sogo.

nondenaturing conditions. Both components are sensitive to digestion by pancreatic ribonuclease, but resistant to snake venom phosphodiesterase.

Sänger *et al.* (1976) examined native and denatured CPFV by electron microscopy. Examination of native CPFV revealed rods or dumbbell molecules with an average particle length of 35 nm. Denaturation of CPFV at 60°C for 5 min in the presence of formamide (80%), urea (4.8 M), formaldehyde (0.4%), and benzyldimethylalkylammonium chloride (25 μg/ml) revealed a variety of structures ranging from rodlike molecules to full circles. The majority of the population consisted of intermediate forms with contours like tennis rackets. Linear molecules (0.5–1%) and balloonlike structures were also detected.

5.5. Molecular Structure

For a number of years, the molecular structure of viroids remained enigmatic, because in some analytical systems they display properties typical of double-stranded RNA, in others properties of single-stranded RNA.

Thus the elution pattern of PSTV from columns of methylated serum albumin suggests double strandedness (Diener and Raymer, 1969), whereas the elution pattern from CF-11 cellulose columns (Franklin, 1966) is consistent with both single- and double-stranded molecules (Diener and Raymer, 1969). A possible explanation for this observation, however, may be deduced from the work of Engelhardt (1972), who showed that the extent of secondary structure of an RNA has a profound influence on its elution pattern from such columns. He found that the greater the amount of secondary structure of an RNA at the time of addition to the column, the greater is the fraction that will elute in ethanol-free buffer, i.e., in the eluate that formerly was believed to consist solely of double-stranded RNA (Franklin, 1966). Judged by this criterion, native PSTV has an extensive secondary structure.

From hydroxylapatite, on the other hand, PSTV elutes mostly at a phosphate buffer concentration lower than that expected of a double-stranded RNA (Diener, 1971c; Lewandowski *et al.*, 1971). Some PSTV, however, elutes at higher buffer concentration (Diener, 1971c).

Immunological tests made with antisera that react specifically with double-stranded RNA (Schwartz and Stollar, 1969) gave no evidence for the presence of double-stranded RNA in highly infectious PSTV preparations (Stollar and Diener, 1971). The thermal denaturation properties of PSTV clearly rule out a regularly base-paired double helix; yet, in electron micrographs, PSTV appears definitely thicker than single-stranded RNA, and of about equal thickness as double-stranded DNA (Sogo *et al.*, 1973). This would be consistent either with a double-stranded molecule with incomplete base pairing or with a single-stranded molecule folded back on itself in the form of a hairpin. To examine the nature of the double-stranded region in PSTV or CEV, unlabeled PSTV or ^{125}I-labeled CEV preparations were treated with double-strand-specific *Escherichia coli* RNase III (Robertson *et al.*, 1967) under conditions that allow the enzyme to demonstrate its full capacity to cleave RNA (Dickson, 1976). Neither the electrophoretic mobility of PSTV or [^{125}I]CEV (Dickson, 1976) nor the infectivity of PSTV (Diener, unpublished) is affected by RNase III treatment. Because RNase III requires either an extended region of perfect double-stranded RNA (about 25 or more base pairs) or a highly specialized RNA sequence (Robertson and Hunter, 1975; Robertson and Dunn, 1975) to cleave RNA, it appears that neither PSTV nor CEV contain such regions.

Thermal denaturation studies of circular molecules of CPFV revealed that the complementary sequences may form one long (>60 base pairs) and fairly regular double helix and not only short hairpins like tRNA, 5 S RNA, and 6 S RNA (Sänger *et al.*, 1976).

Recently, McClements and Kaesberg (1977) studied the structure of PSTV by electron microscopy and detected the presence of linear and circular forms of PSTV which exhibit extensive base pairing and appear as collapsed double-stranded rods under non-denaturing conditions. Both components are sensitive to digestion by pancreatic ribonuclease but resistant to snake venom phosphodiesterase. Diener (1971*c*) reported that incubation of PSTV with snake venom phosphodiesterase had no effect on the infectivity of PSTV, which indicates that PSTV either is circular or is "masked" at the 3′ terminus in such a fashion that the enzyme cannot attack the terminal nucleotide. Since incubation of PSTV with a mixture of snake venom phosphodiesterase and alkaline phosphatase did not reduce PSTV infectivity (Diener, 1971*c*), this masking cannot be due to a phosphorylated 3′ terminus.

Recent detection of circular forms of PSTV partially explains the resistance of PSTV to degradation by snake venom phosphodiesterase. However, linear PSTV molecules were also shown to be resistant to degradation with snake venom phosphodiesterase (McClements and Kaesberg, 1977). Incubation of PSTV with bovine spleen phosphodiesterase, which attacks the nucleic acid from the 5′ terminus, similarly had no effect on the infectivity of PSTV (Diener, 1971c).

In situ, the viroid probably exists as an almost completely but not entirely double-stranded structure. Such a structure could confer the ribonuclease resistance reported by Diener and Raymer (1969). The double-stranded linear form resembles a hairpin. The base-paired form of the circle is hairpinlike, with closures at both ends. This structure conforms to the prediction of Diener and Smith (1973) and explains prior difficulty in determining the strandedness of PSTV.

McClements and Kaesberg (1977) found that the denaturation of (at least) the linear molecule always begins at the closed or loop end of the hairpin and proceeds toward the open end. No "Y"-shaped molecules have ever been detected. These results suggest that the double-helical structure is less stable at the loop end than at the open end of the hairpin. This susceptibility to denaturation may be the result of a lower proportion of $G+C$ type base pairs, or generally fewer base pairs at the loop end. Physical studies of a similar viroid (CEV), which suggest that the loop end may be enriched for $A+U$ type base pairs (Semancik *et al.*, 1975), support the former proposal. Since no protein has been detected in association with purified PSTV (Diener, 1971a, Sänger *et al.*, 1976), it is unlikely that the double-stranded form is stabilized by a protein.

The suggestion that PSTV may be composed of more than one component was first made by Diener and Smith (1973), who showed that formylated PSTV could be resolved into two bands in gels of high polyacrylamide concentration. Whether these two components represent the circular and linear forms described by McClements and Kaesberg remains to be determined. The two structures may be two distinct RNA components or may represent two stages of maturity of a single RNA species. Preliminary sequencing data from a mixture of the two components are consistent with a single RNA sequence containing 250–350 bases (Dickson *et al.*, 1975). It seems likely, therefore, that the two structures are two forms of the same RNA. A tempting, but speculative, scheme is that the linear molecule arises from the circular molecule by a specific double-strand cut about 40 base pairs in from one loop of the native circular PSTV, with subsequent loss of the small fragment.

Randles *et al.* (1976) reported that the kinetics of digestion of the low molecular weight RNA associated with cadang-cadang disease (ccRNA-1) with RNase A and with single-strand-specific S_1 endonuclease, as well as thermal denaturation studies, indicate that ccRNA-1 has both double- and single-stranded regions. A comparative study with PSTV showed that the kinetics of digestion with S_1 nuclease of ccRNA-1 and PSTV are similar. Because disruption of base pairing by melting or hot formamide treatment failed to affect the apparent molecular weight of ccRNA-1, Randles *et al.* (1976) concluded that ccRNA-1 has a looped or "hairpin" secondary structure, stabilized by base pairing. Its buoyant density (1.62 g/ml) falls between the expected values for a single-stranded and a double-stranded viral RNA.

5.6. Composition and Primary Sequence

The base composition of purified PSTV, as determined by the procedure of Randerrath *et al.* (1972), is as follows: G, 28.9%; C, 28.3%; A, 21.7%; U, 20.9% (Niblett *et al.*, 1976). The G + C content is 57.2%, and AMP/UMP and GMP/CMP ratios approach unity. Pure ^{32}P-labeled PSTV, hydrolyzed with alkali and chromatographed on a Dowex formate column, contains 55% G + C (Hadidi, 1976). The base composition of CEV has been determined by polyacrylamide gel electrophoresis of nucleotides obtained from purified CEV by hydrolysis with KOH (Morris and Semancik, 1974; Semancik *et al.*, 1975). CEV base composition is similar to that of PSTV with molar nucleotide composition of CMP, 29.4%; AMP, 21.5%; GMP, 28.8%; UMP, 19.9%. CEV has a high G + C content (58.2%), and AMP/UMP and GMP/CMP ratios approach unity, as is the case with PSTV.

Attempts have been made (Hadidi *et al.*, 1976*b*) to detect poly(A) or poly(C) stretches in PSTV using the *E. coli* DNA polymerase I system in the presence of oligo(dT)$_{10}$ or oligo(dG)$_{12-18}$ primer as described by Modak *et al.* (1975). Addition of either primer to the DNA-synthesizing system did not result in increased synthesis of DNA complementary to PSTV, which indicates absence of poly(A) or poly(C) in PSTV (Hadidi *et al.*, 1976*b*). It is also reported that CEV does not contain poly(A) sequences (Semancik, 1974), as shown by the inability of CEV to hybridize with ^{3}H-labeled poly(U).

Some viral RNAs are known to bind a specific amino acid in a tRNA-like manner, but no such binding to CEV has been observed for any of the 20 amino acids typically found in proteins (Hall *et al.*, 1974; Hall and Davies, 1975).

Dickson *et al.* (1975) have shown by comparative two-dimensional fingerprinting analyses of ^{125}I-labeled PSTV and CEV that the major components of these two viroids are not identical. The minimum dif-

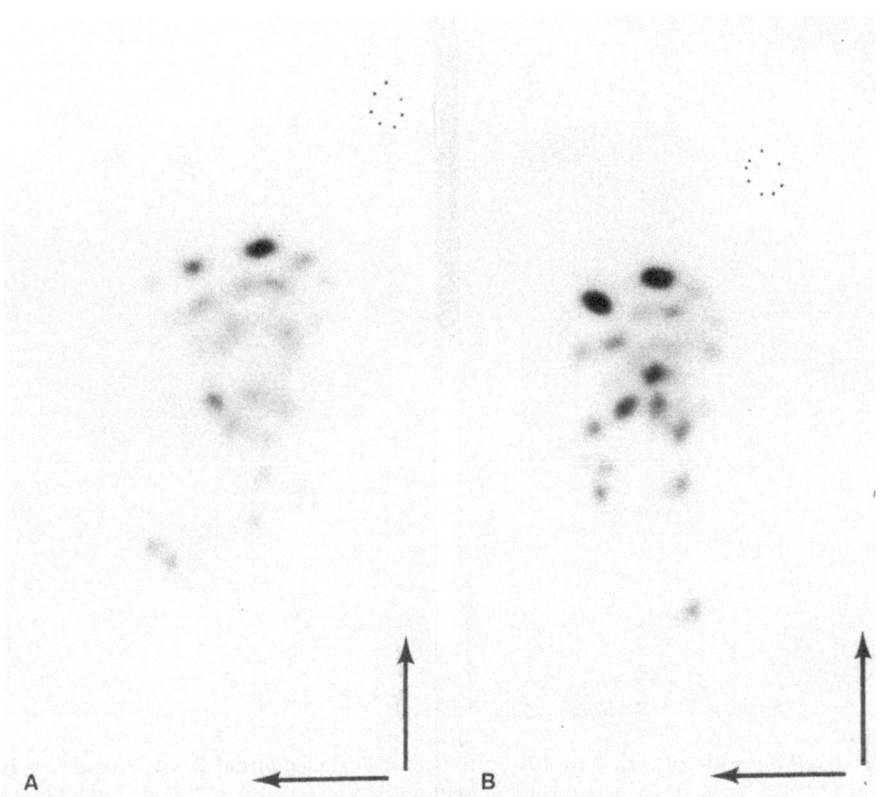

Fig. 7.   Ribonuclease T_1 fingerprints of ^{125}I-labeled viroid RNAs. About 1×10^4 dpm of ^{125}I-labeled RNA was mixed with 10 μg of bacteriophage f2 RNA and digested with 2 μg of RNase T_1 in 2 μl of 0.01 M tris-HCl (pH 7.5)–1 mM EDTA for 40 min at 37°C. Reaction mixtures were applied to cellulose acetate strips (Schleicher and Schuell, Keene, N.H.; 2.5 by 57 cm) soaked with 5% glacial acetic acid containing 5 mM EDTA in 7 M urea, and subjected to high-voltage electrophoresis (25 min, 6 kV). The oligonucleotides were transferred to Machery-Nagel 20- by 40-cm DEAE-cellulose thin-layer chromatography plates by standard procedures (Brownlee and Sanger, 1969). Second dimensions consisted of thin-layer homochromatography, a procedure carried out at 60°C, in which a partially hydrolyzed solution of yeast RNA (BDH) in 7 M urea moves upward over the DEAE-cellulose thin-layer plate, causing the oligonucleotides to separate according to size, with the smallest ones moving the longest way up the plate. In the configuration shown here, the first dimension was from right to left and the second was from bottom to top as shown by the arrows. A: PSTV RNA iodinated *in vitro* to a specific activity of 12×10^6 dpm/μg. B: CEV RNA iodinated *in vitro* to a specific activity of 18×10^6 dpm/μg. From Dickson *et al.* (1975).

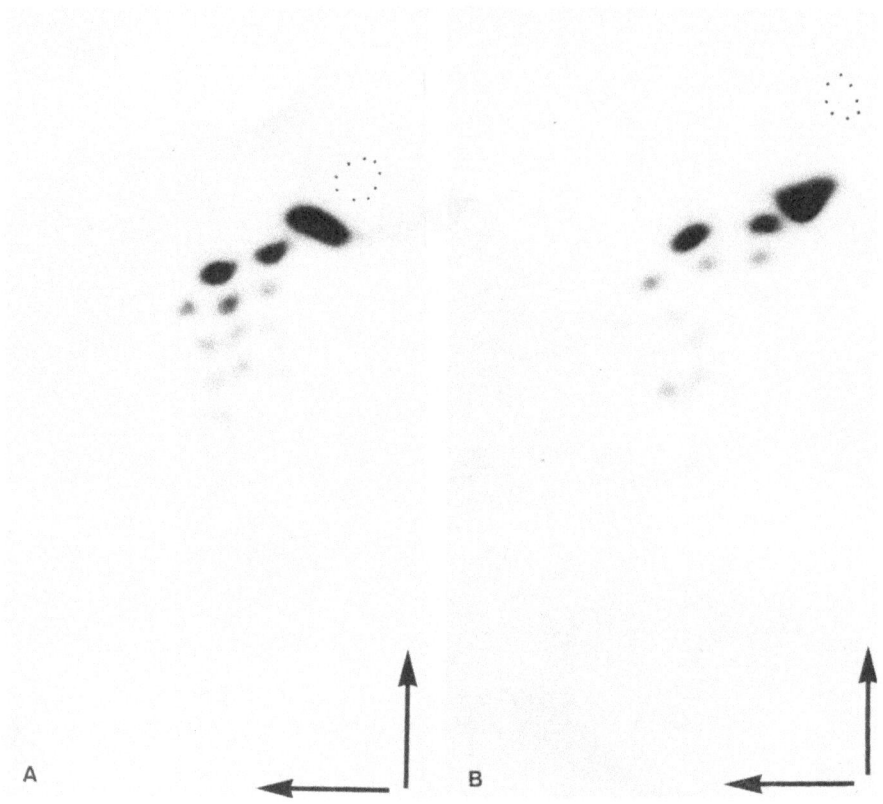

Fig. 8. Pancreatic ribonuclease fingerprints of ^{125}I-labeled viroid RNA. About 1×10^6 dpm of ^{125}I-labeled RNA was mixed with 10 μg of bacteriophage f2 RNA and digested with 2 μg of pancreatic ribonuclease in 2 μl of 0.01 M tris-HCl (pH 7.5)–1 mM EDTA for 30 min at 37°C. Two-dimensional finger-printing analyses were carried out exactly as detailed in the caption of Fig. 7. The origin is at the lower right: the electrophoretic first dimension was from right to left, and the second dimension (homochromatography) was from the bottom of the picture to the top. A: PSTV iodinated *in vitro* to a specific activity of 12×10^6 dpm/μg. B: CEV RNA iodinated *in vitro* to a specific activity of 18×10^6 dpm/μg. From Dickson *et al.* (1975).

ference between the primary structures of the two major components is about 13% as estimated from a comparison of fingerprints of RNase T_1 digests (Fig. 7) and about 10% as estimated from fingerprints of pancreatic RNase digests (Fig. 8). These estimates are based on the assumption that oligonucleotides which contain C are representative of the whole molecule. While the technique of comparative fingerprinting analysis is extremely sensitive for detecting minor differences in closely related RNA molecules, i.e., those differing by less than 10% in sequence (Robertson and Jeppesen, 1972), it is not possible to determine by this technique alone what, if any, is the actual percentage of relatedness of two RNA species. Further study will be required to reveal whether PSTV and CEV contain regions of partial homology or whether they are entirely unrelated in sequence.

Two-dimensional fingerprinting analyses of ^{125}I-labeled CSV and ccRNA-1 digested with T_1 or pancreatic RNase (Dickson, 1976) showed that each RNA has a complexity compatible with the size estimate of about 250–350 nucleotides. In addition, the fingerprint patterns of the four viroids analyzed indicate that each has a different primary structure.

6. REPLICATION

PSTV is able to systemically infect plants of several families (see above). Replication of this low molecular weight RNA could be understood if it were dependent on a helper virus or if PSTV were composed of a population of several RNA molecules of similar length but of different nucleotide sequences, which together might compose a viral genome of more or less conventional size. Existing knowledge, however, does not support the latter scheme (Diener, 1972b, 1973a; Diener et al., 1974; Dickson et al., 1975), and no helper virus appears to be involved in PSTV replication (Diener, 1971b; Diener et al., 1972). Hence PSTV, in spite of its small size, seems to replicate autonomously in susceptible cells.

6.1. Messenger RNA Properties

The question arises as to whether viroids code for novel enzymes (or enzyme subunits) in infected cells or whether they depend on preexisting host enzymes for their replication.

PSTV and CEV are of sufficient chain length to code for a polypeptide of about 1×10^4 daltons. The *in vitro* messenger function of PSTV and CEV in cell-free protein-synthesizing systems has been investigated (Davies et al., 1974; Hall et al., 1974; Hall and Davies, 1975). Extracts from wheat germ, wheat embryo, E. coli, and Pseudomonas aeruginosa were active with plant viral RNAs; however, no messenger function could be detected with either viroid. Incubation at 60°C with extracts from the thermophilic Bacillus stearothermophilus and dimethylsulfoxide denaturation were used in the hope that these procedures might permit ribosome recognition of RNA regions normally inaccessible *in vitro*; but no viroid messenger activity was induced. Viroids have no inhibitory effect on the translation of RNAs known to be messengers.

None of these experiments rules out the possibility that viroids might be transcribed by preexisting host enzymes into a complementary (minus) strand and that this RNA might act as a messenger, possibly coding for a replicase subunit. Comparison of proteins isolated from PSTV-infected tissue with those isolated from healthy tissue, however, gave no evidence for the synthesis in infected leaves of a viroid-specific polypeptide of about 1×10^4 daltons (Zaitlin and Hariharasubramanian, 1972). This finding is in contrast to the detection of a polypeptide (3.45×10^4 daltons) of the viral-induced replicase of brome mosaic virus when proteins from virus-infected and uninfected tissue were compared (Hariharasubramanian *et al.*, 1973; Hadidi and Fraenkel-Conrat, 1973).

6.2. RNA-Directed RNA Synthesis

In light of these results, the possibility must be considered that a preexisting replicase enzyme which accepts a wide variety of RNA species, including viroids, as templates occurs in uninfected plants. Such an enzyme was indeed detected in healthy young tomato leaves; enzyme activity is greatly enhanced by the addition of PSTV (Fig. 9), as well as by several other species of RNA, but not by addition of DNA species (Hadidi, unpublished). It is worth noting that Owens (1976) used PSTV as a template for bacteriophage Qβ replicase-directed RNA synthesis in the presence of Mg^{2+} and Mn^{2+} (Palmenberg and Kaesberg, 1974). Although the reaction products were heterogeneous, the largest product had a molecular weight of approximately 1×10^5.

To search for RNA sequences complementary to PSTV, molecular hybridization experiments between [125I]PSTV and cellular RNA from PSTV-infected or uninfected tomato were performed. In all tests, hybrid yields were small, but the percentage of hybridization in hybrids formed between [125I]PSTV and RNA from PSTV-infected tomato was consistently higher than that obtained between [125I]PSTV and RNA of uninfected tomato. This difference was, however, not large enough to account for cell RNA sequences complementary to a large portion of PSTV. Furthermore, hybrid formed between [125I]PSTV and cellular RNA was shown to contain mismatched duplexes (Hadidi *et al.*, 1976*a*).

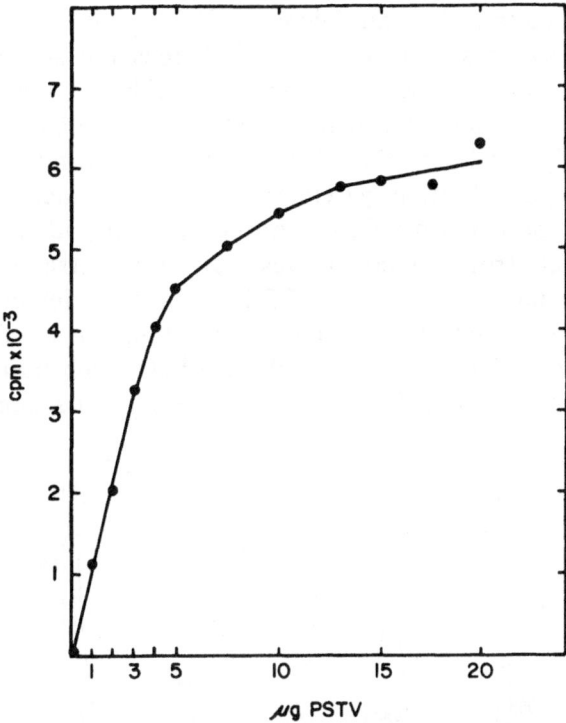

Fig. 9. Dependence of [³H]UMP incorporation by solubilized RNA-directed RNA polymerase from tomato leaves on amount of PSTV added. PSTV concentration is expressed as micrograms per assay of 0.10 ml. Enzyme activity is expressed as the net counts of [³H]UMP incorporated, which is calculated as the difference between trichloroacetic acid-insoluble radioactivity in the samples containing added PSTV and those lacking added PSTV, obtained after 1 h incubation of these samples at 30°C. [³H]UMP incorporated in samples lacking PSTV averaged 985 cpm. At 0 time, in the absence or presence of added PSTV, radioactivity incorporation averaged about 964 cpm. The assay mixture in a total volume of 0.10 ml contained 50 mM tris-HCl (pH 8.0), 10 mM $MgCl_2$, 1.25 µg actinomycin D, 4 mM dithiothreitol, 0.25 mM each of ATP, CTP, and GTP, 1 µM UTP and 5 µl [³H]UTP (specific activity 13 Ci/mmol), 50 µg phosphocreatine, 5 µg creatine phosphokinase, 10% glycerin, 20 µl enzyme, and the desired concentration of PSTV. From Hadidi (unpublished).

6.3. DNA-Directed RNA Synthesis

Alternatively, viroids might be replicated on DNA templates which either are already present in repressed form in uninfected hosts or are synthesized as a consequence of infection with viroids.

Evidence for the involvement of host DNA in PSTV replication has been obtained by inhibiting isotopically labeled PSTV synthesis in tomato leaf strips or tomato nuclei with actinomycin D (Diener and

Smith, 1975; Takahashi and Diener, 1975). This antibiotic inhibits cellular RNA synthesis in plant cells but does not seriously interfere with the replication of several plant viral RNAs. Leaf strips from healthy or PSTV-infected tomato plants were incubated in solutions containing [³H]uracil or [³H]UTP. Extraction of nucleic acids and analysis by polyacrylamide gel electrophoresis revealed ³H incorporation into a component with electrophoretic mobility identical to that of PSTV in extracts from infected leaves, but not in extracts from healthy leaves. No ³H incorporation into PSTV could be detected when leaf strips were pretreated with actinomycin D under conditions which reduced uptake of [³H]uracil only 10–12% but which inhibited cellular RNA transcription 87–99% (Fig. 10). These results suggest that, in

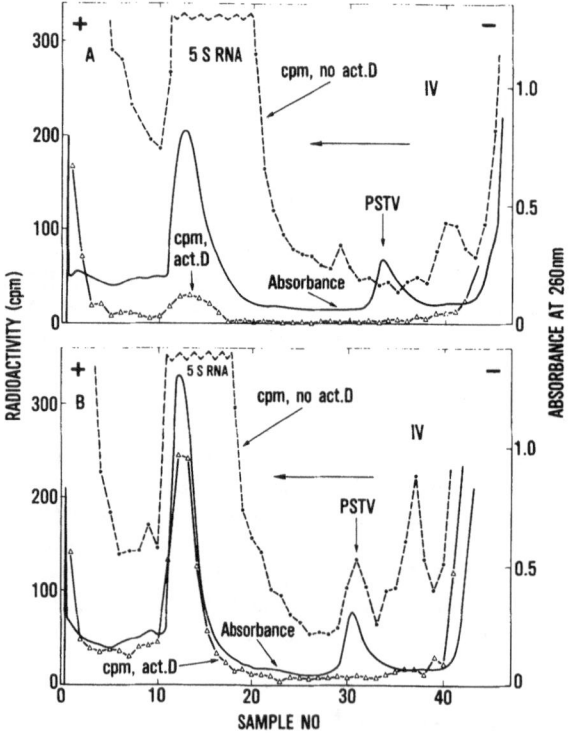

Fig. 10. Ultraviolet absorption (——) and radioactivity profiles of low molecular weight RNA preparations from healthy or PSTV-infected tomato leaves after electrophoresis in 20% polyacrylamide gels for 7.5 h at 4°C. Electrophoretic movement is from right to left. A: Leaf strips from healthy plants infiltrated with water (●---●) or with 30 μg/ml of actinomycin D (△-△-△), followed by incubation for 8 h at 25°C with 125 μCi of [³H]uracil; unlabeled partially purified PSTV was added as internal marker. B: Leaf strips from PSTV-infected leaves treated as described under A. IV, unidentified minor component of cellular RNA (see Diener, 1972a). From Diener and Smith (1975).

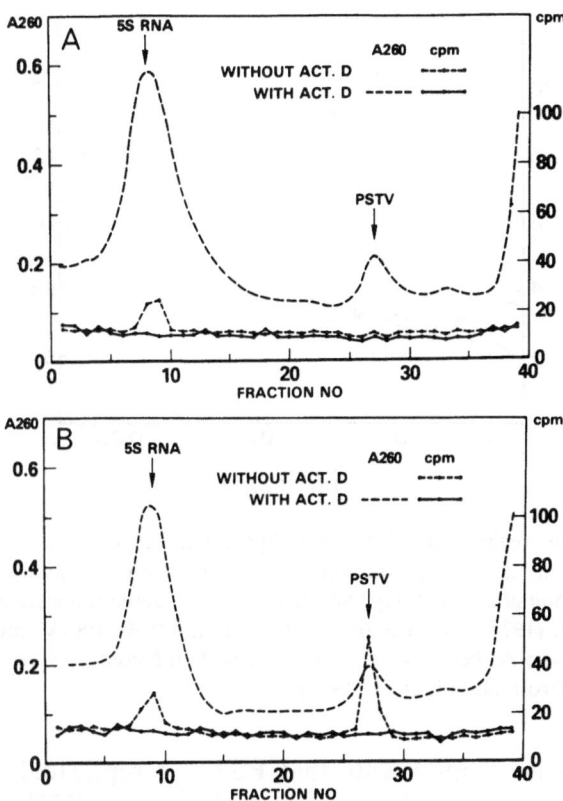

Fig. 11.   Ultraviolet absorption and radioactivity distribution of low molecular weight RNAs isolated from incubation mixtures, each containing 8 μCi of [³H]UTP and nuclei equivalent to 20 μg of DNA, pretreated with either water or 50 μg/ml of actinomycin D, after electrophoresis in 20% polyacrylamide gels for 7.5 h at 4°C. Migration of RNAs is from right to left. DNA and high molecular weight RNAs were removed prior to electrophoresis. Conditions of electrophoresis were such that transfer RNA was run off the gels. Incorporation of [³H]UMP into 5 S RNA and PSTV amounted to 0.05–0.2% of total incorporation into RNA. A: Nuclei isolated from uninfected leaves. B: Nuclei isolated from PSTV-infected leaves. Arrow indicates the position of added PSTV marker. From Takahashi and Diener (1975).

infected tomato leaves, PSTV replication may require the continued synthesis of one or more cellular RNA species or that PSTV replication may proceed via a DNA intermediate (Diener and Smith, 1975). Similar results were obtained with an *in vitro* RNA-synthesizing system, using purified cell nuclei from healthy or PSTV-infected tomato leaves as an enzyme source (Takahashi and Diener, 1975). Isolation of low molecular weight RNAs from the *in vitro* reaction mixtures and analysis by gel electrophoresis revealed that PSTV replication is sensitive to incubation with actinomycin D (Fig. 11).

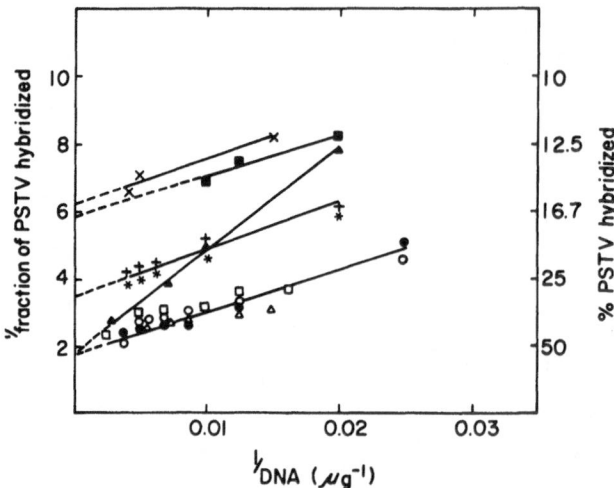

Fig. 12. Double reciprocal plot from hybridization of a constant amount of [^{125}I]PSTV with an increasing amount of cellular DNA of phylogenetically diverse plants at a C_0t value of 2×10^4. Hybrid formation and detection were done as described by Gillespie *et al.* (1975). Sources of DNA: ○, tomato; ●, PSTV-infected tomato; □, potato; △, *Physalis*; ▲, bean; +, *Gynura*; *, PSTV-infected *Gynura*; ■, Chinese cabbage; ×, barley. From Hadidi *et al.* (1976a).

These results also demonstrate that PSTV is replicated in the nucleus of infected cells. The observed sensitivity of PSTV replication to actinomycin D, in both an *in vitro* and an *in vivo* system, suggests that PSTV may be transcribed from a DNA template.

Molecular hybridization of [^{125}I]PSTV to cellular DNA from PSTV-infected or uninfected tomato indeed revealed that at least 60% of PSTV is represented by sequences in the host DNA (Fig. 12) and that infection of tomato with PSTV does not result in the appearance of detectable new sequences complementary to PSTV (Hadidi *et al.*, 1976a).

Synthetic oligonucleotides and polynucleotides have been widely used as primer–template complexes to assay and differentiate DNA polymerases. In particular, the combination of oligo(dT)·poly(rA) and oligo(dG)·poly(rC) has proven invaluable in studies of RNA-directed DNA polymerase (reverse transcriptase). However, other cytoplasmic and nuclear DNA polymerases also use these substrates (Spadari and Weissbach, 1974; Gerard, 1975), so careful interpretation of results is necessary. We detected an enzyme activity in extracts of normal tomato leaves which can efficiently utilize oligo(dT)·poly(rA) as primer-template (Hadidi, unpublished); the identification of that enzyme has not been completed, nor has the role of the enzyme in PSTV replication been elucidated. However, Hadidi *et al.* (1976*b*) reported that a specific cDNA copy of PSTV could be synthesized *in vitro* using DNA polymerase I of *E. coli* but not with reverse transcriptase of avian myeloblastosis virus. These results suggest that the tomato enzyme could be a DNA polymerase similar to the *E. coli* enzyme. At present, no reverse transcriptase enzyme has been isolated from higher plants.

Because no new DNA sequences related to PSTV were found as a consequence of infection with PSTV (Hadidi *et al.*, 1976*a*) and since involvement of DNA in PSTV replication is indicated, preexisting host cell DNA sequences may be utilized during PSTV replication. Possibly, as discussed previously (Diener, 1971*b*), PSTV introduced into cells acts as a regulatory signal, derepressing PSTV-specifying DNA sequences and leading to viroid replication and disease development.

6.4. *De Novo* Synthesis of Viroids

De novo synthesis of PSTV as measured by ^{32}P incorporation into PSTV-infected tomato plants has been investigated recently (Hadidi,

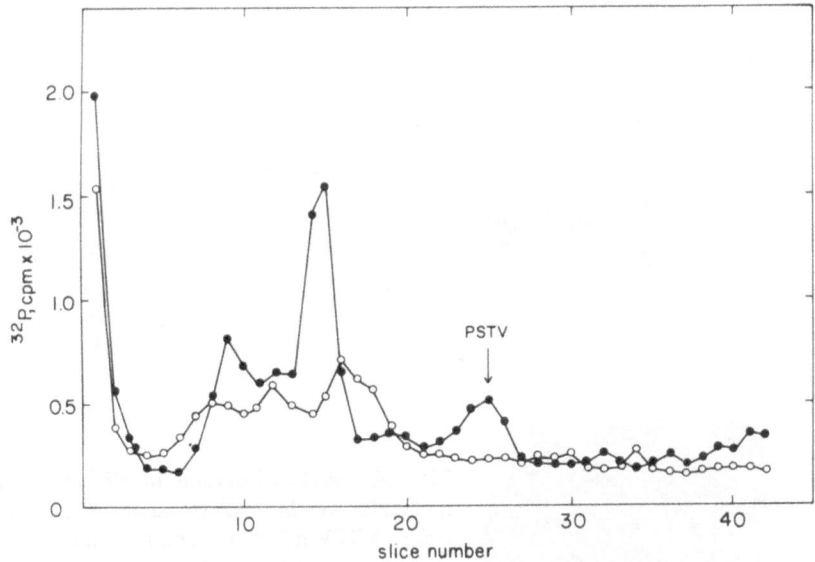

Fig. 13. Electropherograms of ^{32}P-labeled low molecular weight RNA species from uninfected and PSTV-infected tomato leaves in 20% polyacrylamide gels electrophoresed for 14 h at 5 mA/gel. About 250–300 × 10^3 cpm of each ^{32}P-labeled RNA sample was used per gel. O, Uninfected tomato; ●, PSTV-infected tomato; ^{32}P was introduced 2 weeks after inoculation. From Hadidi (unpublished).

1976). ^{32}P was incorporated into RNA with the electrophoretic properties of PSTV (Figs. 13 and 14) at the time when it was introduced into infected tomato plants 2 weeks after inoculation, when systemic PSTV symptoms began to appear. *De novo* synthesis of ^{32}P-labeled PSTV was not observed when ^{32}P was introduced into infected plants 1 or 3 weeks after inoculation.

The rate of synthesis of ^{32}P-labeled PSTV was higher in plants which incorporated ^{32}P for 2 days than in plants which incorporated the isotope for 1 day. After 2 days, the rates of [^{32}P]PSTV synthesis were similar, irrespective of whether the isotope had been incorporated for 2, 3, or 5 days. However, the amount of [^{32}P]PSTV synthesized increased by increasing time of incorporation. The concentration of [^{32}P]PSTV synthesized in infected plants was very small (0.4% of total low molecular weight RNAs) (Table 5).

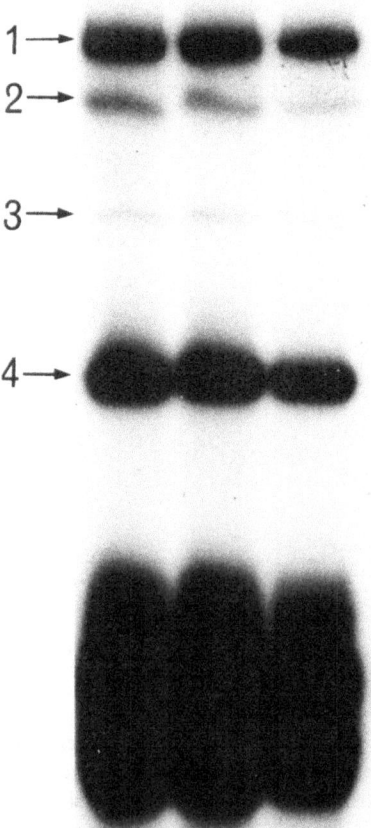

Fig. 14. Autoradiograph of ^{32}P-labeled low molecular weight RNA (total of 8.8×10^6 cpm) from PSTV-infected tomato plants which incorporated ^{32}P 2 weeks after inoculation on 20% polyacrylamide slab gel electrophoresed for 24 h at 100 V. (1) High molecular weight RNA which did not penetrate the gel; (2) 9 S RNA; (3) PSTV; (4) 5 S RNA. From Hadidi (unpublished).

TABLE 5

**Distribution of ^{32}P-Labeled RNAs after Electrophoresis
of 8.8 × 10^6 cpm of a 2 M LiCl-Soluble RNA
Preparation in a 20% Slab Gel for 24 h**[a]

RNA fraction	cpm	Percent of total low molecular weight RNAs
5 S	294,680	3.34
PSTV	35,000	0.39
9 S	64,720	0.70
Top of gel	102,240	1.16
Other RNAs		94.41

[a] Each RNA was extracted from the gel and its total radioactivity
determined.

7. POSSIBLE ORIGIN OF VIROIDS

At present, only the origin of PSTV has been investigated. Hadidi
et al. (1976*a*) reported that PSTV hybridizes with cellular DNA of
several uninfected host species (Solanaceae) and that infection with
PSTV has no detectable effect on the hybridization pattern. PSTV
exhibits less complementarity with DNA of nonsolanaceous plants, and
PSTV sequences are not introduced into one of these plants (*Gynura
aurantiaca*) upon infection (Fig. 12). These results suggest a cellular
origin for PSTV and indicate that PSTV replication does not involve *de
novo* synthesis of a stable DNA copy of PSTV.

These results are at variance with those in a report on citrus
exocortis viroid (CEV), in which the authors claimed that [^{125}I]CEV
hybridizes specifically with DNA-rich preparations from CEV-infected
tomato or *Gynura aurantiaca,* but not with DNA-rich preparations
from uninfected hosts (Semancik and Geelen, 1975). The significance
of this report, however, is uncertain because (1) hybridization reactions
were made with RNA-DNA mixtures and not with purified DNA, (2)
the percentage of input CEV hybridized was small (3.5% and 2.9%, for
DNA-rich preparations from CEV-infected tomato and *Gynura,*
respectively), and (3) neither C_0t values for hybrid formation nor
thermal denaturation properties of the hybrids were reported.

Hybridization of [^{125}I]PSTV to DNA from PSTV-infected or
uninfected tomato revealed a $C_0t_{1/2}$ of 6 × 10^3, which indicates that
PSTV hybridizes to infrequent, possibly unique DNA sequences.

At least 60% of PSTV is represented by sequences in the DNA of the solanaceous host species tomato, potato, and *Physalis peruviana* (Fig. 12). The DNA of a nonsolanaceous host, *Gynura aurantiaca,* contains sequences related to about 30% of the PSTV molecule; however, in this case, mismatched hybrids were formed. The DNAs of Chinese cabbage and barley, plants not known to be hosts of PSTV, contain sequences related to only a small portion of PSTV. Surprisingly, the DNA of Black Valentine bean, which also is resistant to infection by PSTV, contains sequences complementary to a large portion of the PSTV molecule. The frequency of PSTV-related DNA sequences, however, appears to be much lower in DNA of beans than in DNA from the solanaceous hosts. In general, the phylogenetically more distant the plant species are from solanaceous plants, the fewer PSTV-related sequences their DNAs contain and the more distant they are from PSTV. These results support the hypothesis that PSTV originated from genes in normal solanaceous plants.

Evidently, an analogy exists between PSTV, and presumably other viroids, and the endogenous (class 1) RNA tumor viruses, whose genomes are closely related to DNA sequences in their uninfected natural hosts. To our knowledge, PSTV is the first infectious RNA agent of plants which possesses complementarity to its host DNA.

8. CONCLUSIONS AND SPECULATIONS

The evidence now available leaves little doubt that viroids are pathogens which drastically differ from any other pathogenic agents, including viruses. They are the smallest known agents of infectious disease. Although viroids so far identified cause diseases of higher plants, similar agents may exist in other forms of life. It appears reasonable to search for viroids in the many instances where viral etiology of an infectious disease has been assumed, but where no causative agent has ever been identified.

One case in point is the agent of the scrapie disease of sheep, but there are undoubtedly many more. Based on comparisons of known properties of PSTV with those of the scrapie agent, the hypothesis has been advanced that the latter may also be a viroid (Diener, 1972c). So far, however, efforts to isolate infectious nucleic acid from brain preparations of scrapie-infected animals have been fruitless (Marsh *et al.,* 1974). Evidently, only future work will determine whether or not certain infectious diseases of obscure etiology are caused by agents resembling presently known viroids affecting higher plants.

Recent results indicate that, in its native form, PSTV (and presumably other viroids) has a rather unique molecular structure. Although the RNA is single stranded, it assumes a highly structured, hairpinlike configuration in which relatively short base-paired regions appear to alternate with short single-stranded loops. Such a structure explains the characteristic enzymatic susceptibilities of PSTV, its thermal denaturation properties, its peculiar chromatographic behavior, its appearance in electron micrographs, and difficulties in ascribing to the RNA a single- or double-stranded character. The biological significance of this type of RNA structure is unknown.

By what mechanisms viroids replicate is still not known. However, our finding that PSTV replication is sensitive to actinomycin D and our identification of DNA sequences complementary to PSTV in uninfected and infected hosts suggest that PSTV may be transcribed from preexisting DNA templates by preexisting host enzymes. If so, PSTV introduced into cells may act as a specific derepressor of PSTV-specifying DNA sequences. Viroid replication would be analogous to cellular RNA transcription from DNA. Regulatory molecules which are capable of activating their own synthesis have been postulated on theoretical grounds by Gierer (1973), and it is possible that viroids constitute the first known examples of such molecules.

One corollary of these ideas is the possibility that a viroid infecting a species other than its normal host species may derepress a DNA sequence which specifies an RNA molecule whose primary sequence is different from that of the infecting viroid. No conclusive evidence for or against such a possibility exists at present, but preliminary results (Diener and Smith, unpublished) indicate that PSTV, when introduced into chrysanthemum plants, causes the typical syndrome of chrysanthemum stunt disease, a disease which had previously been shown to be caused by a viroid distinct from PSTV (Diener and Lawson, 1973).

9. APPENDIX: DETERMINATION OF VIROID NATURE OF UNKNOWN PATHOGEN

To determine whether the agent of an infectious disease of unknown etiology has properties typical of viroids, several simple exploratory tests may be performed. By necessity, these tests are based on the properties of presently known viroids, and it must be stressed that newly discovered viroids may differ in some of their properties from the few viroids so far investigated. It is by no means certain, for example, whether all viroids are mechanically transmissible or whether all are composed of RNA. Also, depending on the host in which viroids replicate, they may exhibit different characteristics in crude extracts.

9.1. Criteria for Suspecting Viroid Nature of Pathogen

Viroid etiology of an infectious disease of unknown causation should be considered if all of the following observations have been made:

1. No microorganisms are consistently associated with the disease.
2. No viruslike particles are identifiable by electron microscopy of extracts or in sections from infected tissue.
3. Much of the pathogen in extracts cannot be pelleted by ultracentrifugation.
4. The agent is inactivated by either ribonuclease or deoxyribonuclease.

Evidently, the last two tests presuppose that the pathogen is mechanically transmissible and that a suitable assay host is available.

None of these observations constitutes conclusive evidence for viroid etiology. The first two observations are negative evidence and improved techniques may lead to opposite conclusions; the third observation may indicate the presence of virus particles of low density, such as lipid-containing virions; and the fourth observation could indicate the presence of virus particles with a loose protein shell which permits access of nucleases [such as cherry necrotic ringspot (Diener and Weaver, 1959), cucumber mosaic (Francki, 1968), or apple chlorotic leaf spot (Lister and Hadidi, 1971) viruses].

On the other hand, detection of viruslike particles in sections from infected tissue does not necessarily rule out viroid etiology of the disease in question; plants may be infected with a latent virus unrelated to the disease syndrome.

Also, some viroids are not readily released from host constituents or occur in extracts as aggregates of varying size (Diener, 1971a). In either case, much of the infectious material sediments faster than expected.

9.2. Sedimentation Properties

Assuming that infectious extracts can be prepared from infected tissue and that a suitable bioassay host is available, accurate determination of the sedimentation properties of the infectious agent in such extracts should have high priority. This may conveniently be accomplished by subjecting an infectious extract together with markers of known sedimentation coefficients to velocity density gradient centrifugation, followed by fractionation of the gradient and bioassay of all fractions. Tissue extracts should be made with buffers of low and high ionic strength, such as 0.005 M and 0.5 M phosphate buffers, because some viroids are released from subcellular components only in high ionic strength medium (Raymer and Diener, 1969). Viroids usually are more stable in slightly alkaline than in acid media; thus buffers of pH 8–9 are recommended.

A sedimentation coefficient of 6–15 S of the bulk of the infectious material suggests that the unknown pathogen may be a viroid. In crude preparations of this type, however, some infectivity often is found in lower portions of the gradient; and it is not uncommon to find low levels of infectivity in most fractions. For this reason, it is important to assay tenfold dilutions of the inoculum and to determine where in the gradient the bulk of the infectious material is located.

9.3. Nuclease Sensitivity

All known viroids are composed of RNA and are inactivated by incubation with pancreatic ribonuclease. At high ionic strength, some viroids are partially ribonuclease resistant; thus incubation should be made in buffers of low and high ionic strength. Sensitivity should be investigated in the range of 0.1–1.0 μg/ml of ribonuclease with incubations for 1 h at 25°C.

9.4. Insensitivity to Treatment with Phenol

Treatment of buffer extracts from viroid-infected tissue with phenol or with phenol and SDS has little if any effect on the infectivity level of such preparations, or on the sedimentation properties of the infectious material. This is in contrast to extracts containing conventional viruses, which, after such treatments, usually are much less infectious and in which the infectious material sediments at lower rates than before treatment with phenol.

9.5. Electrophoretic Mobility

If the above tests give results consistent with a viroid nature of the pathogen, infectious extracts should be subjected to polyacrylamide gel electrophoresis. This can be accomplished by analyzing partially purified preparations in gels of low and high concentration. Viroid nature of the pathogen is indicated by the position of the infectious entity in the low molecular weight region of gels and by its ability to enter gels of high acrylamide concentration (small pore size), from which high molecular weight RNAs are excluded.

Alternatively, preparations may be more thoroughly purified before electrophoresis and the gels stained to detect the suspected viroid band.

10. REFERENCES

Adams, D. H., 1970, The nature of the scrapie agent: A review of recent progress, *Pathol. Biol.* **18**:559.

Altenburg, E., 1946, The viroid theory in relation to plasmagenes, viruses, cancer, and plastids, *Am. Nat.* **80**:559.

Bailey, L. H., 1969, *Manual of Cultivated Plants,* 11th ed., 1116 p., Macmillan New York.

Boedtker, H., 1971, Conformation independent molecular weight determinations of RNA by gel electrophoresis, *Biochim. Biophys. Acta* **240**:448.

Brakke, M. K., 1970, Systemic infections for the assay of plant viruses, *Annu. Rev. Phytopathol.* **8**:61.

Brierley, P., 1953, Some experimental hosts of the chrysanthemum stunt virus, *Plant Dis. Rep.* **37**:343.

Brownlee, G. G., and Sanger, F., 1969, Chromatography of ^{32}P-labeled oligonucleotides on thin layers of DEAE-cellulose, *Eur. J. Biochem.* **11**:395.

Childs, J. F. L., Norma, G. G., and Eichorn, J. L., 1958, A color test for exocortis infection in *Poncirus trifoliata, Phytopathology* **48**:426.

Davies, J. W., Kaesberg, P., and Diener, T. O., 1974, Potato spindle tuber viroid. XII. An investigation of viroid RNA as a messenger for protein synthesis, *Virology* **61**:281.

Dickson, E., 1976, Studies of plant viroid RNA and other RNA species, Ph.D. thesis, Rockefeller University, New York.

Dickson, E., Prensky, W., and Robertson, H. D., 1975, Comparative studies of two viroids: Analysis of potato spindle tuber and citrus exocortis viroids by RNA finger-printing and polyacrylamide gel electrophoresis, *Virology* **68**:309.

Diener, T. O., 1971a, Potato spindle tuber virus: A plant virus with properties of a free nucleic acid. III. Subcellular location of PSTV-RNA and the question of whether virions exist in extracts or *in situ, Virology* **43**:75.

Diener, T. O., 1971b, Potato spindle tuber "virus." IV. A replicating, low molecular weight RNA, *Virology* **45**:411.

Diener, T. O., 1971c, A plant virus with properties of a free ribonucleic acid: Potato spindle tuber virus, in: *Comparative Virology* (K. Maramorosch and E. Kurstak, eds.), pp. 433–478, Academic Press, New York.

Diener, T. O., 1972a, Potato spindle tuber viroid. VIII. Correlation of infectivity with a

UV-absorbing component and thermal denaturation properties of the RNA, *Virology* **50**:606.

Diener, T. O., 1972*b*, Viroids, in: *Advances in Virus Research,* Vol. 17 (K. M. Smith, M. A. Lauffer, and F. B. Bang, eds.), pp. 295–313, Academic Press, New York.

Diener, T. O., 1972*c*, Is the scrapie agent a viroid? *Nature (London) New Biol.* **235**:218.

Diener, T. O., 1973*a*, Potato spindle tuber viroid. A novel type of pathogen, in: *Perspectives in Virology,* Vol. 8 (M. Pollard, ed.), pp. 7–30, Academic Press, New York.

Diener, T. O., 1973*b*, Virus terminology and the viroid: A rebuttal, *Phytopathology* **63**:1328.

Diener, T. O., 1973*c*, A method for the purification and reconcentration of nucleic acids eluted or extracted from polyacrylamide gels, *Anal. Biochem.* **55**:317.

Diener, T. O., and Lawson, R. H., 1973, Chrysanthemum stunt: A viroid disease, *Virology* **51**:94.

Diener, T. O., and Raymer, W. B., 1967, Potato spindle tuber virus: A plant virus with properties of a free nucleic acid, *Science* **158**:378.

Diener, T. O., and Raymer, W. B., 1969, Potato spindle tuber virus: A plant virus with properties of a free nucleic acid. II. Characterization and partial purification, *Virology* **37**:351.

Diener, T. O., and Raymer, W. B., 1971, Potato spindle tuber "virus," in: C.M.I./A.A.B. Descriptions of Plant Viruses, No. 66, Commonwealth Mycol. Inst. Assoc. Appl. Biol., 4 pp.

Diener, T. O., and Smith, D. R., 1971, Potato spindle tuber viroid. VI. Monodisperse distribution after electrophoresis in 20% polyacrylamide gels, *Virology* **46**:498.

Diener, T. O., and Smith, D. R., 1973, Potato spindle tuber viroid. IX. Molecular weight determination by gel electrophoresis of formylated RNA, *Virology* **53**:350.

Diener, T. O., and Smith, D. R., 1975, Potato spindle tuber viroid. XIII. Inhibition of replication by actinomycin D, *Virology* **63**:421.

Diener, T. O., and Weaver, M. L., 1959, Reversible and irreversible inhibition of necrotic ringspot virus in cucumber by pancreatic ribonuclease, *Virology* **7**:419.

Diener, T. O., Smith, D. R., and O'Brien, M. J., 1972, Potato spindle tuber viroid. VII. Susceptibility of several solanaceous plant species to infection with low-molecular-weight RNA, *Virology* **48**:844.

Diener, T. O., Schneider, I. R., and Smith, D. R., 1974, Potato spindle tuber viroid. XI. A comparison of the ultraviolet light sensitivities of PSTV, tobacco ringspot virus, and its satellite, *Virology* **57**:577.

Diener, T. O., Hadidi, A., and Owens, R. A., 1977, Methods for studying viroids, in: *Methods in Virology,* Vol. 6 (K. Maramorosch and H. Koprowski, eds), Academic Press, New York.

Dorland's Illustrated Medical Dictionary, 1944, 20th ed., 1725 pp., Saunders, Philadelphia.

Engelhardt, D. L., 1972, Assay for secondary structure in ribonucleic acid, *J. Virol.* **9**:903.

Fernow, K. H., 1967, Tomato as a test plant for detecting mild strains of potato spindle tuber virus, *Phytopathology* **57**:1347.

Francki, R. I. B., 1968, Inactivation of cucumber mosaic virus (Q strain) nucleoprotein by pancreatic ribonuclease, *Virology* **34**:694.

Franklin, R. M., 1966, Purification and properties of the replicative intermediate of the RNA bacteriophage R17, *Proc. Natl. Acad. Sci. USA* **55**:1504.

Garnsey, S. M., and Whidden, R., 1970, Transmission of exocortis virus to various citrus plants by knife-cut inoculation, *Phytopathology* **60**:1292.

Garnsey, S. M., and Whidden, R., 1974, Effects of RNase and UV light on transmission of citrus exocortis virus (CEV) by contaminated knife blades, *Proc. Am. Phytopathol. Soc.* **1**:50.

Gerard, G. F., 1975, Poly(2′-*O*-methylcytidylate)-oligodeoxyguanylate, a template-primer specific for reverse transcriptase, is not utilized by HeLa cell γ DNA polymerases, *Biochem. Biophys. Res. Commun.* **63**:706.

Gierer, A., 1973, Molecular models and combinatorial principles in cell differentiation and morphogenesis, *Cold Spring Harbor Symp. Quant. Biol.* **38**:951.

Gillespie, D., Gillespie, S., and Wong-Staal, F., 1975, RNA-DNA hybridization applied to cancer research: Special reference to RNA tumor viruses, in: *Methods in Cancer Research,* Vol. 11 (H. Bush, ed.), pp. 205–245, Academic Press, New York.

Hadidi, A., 1976, ^{32}P-labelling of potato spindle tuber viroid in infected tomato plants, in: *Beltsville Symposium on Virology in Agriculture,* p. 24, U.S.D.A., Beltsville, Md.

Hadidi, A., and Fraenkel-Conrat, H., 1973, Characterization and specificity of soluble RNA polymerase of brome mosaic virus, *Virology* **52**:363.

Hadidi, A., and Fraenkel-Conrat, H., 1974, Host-range and structural data on common plant viruses, in: *Handbook of Genetics* (R. C. King, ed.), pp. 381–413, Plenum Press, New York.

Hadidi, A., Jones, D. M., Gillespie, D. H., Wong-Staal, F., and Diener, T. O., 1976a, Hybridization of potato spindle tuber viroid to cellular DNA of normal plants, *Proc. Natl. Acad. Sci. USA* **73**:2453.

Hadidi, A., Modak, M. J., and Diener, T. O., 1976b, Preparation and characterization of DNA complementary to potato spindle tuber viroid, in: *Beltsville Symposium on Virology in Agriculture,* p. 30, U.S.D.A., Beltsville, Md.

Hall, T. C., and Davies, J. W., 1975, Viroid RNA lacks messenger and transfer functions, *Third International Congress for Virology,* p. 81, Madrid, Spain.

Hall, T. C., Wepprich, R. K., Davies, J. W., Weathers, L. G., and Semancik, J. S., 1974, Functional distinctions between the ribonucleic acids from citrus exocortis viroid and plant viruses. 1. Cell-free translation and aminoacylation reactions, *Virology* **61**:486.

Hariharasubramanian, V., Hadidi, A., Singer, B., and Fraenkel-Conrat, H., 1973, Possible identification of a protein in brome mosaic virus infected barley as a component of viral RNA polymerase, *Virology* **54**:190.

Hollings, M., and Stone, O. M., 1973, Some properties of chrysanthemum stunt, a virus with the characteristics of an uncoated ribonucleic acid, *Ann. Appl. Biol.* **74**:333.

Horst, R. K., 1975, Detection of a latent infectious agent that protects against infection by chrysanthemum chlorotic mottle viroid, *Phytopathology* **65**:1000.

Hunter, D. E., Darling, H. M., and Beale, W. L., 1969, Seed transmission of potato spindle tuber virus, *Am. Potato J.* **46**:247.

Inman, R. B., and Schnös, M., 1970, Partial denaturation of thymine- and 5-bromouracil-containing λ DNA in alkali, *J. Mol. Biol.* **49**:93.

Kaper, J. M., and Waterworth, H. E., 1973, Comparisons of molecular weights of single-stranded viral RNAs by two empirical methods, *Virology* **51**:183.

Kelsey, H. P., and Dayton, W. A., eds, 1942, *Standardized Plant Names,* 2nd ed., 675 pp., J. Horace McFarland, Harrisburg, Pa.

Kleinschmidt, A. K., and Zahn, R. K., 1959, Ueber Desoxyribonucleinsäure-Molekeln in Protein-Mischfilmen, *Z. Naturforsch.* **14b**:770.

Kuehl, L., 1964, Isolation of plant nuclei, *Z. Naturforsch.* **19b**:525.

Lang, D., 1970, Molecular weights of coliphages and coliphage DNA. III. Contour length and molecular weight of DNA from bacteriophages T$_4$, T$_5$, and T$_7$ and from bovine papilloma virus, *J. Mol. Biol.* **54**:557.

Lawson, R. H., 1968, Some properties of chrysanthemum stunt virus, *Phytopathology* **58**:885.

Lewandowski, L. J., Kimball, P. C., and Knight, C. A., 1971, Separation of the infectious ribonucleic acid of potato spindle tuber virus from double-stranded ribonucleic acid of plant tissue extracts, *J. Virol.* **8**:809.

Lister, R. M., and Hadidi, A. F., 1971, Some properties of apple chlorotic leaf-spot virus and their relation to purification problems, *Virology* **45**:240.

Loening, U. E., 1967, The fractionation of high-molecular-weight ribonucleic acid by polyacrylamide-gel electrophoresis, *Biochem. J.* **102**:251.

Marsh, R. F., Semancik, J. S., Medappa, K. C., Hanson, R. P., and Rueckert, R. R., 1974, Scrapie and transmissible mink encephalopathy: Search for infectious nucleic acid, *J. Virol.* **13**:993.

McClements, W. L., and Kaesberg, P., 1977, Size and secondary structure of potato spindle tuber viroid, *Virology* **76**:477.

Miura, K., Kimura, I., and Suzuki, N., 1966, Double-stranded ribonucleic acid from rice dwarf virus, *Virology* **28**:571.

Modak, M. J., Marcus, S. L., and Cavalierie, L. F., 1975, A new sensitive method for detecting polyadenylate in viral and other ribonucleic acids using *Escherichia coli* deoxyribonucleic acid polymerase I, *J. Biol. Chem.* **249**:7373.

Morris, T. J., and Semancik, J. S., 1974, Nucleotide composition of RNA by polyacrylamide gel electrophoresis, *Anal. Biochem.* **61**:48.

Niblett, C. L., Hedgcoth, C., and Diener, T. O., 1976, Base composition of potato spindle tuber viroid, in: *Beltsville Symposium on Virology in Agriculture,* p. 27, U.S.D.A., Beltsville, Md.

O'Brien, M. J., and Raymer, W. B., 1964, Symptomless hosts of the potato spindle tuber virus. *Phytopathology* **54**:1045.

Olson, E. O., and Shull, A. V., 1956, Exocortis and xyloporosis-bud transmission virus disease of rangpur and other mandarin-lime rootstocks, *Plant Dis. Rep.* **40**:939.

Owens, R. A., 1976, Potato spindle tuber viroid as a template for RNA synthesis by Qβ replicase, in: *Beltsville Symposium on Virology in Agriculture,* p. 31, U.S.D.A., Beltsville, Md.

Palmenberg, A., and Kaesberg, P., 1974, Synthesis of complementary strands of heterologous RNAs with Qβ replicase, *Proc. Natl. Acad. Sci. USA* **71**:1371.

Randerrath, E., Yu, C.-T., and Randerrath, K., 1972, Base analysis of ribopolynucleotides by chemical tritium labelling: A methodological study with model nucleosides and purified tRNA species, *Anal. Biochem.* **48**:172.

Randles, J. W., 1975, Association of two ribonucleic acid species with cadang-cadang disease of coconut palm, *Phytopathology* **65**:163.

Randles, J. W., Rillo, E. P., and Diener, T. O., 1976, The viroid like structure and cellular location of anomalous RNA associated with cadang-cadang disease. *Virology* **74**:128.

Raymer, W. B., and Diener, T. O., 1969, Potato spindle tuber virus: A plant virus with properties of a free nucleic acid. I. Assay, extraction, and concentration, *Virology* **37**:343.

Raymer, W. B., and O'Brien, M. J., 1962, Transmission of potato spindle tuber virus to tomato, *Am. Potato J.* **39**:401.

Robertson, H. D., and Dunn, J. J., 1975, Ribonucleic acid processing activity of *Escherichia coli* ribonuclease III, *J. Biol. Chem.* **250**:3050.

Robertson, H. D., and Hunter, T., 1975, Sensitive methods for the detection and characterization of double helical ribonucleic acid, *J. Biol. Chem.* **250**:418.

Robertson, H. D., and Jeppesen, P. G. N., 1972, Extent of variation in three related bacteriophage RNA molecules, *J. Mol. Biol.* **68**:417.

Robertson, H. D., Webster, R. E., and Zinder, N. D., 1967, A nuclease specific for double-stranded RNA, *Virology* **32**:718.

Romaine, C. P., and Horst, R. K., 1975, Suggested viroid etiology for chrysanthemum chlorotic mottle disease, *Virology* **64**:86.

Sänger, H. L., 1972, An infectious and replicating RNA of low molecular weight. The agent of exocortis disease of citrus, *Adv. Biosci.* **8**:103.

Sänger, H. L., Klotz, G., Riesner, D., Gross, H. J., and Kleinschmidt, A. K., 1976, Viroids are single-stranded covalently closed circular RNA molecules existing as highly base-paired rod-like structures, *Proc. Natl. Acad. Sci. USA* **73**:3852.

Schneider, I. R., 1971, Characteristics of a satellite-like virus of tobacco ringspot virus, *Virology* **45**:108.

Schwartz, E. F., and Stollar, B. D., 1969, Antibodies to polyadenylate–polyuridylate copolymers as reagents for double stranded RNA and DNA:RNA hybrid complexes, *Biochem. Biophys. Res. Commun.* **35**:115.

Semancik, J. S., 1974, Detection of polyadenylic acid sequences in plant pathogenic RNA, *Virology* **62**:288.

Semancik, J. S., and Geelen, J. L. M. C., 1975, Detection of DNA complementary to pathogenic viroid RNA in exocortis disease, *Nature (London)* **256**:753.

Semancik, J. S., and Vanderwoude, W. J., 1976, Exocortis viroid: Cytopathic effects at the plasma membrane in association with pathogenic RNA, *Virology* **69**:719.

Semancik, J. S., and Weathers, L. G., 1968, Exocortis virus of citrus: Association of infectivity with nucleic acid preparations, *Virology* **36**:326.

Semancik, J. S., and Weathers, L. G., 1972a, Pathogenic 10 S RNA from exocortis disease recovered from tomato bunchy-top plants similar to potato spindle tuber virus infection, *Virology* **49**:622.

Semancik, J. S., and Weathers, L. G., 1972b, Exocortis disease: Evidence for a new species of "infectious" low molecular weight RNA in plants, *Nature (London) New Biol.* **237**:242.

Semancik, J. S., and Weathers, L. G., 1972c, Exocortis virus: An infectious free-nucleic acid plant virus with unusual properties, *Virology* **47**:456.

Semancik, J. S., Magnuson, D. S., and Weathers, L. G., 1973a, Potato spindle tuber disease produced by pathogenic RNA from citrus exocortis disease: Evidence for the identity of the causal agents, *Virology* **52**:292.

Semancik, J. S., Morris, T. J., and Weathers, L. G., 1973b, Structure and conformation of low molecular weight pathogenic RNA from exocortis disease, *Virology* **53**:448.

Semancik, J. S., Morris, T. J., Weathers, L. G., Rodorf, B. F., and Kearns, D. R.,

1975, Physical properties of a minimal infectious RNA (viroid) associated with the exocortis disease, *Virology* **63**:160.

Semancik, J. S., Tsuruda, D., Zaner, L., Geelen, J. L. M. C., and Weathers, L. G., 1976, Exocortis disease. Subcellular distribution of pathogenic (viroid) RNA, *Virology* **69**:669.

Singh, R. P., 1970, Seed transmission of potato spindle tuber virus in tomato and potato, *Am. Potato J.* **47**:225.

Singh, R. P., 1971, A local lesion host for potato spindle tuber virus, *Phytopathology* **61**:1034.

Singh, R. P., 1973, Experimental host range of the potato spindle tuber "virus," *Am. Potato J.* **50**:111.

Singh, R. P., and Bagnall, R. H., 1968, Infectious nucleic acid from host tissues infected with the potato spindle tuber virus, *Phytopathology* **58**:696.

Singh, R. P., and Clark, M. C., 1971, Infectious low-molecular-weight ribonucleic acid from tomato, *Biochem. Biophys. Res. Commun.* **44**:1077.

Singh, R. P., and Clark, M. C., 1973, Similarity of host response to both potato spindle tuber and citrus exocortis viruses, *FAO Plant Prot. Bull.* **21**:121.

Singh, R. P., and O'Brien, M. J., 1970, Additional indicator plants for potato spindle tuber virus, *Am. Potato J.* **47**:367.

Singh, R. P., Finnie, R. E., and Bagnall, R. H., 1970, Relative prevalence of mild and severe strains of potato spindle tuber virus in Eastern Canada, *Am. Potato J.* **47**:289.

Singh, R. P., Finnie, R. E., and Bagnall, R. H., 1971, Losses due to the potato spindle tuber virus, *Am. Potato J.* **48**:262.

Singh, R. P., Michniewicz, J. J., and Narang, S. A., 1974, Multiple forms of potato spindle-tuber metavirus ribonucleic acid, *Can. J. Biochem.* **52**:809.

Sogo, J. M., Koller, T., and Diener, T. O., 1973, Potato spindle tuber viroid. X. Visualization and size determination by electron microscopy, *Virology* **55**:70.

Spadari, S., and Weissbach, A., 1974, HeLa cell R-deoxyribonucleic acid polymerases. Separation and characterization of two enzymatic activities, *J. Biol. Chem.* **249**:5809.

Stedman's Medical Dictionary, 1942, 15th ed., Rev., 1257 pp., William Wood and Co., Division of Williams and Wilkins, Baltimore.

Stollar, B. D., and Diener, T. O., 1971, Potato spindle tuber viroid. V. Failure of immunological tests to disclose double-stranded RNA or RNA-DNA hybrids, *Virology* **46**:168.

Takahashi, T., and Diener, T. O., 1975, Potato spindle tuber viroid. XIV. Replication in nuclei isolated from infected leaves, *Virology* **64**:106.

Van Dorst, H. J. M., and Peters, D., 1974, Some biological observations on pale fruit, a viroid-incited disease of cucumber, *Neth. J. Plant Pathol.* **80**:85.

Waterworth, H. E., and Kaper, J. M., 1972, Purification and some properties of carnation mottle virus and its ribonucleic acid, *Phytopathology* **62**:959.

Weathers, L. G., Greer, Jr., F. C., and Harjung, M. K., 1967, Transmission of exocortis virus of citrus to herbaceous hosts, *Plant. Dis. Rep.* **51**:868.

Zaitlin, M., and Hariharasubramanian, V., 1972, A gel electrophoretic analysis of proteins from plants infected with tobacco mosaic and potato spindle tuber viruses, *Virology* **47**:296.

Index